Cardiology

Editor

DANIEL T. THIBODEAU

PHYSICIAN ASSISTANT CLINICS

www.physicianassistant.theclinics.com

Consulting Editor
JAMES A. VAN RHEE

October 2017 • Volume 2 • Number 4

ELSEVIER

1600 John F. Kennedy Boulevard • Suite 1800 • Philadelphia, Pennsylvania, 19103-2899

http://www.theclinics.com

PHYSICIAN ASSISTANT CLINICS Volume 2, Number 4
October 2017 ISSN 2405-7991, ISBN-13: 978-0-323-54682-9

Editor: Jessica McCool
Developmental Editor: Casey Potter

Physician Assistant Clinics (ISSN: 2405–7991) is published quarterly by Elsevier Inc., 360 Park Avenue South, New York, NY 10010-1710. Months of issue are January, April, July, and October. Periodicals postage paid at New York, NY and additional mailing offices. Subscription prices are $150.00 per year (US individuals), $205.00 (US institutions), $100.00 (US students), $210.00 (Canadian individuals), $257.00 (Canadian institutions), $100.00 (Canadian students), $150.00 (international individuals), $257.00 (international institutions), and $100.00 (international students). Foreign air speed delivery is included in all *Clinics* subscription prices. All prices are subject to change without notice. POSTMASTER: Send address changes to *Physician Assistant Clinics*, Elsevier Periodicals Customer Service, 11830 Westline Industrial Drive, St. Louis, MO 63146. Customer Service Health Sciences Division, Subscription Customer Service, 3251 Riverport Lane, Maryland Heights, MO 63043. **Customer Service: 1-800-654-2452 (U.S. and Canada); 314-447-8871 (outside U.S. and Canada). Fax: 314-447-8029. E-mail: journalscustomerservice-usa@elsevier.com (for print support); journalsonlinesupport-usa@elsevier.com (for online support).**

Reprints. For copies of 100 or more, of articles in this publication, please contact the Commercial Reprints Department, Elsevier Inc., 360 Park Avenue South, New York, NY 10010-1710. Tel. 212-633-3874; Fax: 212-633-3820; E-mail: reprints@elsevier.com.

Physician Assistant Clinics is covered in *MEDLINE/PubMed (Index Medicus)* and *EMBASE/Excerpta Medica, Current Contents/Clinical Medicine, and ISI/BIOMED.*

PROGRAM OBJECTIVE
The goal of the *Physician Assistant Clinics* is to keep practicing physician assistants up to date with current clinical practice by providing timely articles reviewing the state of the art in patient care.

TARGET AUDIENCE
Physician Assistants and other healthcare professionals.

LEARNING OBJECTIVES
Upon completion of this activity, participants will be able to:
1. Review current guidelines for management of common cardiovascular conditions.
2. Discuss long term management of cardiologic conditions in the primary care office.
3. Recognize evolving strategies in the evaluation and diagnosis of cardiac conditions in primary care.

ACCREDITATION
The Elsevier Office of Continuing Medical Education (EOCME) is accredited by the Accreditation Council for Continuing Medical Education (ACCME) to provide continuing medical education for physicians.

The EOCME designates this enduring material for a maximum of 15 *AMA PRA Category 1 Credit*(s)™. Physicians should claim only the credit commensurate with the extent of their participation in the activity.

All other healthcare professionals requesting continuing education credit for this enduring material will be issued a certificate of participation.

DISCLOSURE OF CONFLICTS OF INTEREST
The EOCME assesses conflict of interest with its instructors, faculty, planners, and other individuals who are in a position to control the content of CME activities. All relevant conflicts of interest that are identified are thoroughly vetted by EOCME for fair balance, scientific objectivity, and patient care recommendations. EOCME is committed to providing its learners with CME activities that promote improvements or quality in healthcare and not a specific proprietary business or a commercial interest.

The planning committee, staff, authors and editors listed below have identified no financial relationships or relationships to products or devices they or their spouse/life partner have with commercial interest related to the content of this CME activity:
Eric W. Cucchi, MS, PA-C; Joseph Daniel; Jane Davis, DNP; Harvey A. Feldman, MD, FACP; Anjali Fortna; Trent Honda, PhD, MMS, PA-C; Craig Hricz, MPAS, PA-C; Casey Jackson; Jillian Levy, MS, PA-C; Andrew Mackie, MPAS, PA-C; Nicholas Marshall, MS, PA-C; Jessica McCool; James A. Van Rhee, MS, PA-C, DFAAPA; Daniel T. Thibodeau, MHP, PA-C, DFAAPA; Dan Tzizik, MPAS, PA-C; Amy Williams; Kim Zuber, PA-C.

UNAPPROVED/OFF-LABEL USE DISCLOSURE
The EOCME requires CME faculty to disclose to the participants:
1. When products or procedures being discussed are off-label, unlabelled, experimental, and/or investigational (not US Food and Drug Administration [FDA] approved); and
2. Any limitations on the information presented, such as data that are preliminary or that represent ongoing research, interim analyses, and/or unsupported opinions. Faculty may discuss information about pharmaceutical agents that is outside of FDA-approved labelling. This information is intended solely for CME and is not intended to promote off-label use of these medications. If you have any questions, contact the medical affairs department of the manufacturer for the most recent prescribing information.

TO ENROLL
The CME program is available to all *Physician Assistant Clinics* subscribers at no additional fee. To subscribe to the *Physician Assistant Clinics*, call customer service at 1-800-654-2452 or sign up online at www.physicianassistant.theclinics.com.

METHOD OF PARTICIPATION
In order to claim credit, participants must complete the following:
1. Complete enrolment as indicated above.
2. Read the activity.
3. Complete the CME Test and Evaluation. Participants must achieve a score of 70% on the test. All CME Tests and Evaluations must be completed online.

CME INQUIRIES/SPECIAL NEEDS
For all CME inquiries or special needs, please contact elsevierCME@elsevier.com.

Contributors

CONSULTING EDITOR

JAMES A. VAN RHEE, MS, PA-C
Associate Professor, Program Director, Yale School of Medicine, Yale Physician Assistant
Online Program, New Haven, Connecticut

EDITOR

DANIEL T. THIBODEAU, MHP, PA-C, DFAAPA
Associate Professor, Physician Assistant Program, Director, Clinical Education
Recruitment and Support, Eastern Virginia Medical School, Norfolk, Virginia;
Cardiovascular Specialists Inc, Suffolk, Virginia

AUTHORS

ERIC W. CUCCHI, MS, PA-C
Director, Affiliate Practitioner Critical Care Residency Program, Critical Care, UMass
Memorial Medical Center, Instructor of Nursing, The Graduate School of Nursing,
University of Massachusetts Medical School, Worcester, Massachusetts; Clinical
Assistant Professor, Physician Assistant Studies, Bay Path University, Longmeadow,
Massachusetts

JANE DAVIS, DNP
Communication Chair, National Kidney Foundation of Advanced Practitioners, Division of
Nephrology, UAB Hospital, Birmingham, Alabama

HARVEY A. FELDMAN, MD, FACP
Physician Assistant Program, Nova Southeastern University, Fort Lauderdale, Florida

TRENT HONDA, PhD, MMS, PA-C
Program Director, Assistant Clinical Professor, Physician Assistant Program, Northeastern
University, Boston, Massachusetts

CRAIG HRICZ, MPAS, PA-C
Assistant Professor, School of Physician Assistant Studies, Massachusetts College of
Pharmacy and Health Sciences, Manchester, New Hampshire; Physician Assistant,
Emergency Department, Wentworth-Douglass Hospital, Dover, New Hampshire

JILLIAN LEVY, MS, PA-C
Staff Physician Assistant, Critical Care Unit, Critical Care, UMass Memorial Medical
Center, Worcester, Massachusetts

ANDREW MACKIE, MPAS, PA-C
Director of Didactic Education, Assistant Clinical Professor, Northeastern University,
Boston, Massachusetts

NICHOLAS MARSHALL, MS, PA-C
Physician Assistant, University of Massachusetts Medical School, Worcester, Massachusetts

DANIEL T. THIBODEAU, MHP, PA-C, DFAAPA
Associate Professor, Physician Assistant Program, Director, Clinical Education Recruitment and Support, Eastern Virginia Medical School, Norfolk, Virginia; Cardiovascular Specialists Inc, Suffolk, Virginia

DAN TZIZIK, MPAS, PA-C
Assistant Professor, Department of Physician Assistant Studies, Massachusetts College of Pharmacy and Health Sciences, Manchester, New Hampshire

KIM ZUBER, PA-C
American Academy of Nephrology PAs, Oceanside, California; Past Chair, National Kidney Foundation of Advanced Practitioners, New York, New York

Contents

> Despite longstanding knowledge of the consequences of uncontrolled hypertension and the availability of effective classes of antihypertensives, the understanding of optimal management remains incomplete, and the benefit of full implementation of existing evidence remains elusive. Guidelines face the challenge of providing clinicians with practical guidance and balancing evolving evidence, while keeping updates infrequent enough to allow time to be adopted. Supporting and encouraging patients to increase understanding of their chronic illnesses and employment of shared decision making are key to increasing compliance and maximizing benefit, with the ultimate goal of providing benefit while minimizing risks for individual patients.

> Presentation of chest pain in the primary care setting is a challenge for physician assistants. Because of the extensive nature of a differential diagnosis that includes many systems, accurately diagnosing the cause of chest pain is key. Several points lead a practitioner to accurately direct the investigation and treatment plans based on sound fundamental practices when the patient presents to their practice. It is important for the physician assistant to start the encounter with the patient in an organized, practical, directed fashion. Failure to do so may lead the physician assistant to prolong treatment and not find an accurate diagnosis.

> Cardiac arrhythmias are routinely seen in clinical patients, ranging from the benign and latent to the lethal and acutely obvious. Atrial fibrillation, atrioventricular block, long QT syndrome, sinus arrhythmia, and sick sinus syndrome are discussed. Understanding their mechanisms, presenting symptoms, diagnostic properties, and current therapy guideline will enhance physician assistants' level of patient care.

Vitamin K antagonists such as warfarin have been the mainstay of management for anticoagulation. Two new classes of medications have recently become available: direct thrombin inhibitor and Factor Xa inhibitors. These new classes combined are called direct oral anticoagulants (DOACs), which are being used effectively and safely for the management of venous thromboembolism (VTE) and nonvalvular atrial fibrillation. Choosing the appropriate agent for the treatment of VTE and nonvalvular atrial fibrillation requires an understanding of the differences between the medications. Bleeding while concomitantly taking a DOAC is of particular concern because of risk of fatality or severe disability.

After an ischemic coronary event, it is important for the provider to follow up with the patient at regular intervals and to be knowledgeable about appropriate testing that should occur with each visit. Appropriate medical therapy and lifestyle changes are essential to improving outcomes in these patients but are only effective if the patient is diligent in adhering to the recommendations. The provider should use any and all techniques necessary to improve patient compliance and adherence to the prescribed medication and lifestyle regimen, which, in turn, will result in an improved quality of life.

Dyslipidemia is a major contributor to atherosclerotic cardiovascular disease, and its management is crucial to reducing cardiovascular risk. After years of following the National Cholesterol Education Program Adult Treatment Panel III guidelines for the assessment and management of hypercholesterolemia, clinicians are now faced with new guidelines that are vastly different in several ways. Poor understanding leads to nonadherence by clinicians and patients. This article provides physician assistants with the information needed to make appropriate clinical decisions based on the latest evidence-based lipid management guidelines.

Heart failure is a complex disease with many contributing factors that make the management complicated and multifaceted. With careful examination, collaboration, and education to both the patients and other key stakeholders, the disease can be appropriately managed. Overall goals are directed toward prolonging life, improving adherence, and lengthening survival rates. Frank discussions with patients on expectations and limitations must be done to achieve realistic goals, and eventually preparing for end-of-life discussions is paramount.

Selecting an appropriate diagnostic modality for a patient with chest pain can seem daunting given the variety of options available. Understanding the basic premise of each modality and which is most appropriate for a patient can greatly increase the diagnostic accuracy and reduce costs. Once a diagnosis has been made, aggressive medical management should be initiated according to the most recent guidelines. Early recognition of symptoms concerning for coronary artery disease, selecting appropriate testing, and vigilant management through medications and lifestyle changes will improve outcomes and quality of life for patients.

Valvular heart disease (VHD) is commonly encountered in primary care practice. Involvement of the aortic and mitral valves is more common than right-sided involvement and can present with classic history and physical findings. Cardiac remodeling and adaptation often precede symptom onset and can become maladaptive and irreversible. Treatment often involves valve repair or replacement and progress has been made in minimally invasive transcatheter intervention, which has benefited many patients who otherwise would not be candidates for surgical repair or replacement. Identification of patients with VHD, to include accurate staging, is essential to responsibly counsel and refer for further evaluation.

Syncope is defined as a transient, abrupt, and brief loss of consciousness due to impaired cerebral blood flow. Possible causes for an episode of syncope are numerous and generally grouped into 3 categories: cardiovascular, neutrally mediated, and orthostatic. These can range from benign to life-threatening and frequently be distinguished by history alone. If there is doubt or the cause is suspected to be highly acute, a minimum of basic blood tests and an electrocardiogram should be performed with further testing considered based on prioritization of the differential diagnosis.

Pulmonary arterial hypertension has many causes, all of which are treated with specific therapies. Managing the underlying cause of pulmonary hypertension often secondarily improves the pulmonary hypertension. Pulmonary arterial hypertension is associated with increased thrombosis and disrupted coagulation and fibrinolysis, making anticoagulation an attractive and frequently used therapeutic modality. At the present time, pulmonary vasodilator therapy and oral anticoagulation are the main tools of long-term medical therapy.

Over the past century there has been a shift in the main causes of death from infectious to cardiovascular. Strategies to prevent morbidity and mortality have evolved, and there are now well-described atherosclerotic risk factors available to help target preventative efforts before and after a patient has suffered an event. Current risk calculators help identify those who would most benefit from preventative efforts but remain suboptimal because they do not adequately reflect risk in several large minority populations. Understanding the pathogenesis of atherosclerosis and the different levels of prevention will position clinicians to best maintain patient health.

PHYSICIAN ASSISTANT CLINICS

RELATED INTEREST

Medical Clinics of North America
January 2017 (Vol. 101, Issue 1)
Hypertension
Edward D. Frohlich, *Editor*

THE CLINICS ARE AVAILABLE ONLINE!
Access your subscription at:
www.theclinics.com

Foreword
Getting Ready for Boards?

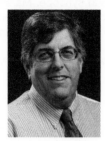

James A. Van Rhee, MS, PA-C
Consulting Editor

Like many Physician Assistants every year, you may be getting ready to take the Physician Assistant National Certifying Exam (PANCE) for the first time or getting ready to recertify with the Physician Assistant Recertifying Exam (PANRE). You may be looking at review courses, review books (no I am not promoting my review book), pulling out old textbooks and school notes (please don't use these to prepare), and setting aside many hours to study. I would like to point out to you that this publication, *Physician Assistant Clinics*, is an excellent source of information for the boards and can provide you with continuing medical education (CME) credit.

Over the eight issues we have published, we have covered the following systems: nephrology, dermatology, oncology, pediatrics, endocrinology, infectious disease, emergency medicine, and this issue, cardiology. Urology and otolaryngology are coming soon.

Throughout all these issues, we have covered a wide variety of topics that you will also see on the PANCE or PANRE. We have covered everything from acute and chronic kidney injury to kidney stones in the very first issue. In subsequent issues, we have covered skin cancer to nail disorders, ovarian cancer to graft-versus-host disease, epilepsy to attention-deficit disorders, diabetes to pheochromocytoma, community-acquired pneumonia to tick-borne infections, anaphylaxis to headache emergencies. And this month's issue covers twelve topics in cardiology. Just doing a quick review of all the topics, we have covered over 120 of the various topics on the PANCE and PANRE exam blueprint. All of this in only eight issues, with more to come.

So, *Physician Assistant Clinics* provides you not only with the latest review of a wide variety of topics but also with coverage of a wide range of topics seen on the exam. So, in one location you can keep up-to-date on medical information, obtain CME, and prepare for the boards. One-stop shopping.

In this issue, we are focusing on cardiology. Guest editor, Daniel Thibodeau, has put together an excellent issue covering a wide variety of topics. Thibodeau himself

Physician Assist Clin 2 (2017) xiii–xiv
http://dx.doi.org/10.1016/j.cpha.2017.07.002
2405-7991/17/© 2017 Published by Elsevier Inc.

physicianassistant.theclinics.com

provides you with an excellent review on heart failure and the evaluation of chest pain in the primary care setting. Feldman, Zuber, and Davis are back with us again covering the latest in dyslipidemia. Hricz is covering all the bases in acute coronary syndrome and ischemic heart disease. Cucchi covers anticoagulation, and with Levy, applies this information to the topic of pulmonary hypertension and thromboembolism. Tzizik discusses the primary care approach to valvular heart disease and syncope. Marshall covers cardiac arrhythmias, and no issue on cardiology would be complete without Mackie's articles on hypertension and preventive cardiology with co-author Trent Honda.

I hope you enjoy the eighth issue of *Physician Assistant Clinics*. Our next issue will provide you with a review of the latest in urology.

James A. Van Rhee, MS, PA-C
Yale School of Medicine
Yale Physician Assistant Online Program
100 Church Street South, Suite A250
New Haven, CT 06519, USA

E-mail address:
james.vanrhee@yale.edu

Website:
http://www.paonline.yale.edu

Preface
Cardiology

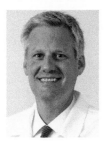

Daniel T. Thibodeau, MHP, PA-C, DFAAPA
Editor

Cardiovascular disease has been, and remains, the number one cause of death in the United States. According to the Centers for Disease Control and Prevention, roughly 610,000 deaths are a result of cardiovascular disease. As physician assistants (PAs), we all encounter patients who either have some cardiovascular condition that is being treated or are at risk. To understand the nature of the most common conditions, how to evaluate and analyze patients is at the very core of what we do. We hope this issue will guide you in your practice, and we certainly hope it gives you improvement with your clinical skills.

Throughout these articles are the essential topics that we as PAs see on a regular basis. Whether you are in primary care, internal medicine, urgent care, or emergency medicine, this issue will help you appreciate the various management strategies and treatment plans. We have taken the time to ensure that the most up-to-date guidelines have been in place, and we have looked for all the latest treatment options that you will find helpful in the care of your patients. We recognize that things change rapidly in medicine, so we have attempted to ensure that all information is as up-to-date as possible.

A little note about our authors. All of them are PAs (and we thank our MD and NP authors for our lipids article contributions), and many of them practice and teach in our best schools. Without them, this issue would not be possible, and I think you will appreciate the care that has been given in each article to provide you with a well-written series of topics that are germane to your clinical life. Because we all teach, we also work to develop and nurture the next generation of PAs that will one day become our professional colleagues. We urge you to do the same, and for those who already teach, thank you. For those who have not, please remember those that taught you and reach out to your local program. They would love your help.

Physician Assist Clin 2 (2017) xv–xvi
http://dx.doi.org/10.1016/j.cpha.2017.07.001
2405-7991/17/© 2017 Published by Elsevier Inc.

physicianassistant.theclinics.com

Thank you for all that you do for our profession. And thank you for all you do for your patients and your community.

Daniel T. Thibodeau, MHP, PA-C, DFAAPA
Physician Assistant Program
Clinical Education Recruitment and Support
Eastern Virginia Medical School
700 W. Olney Road, Lewis Hall 3168
Norfolk, VA 23505, USA

Cardiovascular Specialists Inc
5838 Harbour View Boulevard
Suite 270, Suffolk, VA 23435, USA

E-mail address:
thiboddt@evms.edu

Hypertension: An Evidence Informed, Case Based Approach

Andrew Mackie, MPAS, PA-C

KEYWORDS

- Cardiovascular disease • Hypertension • High Blood Pressure • JNC • Guideline

KEY POINTS

- Despite longstanding knowledge of the consequences of uncontrolled hypertension and the availability of effective classes of antihypertensives, the understanding of optimal management is still incomplete, and the benefit of full implementation of existing evidence remains elusive.
- Guidelines face the challenge of providing busy clinicians with practical guidance and balancing rapidly evolving evidence, while keeping updates infrequent enough to allow time to be adopted.
- Supporting and encouraging patients to increase understanding of their chronic illnesses through employment of shared decision making is key to increasing compliance and maximizing benefit, with the ultimate goal of improving outcomes while minimizing risks for individual patients.
- Antihypertensive agent selection and target blood pressure requires placing an individual patient's comorbidities and characteristics in the context of available guidelines and subsequently published studies, with ultimate clinician and patient shared decision making to determine an optimal regimen.

BACKGROUND

On April 12, 1945, President Franklin D. Roosevelt, who had led the United States out of the Great Depression and guided the nation during World War II, was relaxing in Warm Springs, Georgia. While having his portrait painted, he complained of a severe headache and lost consciousness. Before he died of a cerebral hemorrhage, his cardiologist Dr. Howard G. Bruenn found his blood pressure (BP) to be 300/190 mm Hg.[1] Despite his prominence as the leader of the free world, medical care at this time had no effective treatments for the president's hypertension, contributing to his premature death at age 63 (**Fig. 1**).

Author Disclosure: The author has no conflicts of interest and no disclosures to report.
Physician Assistant Program, Bouvé College of Health Sciences, Northeastern University, 202 Robinson Hall, 360 Huntington Avenue, Boston, MA 02115, USA
E-mail address: a.mackie@neu.edu

Physician Assist Clin 2 (2017) 557–570
http://dx.doi.org/10.1016/j.cpha.2017.06.001
2405-7991/17/© 2017 Elsevier Inc. All rights reserved.

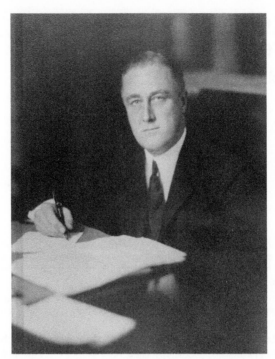

Fig. 1. Franklin D. Roosevelt in 1933, just 12 years prior to his premature death at age 63. (http://www.fdrlibrary.marist.edu/archives/collections/franklin/index.php?p=digitallibrary/digitalcontent&id=2178).

The president's death provides a window into the consequences of untreated hypertension[2] and provides today's clinicians with an appreciation of the wide range of antihypertensives now available. Medicine has progressed, and there are now the tools to prevent premature death and disability from a range of illnesses in which hypertension plays a key role. This article provides an overview of the development of the key evidence for treatment of hypertension, applies the most recent guidelines in a case-based approach, and considers the impact of more recently published studies on management decisions.

Following World War II, the efforts of the scientific community focused on health research rather than treatment of catastrophic injury. In June 1948, President Harry Truman signed the National Heart Act,[3] which lead to the creation of the National Heart, Lung, and Blood Institute and the longitudinal Framingham Heart Study.[4] This landmark study, which continues to this day, identified multiple risk factors associated with the development of cardiovascular disease (CVD) such as cholesterol, smoking, and hypertension.[5,6]

By 1967, a randomized placebo-controlled clinical trial was published demonstrating the cardiovascular benefit of antihypertensives (hydrochlorothiazide, reserpine, and hydralazine) in patients with diastolic hypertension.[7] By the 1970s, additional classes of medication were available, and the need for guidelines became necessary to provide practical recommendations,[8] define the appropriate population to treat, and provide guidance for agent selection.

The first Joint National Commission[8] guidelines (JNC1) were published in 1977 and recommended a 4 step approach to therapy, escalating coverage by adding additional medications if control was not achieved. At that time the first line of treatment was a thiazide diuretic, adding a 2nd drug (propranolol, methyldopa, or reserpine) if necessary. Third and 4th line recommended medications were hydralazine and guanethidine, respectively. At that time, elevated systolic blood pressure (SBP) was thought to be a natural consequence of aging,[9] with a normal systolic blood pressure defined as the patient's age plus 100. As such, the JNC 1 guidelines focused on diastolic hypertension.[8] An additional point of interest is that the JNC 1 guidelines featured only a single reference: the 1970 Veterans Administration Cooperative Study.[10]

Subsequently updates to these guidelines were published every 3 to 6 years,[11–15] with the exception of a 12 year gap between JNC 7 and the most recent JNC 8 guidelines.[16,17] The latest guidelines were also the first to be evidence-based, rather than based on expert opinion. Within a year of the release of JNC 8,[18] the publication of new evidence in the SPRINT trial (Systolic Blood Pressure Intervention Trial)[19] called into question some elements of the latest guidelines, leading a New England Journal of Medicine editorial to state, "Current guidelines and guideline processes require revision.[20]"

JNC 8 was the first set of evidence-based guidelines for hypertension and included a grading process to indicate the level of evidence, based on the relationship of benefit vs. harm. Grade A indicated a high certainty of benefit, grade B moderate, and grade C weak benefit. Grade "D" indicates a recommendation against a particular therapy (harm outweighs benefit), and expert opinion indicates a lack of clear evidence (but a consensus recommendation among experts). The guideline is structured to provide recommendations (**Table 1**). Recommendations 1 to 5 cover the threshold (to start) treatment and the goal (target BP) of treatment. Recommendations 6 to 8 address the choice of antihypertensive agent. Finally, recommendation 9 suggests an overall approach to implementation of the guidelines.

JNC 8 differs from JNC 7[21] in several ways. JNC 7 recommendations were based upon a nonsystematic review of the literature with treatment recommendations decided by expert consensus. On the contrary, JNC 8 used a systematic approach to reviewing the extant literature and determined recommendations based upon a predefined protocol. Importantly, nomenclature such as prehypertension was dropped in JNC 8, but thresholds for initiation of therapy were maintained.

Table 1
Summary of the structure of recommendations in Joint National Commission 8

Recommendation	Type	Population
1	Threshold/goal	Age >60
2	Threshold/goal	Age <60 (diastolic)
3	Threshold/goal	Age <60 (systolic)
4	Threshold/goal	Chronic kidney disease
5	Threshold/goal	Diabetes
6	Agent selection	Nonblack (including diabetes)
7	Agent selection	Black (including diabetes)
8	Agent selection	Chronic kidney disease
9	Approach	All

Data from James PA, Oparil S, Carter BL, et al. 2014 evidence-based guideline for the management of high blood pressure in adults: report from the panel members appointed to the Eighth Joint National Committee (JNC 8). Jama. 2014;311(5):507–520.

CASES

Given the current state of information, how can one best incorporate the existing guidelines and evidence to care for individual patients? To approach this from a practical perspective, the article employs a case-based approach that considers how the evidence might be applied for patients with different, yet frequently encountered characteristics that need to be considered when optimizing antihypertensive therapy for each given individual. The framework for these cases will be several days in a typical week in a primary care clinic, where each day a patient with differing characteristics presents a challenge to adapt one's approach in an informed manner to best care for a particular individual.

Monday

A Caucasian 55-year-old truck driver with no known medical issues and taking no medications, presents for his Department of Transportation routine physical examination. Before you enter the room, you notice that the vital signs documented by the medical assistant are temperature 98.7°F, respiratory rate 14 breaths per minute, heart rate 82 beats per minute, and BP 150/88 mm Hg. He is listed as being 6 feet tall and weighs 210 pounds (body mass index [BMI] 28.5 kg/m^2).

Upon questioning, you find out that he has no current concerns, and that a review of systems form he filled out while waiting is unremarkable. You repeat his BP and find it to be 154/88 mm Hg. You review his chart and find that he had a similar blood pressure when seen in the emergency room for a minor laceration 6 months ago.

You conclude that he likely has hypertension, and several questions come to mind:

- What should the history and physical should cover?
- What other evaluation should be done?
- What lifestyle counseling is appropriate?
- Should pharmacologic treatment be initiated?
- When should you see him to follow up?

His history has already indicated he has no complaints either at present or on his review of systems. You inquire about his family history and find none of his parents, siblings, or children has had atherosclerotic CVD (ASCVD). He is a lifelong nonsmoker and drinks "a beer or two" when watching televised sports every Sunday. He explains, "the rest of the time I'm either working or doing chores, so I don't really drink much".

His physical examination reveals no arteriovenous nicking or other apparent abnormalities on fundoscopy and no thyroid abnormalities or carotid bruit; his heart examination is normal with no S4 gallop to suggest hypertrophy, and his lungs are clear. You are unable to appreciate organomegaly, abdominal bruit, or a palpable abdominal aorta. He has no pedal edema, and his distal pulses are normal.

You decide to perform a routine diagnostic evaluation and see him again in 2 weeks to review the results and discuss possible options. You provide him with a printout designed for patient education and ask him to review this and bring any questions to his next appointment.

Before leaving the room, you order a chemistry panel (to assess electrolytes, renal function, and screen for hyperglycemia), urinalysis (to screen for abnormalities such as proteinuria), a fasting lipid profile, and electrocardiogram (ECG, to screen for left ventricular hypertrophy or evidence of a previously unrecognized cardiac event).

Upon return in 2 weeks, you review his laboratory work and ECG, all of which reveal no abnormalities. His blood pressure on this visit is 156/88. Given the patient's age, habitus, normal physical examination, and blood work, you have little reason to believe his hypertension might be due to a secondary cause. You discuss with the patient the importance of treating hypertension and find that he has reviewed the patient information brochure you provided last visit. He indicates that he understands the risks involved with untreated hypertension and wishes to initiate treatment.

You now consider the latest evidence and guidelines and how they might apply to this patient. On reviewing the Eighth Joint National Committee guidelines on hypertension (JNC 8) you find that the level of evidence for treating systolic hypertension at this level is only expert opinion, while Grade A evidence exists to treat diastolic BP (DBP) above 90 mm Hg (his is 88). You decide to follow the expert recommendations and treat him for systolic hypertension.

Next, you consider therapeutic options. JNC 8 recommends initiation of a thiazide diuretic, angiotensin-converting enzyme (ACE) inhibitor, angiotensin receptor blocker (ARB), or calcium channel blocker. Because of his job as a truck driver, you choose a calcium channel blocker rather than a diuretic (as he will not have easy access to restroom facilities during work). Although an ACE inhibitor or ARB would also have been valid options, you write him a prescription for amlodipine 5 mg and instruct him to take half a tablet daily for a week, then increase to 1 tablet daily. You plan to see him again in a month.

Before you finish your visit with him, you discuss the importance of lifestyle modifications[22] including diet (sodium <2,400 mg daily, avoidance of saturated fat), exercise (goal of 150 minutes per week of brisk walking), and weight reduction (write down food intake, attempt moderate calorie reduction).

His BMI of 28.5 kg/m^2 places him in the overweight (25.0–29.9) category.[23] In order to be within the normal range, he must drop his weight from 210 pounds to 184 pounds. You advise him that the combination of calorie reduction and increased physical activity can help him move toward this range and that when you see him again, you will be looking for progress, not perfection. If more specific direction is desired, providing information about the DASH (Dietary Approaches to Stop Hypertension) diet[24] or a referral to a nutritionist is a reasonable starting point.

When he returns in a month, he has successfully titrated his medications and is having no adverse effects. His blood pressure is now 136/82 mm Hg, and his weight has dropped by 3 lbs. You consider the target blood pressure, keeping in mind that JNC 8 recommended a BP of less than 140/90 for his age group. Having reached the target blood pressure, you recommend follow-up in 6 months. Success!

This is a straightforward case of newly diagnosed hypertension in a patient with no comorbidities. The JNC 8 guidelines help to direct diagnosis and management. It is important to note, however, that the recommendation to treat systolic hypertension in this subpopulation is based upon expert opinion only. This illustrates the limitations clinicians face in terms of evidence to manage diseases even one as prevalent and widely studied as hypertension.

Key points learned from this case include

- Management of the hypertensive patient without comorbidities
- Use multiple measurements to confirm hypertension before initiating therapy
- Elements of initial physical examination
- Elements of initial evaluation
- Awareness of levels of evidence for initiation of therapy at a given level of hypertension
- Agent selection based on guidelines, but individualized for a patient

Tuesday

On Tuesday Mr. Johnson, a 44-year-old Caucasian man, comes in for his biannual evaluation. You diagnosed him with type 2 diabetes mellitus 3 years ago, and he has since dropped his weight from 251 pounds (BMI 36.0 kg/m^2) to 223 pounds (BMI 32.0 kg/m^2). Today his weight is 216 pounds (BMI 31.0 kg/m^2). He reports that he has reduced calorie intake and has been walking his dog for 30 minutes after dinner at least 5 days per week (150 minutes per week). His diabetes has been fairly well controlled; his most recent Hemoglobin A1c (HgbA1c) was 6.6% (goal of <6.5%). Other laboratory work from his last visit included a total cholesterol of 183 mg/dL and a low-density lipoprotein level of 104 mg/dL.

Today he has no complaints. You note that his blood pressure has increased from 136/84 mm Hg to 150/88 mm Hg. At his last visit, you discussed his blood pressure level and the increased risk for cardiovascular issues with diabetes. Using shared decision making, you both agreed that it was reasonable for the patient to pursue lifestyle changes instead of initiating an antihypertensive medication.

Although you feel that this level of hypertension warrants treatment, you wonder about how the guidelines and literature can inform your management. The ACCORD trial (Action to Control Cardiovascular Risk in Diabetes)[25] was published in 2008 and had a primary goal of determining if intensive glycemic management would be beneficial in patients with type 2 diabetes, but also contained an arm to study whether there was benefit to targeting systolic blood pressure to less than 120 mm Hg versus less than 140 mm Hg among diabetics. Guidelines at the time recommended a target blood pressure of less than 130 mm Hg in diabetics.[21] As you look over the study and its results, you note that the inclusion criteria for the ACCORD trial required that those in your patient's age range have preexisting coronary artery disease as well as HgbA1c levels above 7.5%. In addition, the average age of those enrolled in the trial was 62.2. You conclude that findings from this trial cannot be directly extrapolated to your patient.

You next consider the more recently published SPRINT trial. However, you quickly recognize that while the study design is similar to ACCORD, diabetics were excluded. Lastly, you turn to the JNC 8 guidelines and note that several recommendations apply to diabetics, including recommendations 5 to 7.

Recommendation 5 specifically indicates initiation of antihypertensives at a threshold of SBP of at least 140 or DBP of at least 90, and that the target SBP and DBP should be no more than 140 and no more than 90, respectively. Recommendations 6 and 7 both address antihypertensive selection and both include diabetics. They differ in that recommendation 6 applies to the nonblack population and 7 to the black population.

In the nonblack population, JNC 8 recommends initiation of a thiazide-type diuretic, calcium channel blocker, or either an ACE inhibitor or an ARB. In the black population (including those with diabetes), either a thiazide-type diuretic or a calcium channel blocker is recommended.

Mr. Johnson is Caucasian and has no signs/symptoms of chronic kidney disease (CKD) and fits into the population in which an ACE or ARB are first-line choices. You reflect that although you are considering how to manage his hypertension, his health must be considered in the context of all of his comorbidities, particularly his diabetes. Separate from the benefit conferred by control of hypertension, ACE and ARBs have been shown to reduce the incidence of diabetic nephropathy in both type 1[26] and type 2 diabetes.[27] Given this benefit, the American Diabetes Association recommends the use of an ACE inhibitor or ARB for diabetics with hypertension, to a goal of less than 140/90 mm Hg.[28]

Key points from this case include:

- Management of hypertension in diabetics
- Importance of inhibition of the renin-angiotensin system in diabetics for renal protection
- Medication selection is often dependent on comorbidities

Wednesday

Ms. Knowles, a 52-year-old African American woman with type 2 diabetes mellitus for 6 years, presents with viral pharyngitis. Vital signs reveal a blood pressure of 168/96 mm Hg. She reports that her sister, who is a nurse, checked her blood pressure a "month or two ago" and told her it was "too high, 150 something." You repeat a blood pressure after talking with her for a few minutes and find it to be unchanged. You determine that she has hypertension and requires treatment.

You further determine that she has a family history of not only diabetes, but of stroke (her father at age 56, now deceased) and end-stage renal disease requiring dialysis (her mother at 68, now age 74).

You decide to order a routine diagnostic evaluation, as you did in an earlier case, but also check her HgbA1c and urine albumin to creatinine ratio (UACR). While the HgbA1c will provide a sense of the overall control of her diabetes, the KDOQI (Kidney Disease Quality Outcomes Initiative) 2012 guidelines recommend a level of less than 7.0% to delay progression of microvascular complications, including CKD.[29] Before serum creatine rises, microalbuminuria (UACR 30–300 mg/g) may be present, providing an early indication of the development of kidney disease.[30]

Both JNC 8 and the 2016 Americans with Diabetes Association (ADA) standards recommend treating pharmacologically when blood pressure exceeds 140/90 in diabetics,[18,28] while KDIGO (Kidney Disease: Improving Global Outcomes) suggests a target less than 130/80 mm Hg if albuminuria if present.[30] Whether albuminuria is present may influence agent selection.

You explain to the patient your concern of her high blood pressure and the elevated risks for heart attack, stroke, and kidney disease. She agrees to begin treatment.

Diabetic patients are at risk for both macrovascular (coronary heart disease, cerebrovascular disease, and peripheral arterial disease) and microvascular (retinopathy, nephropathy, and neuropathy)[29] complications. African Americans have higher rates of hypertension than other racial/ethnic groups (40.4% incidence, vs 27.4% in whites).[31] In addition, genetic variations have been determined to contribute to differences in the underlying mechanisms for hypertension.[32] In particular, upregulation of renin plays a lesser role for African Americans in both experimental[33] and clinical trials.[34]

There is also a tendency to have increased salt sensitivity in this population.[35] Consequently, African American patients have less of a response to angiotensin blockade compared with medications with other pharmacologic actions, such as thiazide type diuretics.[34] Despite this, there is some evidence that this differential efficacy can be mitigated by concomitant use of a thiazide diuretic or calcium channel blocker with an ACEI or ARB.[36,37]

Although one goal for this patient is blood pressure control to prevent adverse cardiovascular events, such as stroke or myocardial infarction, she also has diabetes, which puts her at additional risk for chronic kidney disease, neuropathy, and retinopathy. Diabetes is the leading cause of chronic kidney disease, causing a glomerulopathy that is associated with progressive proteinuria. Delay in progression of CKD to end-stage renal disease (ESRD) has been demonstrated with both the use of ACEI and ARBs.[29] Given the previously stated reduced responsiveness to renin inhibition, you wonder about the role of these agents in your patient.

One consideration in this scenario is whether the patient has yet developed albuminuria, indicating at least early CKD. If albuminuria is present, angiotensin blockade (ACEI or ARB) is necessary.[28,38]

Some experts advocate initiation of angiotensin blockade before the development of albuminuria. Because the diabetic, hypertensive, African American population has a higher likelihood of developing CKD, the rationale is that using an angiotensin blockade will prevent progression of glomerulonephropathy at its most nascent stages.[39,40]

A further consideration is to have a clear conceptual intent regarding the initiation and maintenance of antihypertensive therapy. Rather than treating hypertension to decrease blood pressure, the primary goal is to prevent ASCVD complications. The addition of hypertension to diabetes further increases the risk of cardiovascular disease and is a risk factor for the development of CKD and retinopathy.[41] Only 54.1% of those with hypertension were controlled according to data from NHANES 2009 to 2012.[42] In the case of diabetes, which is the most frequent cause of end-stage renal failure in the United States,[30] renal protection is a separate but overlapping goal.

JNC 8 recommended initial therapy with a calcium channel blocker or thiazide type diuretic in African American patients, even with diabetes, unless they had signs/symptoms of CKD. Intervention is aimed at preventing atherosclerotic cardiovascular disease (ASCVD). If one looks a bit more closely at recommendation 7 (general black population, including those with diabetes), starting with a CCB or thiazide is given a grade B (moderate recommendation), but for those with diabetes the level is grade C (weak recommendation). Thus, given the available evidence, a shared decision making approach with your patient is appropriate.

Although you feel that this level of hypertension warrants treatment, you wonder about how the guidelines and literature can inform your management. The ACCORD BP trial randomized diabetic patients with either preexisting CVD (or at least 2 CVD risk factors) to a goal BP of 140/90 versus 120/80.[25] Although target BPs were achieved in both groups, the lower target failed to demonstrate a mortality benefit after an average follow-up of 4.7 years. This trial also determined that although there was a lower risk of stroke in those treated to the lower target, there was an increased risk of complications, and a slight rise in serum creatinine.

Although the ACCORD trial,[25] which only enrolled diabetics, did not show a mortality benefit for more intensive blood pressure treatment (to a goal of 120/80), there was a reduction in strokes (number need to treat of 89 over 5 years). Additionally, a meta-analysis[43] that contained a subgroup of 5 trials[25,41,44–46] of diabetics (including the ACCORD trial) demonstrated a reduction in major cardiovascular events, with a non-significant mortality benefit.

Considering the available guidelines for both diabetes and hypertension, as well as the dual goals in this patient of preventing ASCVD (eg, stroke) and complications of diabetes (eg, CKD), you and the patient agree to initiate dual therapy with a low dose of a thiazide -type diuretic as well as an ACE inhibitor and aspirin. You plan to see her again in 2 weeks to assess for adverse effects, ensure there have been no adverse effects on electrolytes or renal function (which might indicate renal artery stenosis), and to assess the efficacy of therapy.

Key points from this case include

- Management of hypertension in African Americans
- Workup for evaluation of hypertension
- Considerations for timing of inhibition of the renin-angiotensin system in diabetics
- Differences in goals of therapy (eg, ASCVD vs renal protection) in agent selection

Thursday

An 83-year-old Caucasian woman with a history of a myocardial infarction at age 65 (which prompted her to quit smoking) and hypertension presented for transfer of her care to your office. She is accompanied by her daughter who explains that she was unsatisfied with her mother's quality of care and cites that her prior practitioner indicated her BP was "good enough given her age" (systolic blood pressure 180 mm Hg). The daughter states her mom's sister recently suffered a stroke related to high BP. The daughter asks you to consider a more aggressive approach to managing her mother's hypertension.

There are no records, and the past medical history is simply what is obtained from the daughter and mother. History shows a hospitalization for community-acquired pneumonia at age 75 (she subsequently received pneumococcal vaccination and has since had annual influenza vaccination), untreated hyperlipidemia, and an appendectomy at age 20.

Physical examination shows her to be afebrile with a respiratory rate of 18, a heart rate of 75, and BP of 178/92 mm Hg. On general appearance, she is a moderately overweight elderly, but otherwise apparently healthy, woman in no distress with a pleasant demeanor and a quick wit. She has no carotid bruits, and her lungs are clear; you do, however, appreciate an early crescendo systolic murmur at the right upper sternal border with a preserved S2 and no radiation to the carotids, which you feel is likely caused by aortic sclerosis. Her cardiac examination is otherwise notable for an S4 but no S3. Her abdominal examination is benign and without a palpable aorta and no bruit. Her peripheral pulses are normal.

She is able to climb 2 flights of stairs with only transient mild dyspnea and has a small dog that she loves, and walks twice a day for about one-half mile each time. She describes a reasonably healthy diet and rarely drinks alcohol. She socializes with friends on a weekly basis and has 2 children, whom she sees "a few times a month." She has been widowed for 10 years and lives in her own home. She still drives, but "not on the highway." She retired from accounting for a small business at age 65.

As you consider how to manage this patient, there are several thoughts you feel are important to consider. Overall, she is relatively healthy and active but is at risk for ASCVD, including stroke, myocardial infarction, and heart failure. You are inclined to treat her hypertension more aggressively, as well as address her hyperlipidemia, but decide to consult the guidelines and literature before making a decision. You order laboratory work and plan to see her again in a week.

Routine laboratory studies show a normal complete blood cell (CBC) count and chemistries, normal liver function tests, and a normal thyroid-stimulating hormone (TSH). Her lipid panel shows a total cholesterol of 190 mg/dL, and her urinalysis is unremarkable. An ECG shows a normal sinus rhythm and is otherwise normal save for borderline left ventricular hypertrophy.

You consult several sources in making your decision, including the JNC 8 guidelines, a study you recall hearing about of "very elderly" patients with hypertension, and the recent SPRINT 75 (those patients above age 75) trial results.

The JNC 8 guidelines recommendation 1 is to initiate therapy in patients over the age of 60 when they have hypertension in excess of either a systolic pressure of 150 mm Hg or a diastolic of 90 mm Hg, with a grade A (strong) level of recommendation.[18] The goal blood pressure is less than 150 mm Hg, with a corollary recommendation indicating if a blood pressure below 140 mm Hg is achieved without adverse consequences no change is necessary.

In 2008, the HYVET trial (Hypertension in the Very Elderly Trial),[47] looking at the management of hypertension in patients above the age of 80 was published. This trial examined 3845 relatively healthy (**Box 1**) patients who were randomly assigned to either placebo or an extended-release thiazide-like diuretic (indapamide), with a

---

Box 1
Overview of Hypertension in the Very Elderly Trial study population

Location

3845 patients in 195 centers in 13 countries
- 2144 from Eastern Europe
- 86 from Western Europe
- 1526 from China
- 19 from Australasia
- 70 from Tunisia

Patient characteristics

- Average age 83
- Women 60%
- Prior cardiovascular disease 11% to 12%
- Diabetes 6.8% to 6.9%
- Current smoker 6.4% to 6.6%
- Average BMI 24.7 kg/m^2

---

goal BP of 150/80 mm Hg. If the goal blood pressure was not achieved, an ACE inhibitor (perindopril) was added, for a stepped care approach.

While the trial had impressive reductions in stroke (30%) and heart failure (64%), an unexpected result was a 21% reduction in death from any cause. Criticisms of the trial included whether the results could be extrapolated to the majority of patients in this age range given the inclusion/exclusion criteria (**Box 2**), the overall good health of the included patients, and the geographic distribution of the patients enrolled (of the 3845 patients, 2144 were from Eastern Europe, and 1526 were from China).[48]

Despite these limitations, it clearly demonstrated that, at least in a subpopulation of healthy elderly patients, treatment of hypertension to a goal of less than 150/80 mm Hg has the potential for significant benefits in terms of: stroke, development of heart failure, and overall mortality. In response to criticisms of the study, the authors pointed

---

Box 2
Selected Hypertension in the Very Elderly Trial inclusion/exclusion criteria

Inclusion criteria

- Age ≥80
- Sustained SBP ≥160

Exclusion criteria

- Hemorrhage stroke less than 6 months ago
- Heart failure on antihypertensive
- Serum creatinine ≥1.7 mg/dL
- Gout
- Dementia
- Requirement of nursing care

---

out that, "the number of 80-year-olds who are healthy is increasing, so it will be important to take steps to ensure that they remain so."[48]

The final study you review is the SPRINT 75 trial,[49] which was published in 2016 as a preplanned subgroup analysis of the original 2015 SPRINT trial. Although this subgroup analysis evaluated even more aggressive target blood pressures (goal systolic of <120 mm Hg vs <140 mm Hg), it demonstrated a 33% relative risk reduction in cardiovascular events, and a 32% reduction in overall mortality.

Although the authors described, "some adverse events occurred significantly more frequently with the lower target," one criticism of the trial elaborated that, "combined serious adverse events of hypotension, syncope, bradycardia, electrolyte abnormality, injurious fall, and acute kidney injury were found significantly more frequently in the intervention group versus the control group among the frail subgroup."[50]

This patient is in overall good health with excellent functional status. The studies described for this demographic generally excluded patients who were frail or required nursing care. This patient is similar enough to the study populations for HYVET and SPRINT 75 that one can reasonably extrapolate she may derive similar benefit.

JNC 8 recommends a target pressure of less than 150/90 mm Hg, the HYVET intervention group had a target of 150/80 mm Hg, and SPRINT 75 had either a systolic target of less than 140 mm Hg in the standard treatment group or less than 120 mm Hg in the intervention group. In this patient, a graded approach may be considered, with an initial target less than 150/90 mm Hg. Functional status and laboratory parameters should be reassessed in subsequent visits before lowering the target to 140 mm Hg. Reduction beyond this initial goal may be considered if the patient is having no adverse consequences and wishes to attempt to further reduce her blood pressure, after fully understanding the potential risks and benefits.

Lastly, the issue of agent selection arises. The JNC 8 guidelines recommend initial therapy with a thiazide-like diuretic, calcium channel blocker, ACE inhibitor, or ARB. HYVET used a stepped approach with indapamide extended release with addition of the ACE inhibitor perindopril if not yet at target. SPRINT 75 recommended (but did not require) chlorthalidone, a thiazide-type diuretic, as the first-line agent, and permitted additional agents based on the patient's comorbidities and preference, including beta adrenergic blockers, calcium channel blockers, loop diuretics, and angiotensin system blockade agents.

You decide to try the HYVET approach of indapamide with re-evaluations monthly for 3 months, then every 3 months subsequently. If needed, you plan to add an ACE inhibitor with the intention of offsetting some of the hypokalemia that may be caused by the thiazide.

Key points from this case include

- Treatment of hypertension in elderly patients
- Considering trial population similarities/differences to your patient
- Synthesizing the available guidelines and evidence for an individual patient
- Importance of shared decision making where evidence becomes less certain

SUMMARY

Despite longstanding knowledge of the consequences of uncontrolled hypertension and the availability of effective classes of antihypertensives, understanding of optimal management is still incomplete, and the benefit of full implementation of existing evidence remains elusive. Guidelines face the challenge of providing busy clinicians with practical guidance and balancing rapidly evolving evidence, while keeping updates infrequent enough to allow time to be adopted. Supporting and encouraging patients to increase understanding of their chronic illnesses and employment of shared decision making are key to increasing compliance and maximizing benefit, with the ultimate goal of providing benefit while minimizing risks for individual patients.

REFERENCES

1. Bruenn HG. Clinical notes on the illness and death of president Franklin D. Roosevelt. Ann Intern Med 1970;72(4):579–91.
2. Moser M. Historical perspectives on the management of hypertension. J Clin Hypertens (Greenwich) 2006;8(8 Suppl 2):15–20 [quiz: 39].
3. Health NIO. Important events in NHLBI history. Available at: https://www.nih.gov/about-nih/what-we-do/nih-almanac/national-heart-lung-blood-institute-nhlbi. Accessed August 31, 2016.
4. Mahmood SS, Levy D, Vasan RS, et al. The Framingham heart study and the epidemiology of cardiovascular disease: a historical perspective. Lancet 2014; 383(9921):999–1008.
5. Kannel WB, Dawber TR, Kagan A, et al. Factors of risk in the development of coronary heart disease–six year follow-up experience. The Framingham study. Ann Intern Med 1961;55:33–50.
6. Kannel WB, Dawber TR, McNamara PM, et al. Vascular disease of the brain—epidemiologic aspects: The Framingham study. Am J Public Health Nations Health 1965;55(9):1355–66.
7. Effects of treatment on morbidity in hypertension. Results in patients with diastolic blood pressures averaging 115 through 129 mm Hg. JAMA 1967;202(11): 1028–34.
8. Report of the Joint National Committee on detection, evaluation, and treatment of high blood pressure. A cooperative study. JAMA 1977;237(3):255–61.
9. Black HR. The paradigm has shifted to systolic blood pressure. J Hum Hypertens 2004;18(Suppl 2):S3–7.
10. Effects of treatment on morbidity in hypertension. II. Results in patients with diastolic blood pressure averaging 90 through 114 mm Hg. JAMA 1970;213(7): 1143–52.
11. The 1980 report of the Joint National Committee on detection, evaluation, and treatment of high blood pressure. Arch Intern Med 1980;140(10):1280–5.
12. The 1984 report of the Joint National Committee on detection, evaluation, and treatment of high blood pressure. Arch Intern Med 1984;144(5):1045–57.
13. The 1988 report of the Joint National Committee on detection, evaluation, and treatment of high blood pressure. Arch Intern Med 1988;148(5):1023–38.
14. The fifth report of the Joint National Committee on detection, evaluation, and treatment of high blood pressure (JNC V). Arch Intern Med 1993;153(2):154–83.
15. The sixth report of the Joint National Committee on prevention, detection, evaluation, and treatment of high blood pressure. Arch Intern Med 1997;157(21): 2413–46.
16. Chobanian AV, Bakris GL, Black HR, et al. The seventh report of the Joint National Committee on prevention, detection, evaluation, and treatment of high blood pressure: the JNC 7 report. JAMA 2003;289(19):2560–72.
17. Krakoff LR, Gillespie RL, Ferdinand KC, et al. 2014 hypertension recommendations from the eighth joint national committee panel members raise concerns for elderly black and female populations. J Am Coll Cardiol 2014;64(4):394–402.

18. James PA, Oparil S, Carter BL, et al. 2014 evidence-based guideline for the management of high blood pressure in adults: report from the panel members appointed to the Eighth Joint National Committee (JNC 8). JAMA 2014;311(5): 507–20.
19. Wright JT Jr, Williamson JD, Whelton PK, et al. A randomized trial of intensive versus standard blood-pressure control. N Engl J Med 2015;373(22):2103–16.
20. Perkovic V, Rodgers A. Redefining blood-pressure targets–SPRINT starts the Marathon. N Engl J Med 2015;373(22):2175–8.
21. Chobanian AV, Bakris GL, Black HR, et al. Seventh report of the Joint National Committee on prevention, detection, evaluation, and treatment of high blood pressure. Hypertension 2003;42(6):1206–52.
22. Eckel RH, Jakicic JM, Ard JD, et al. 2013 AHA/ACC guideline on lifestyle management to reduce cardiovascular risk: a report of the American College of Cardiology/American Heart Association Task Force on practice guidelines. Circulation 2014;129(25 Suppl 2):S76–99.
23. Prevention CfDCa. Healthy weight. 2015. CDC BMI calculator. 2016. Available at: https://www.cdc.gov/healthyweight/assessing/bmi/adult_bmi/english_bmi_calculator/bmi_calculator.html. Accessed September 19, 2016.
24. Sacks FM, Svetkey LP, Vollmer WM, et al. Effects on blood pressure of reduced dietary sodium and the dietary approaches to stop hypertension (DASH) diet. DASH-Sodium Collaborative Research Group. N Engl J Med 2001;344(1):3–10.
25. Group AS, Cushman WC, Evans GW, et al. Effects of intensive blood-pressure control in type 2 diabetes mellitus. N Engl J Med 2010;362(17):1575–85.
26. Lewis EJ, Hunsicker LG, Bain RP, et al. The effect of angiotensin-converting-enzyme inhibition on diabetic nephropathy. The Collaborative Study Group. N Engl J Med 1993;329(20):1456–62.
27. Brenner BM, Cooper ME, de Zeeuw D, et al. Effects of losartan on renal and cardiovascular outcomes in patients with type 2 diabetes and nephropathy. N Engl J Med 2001;345(12):861–9.
28. American Diabetes Association. Standards of medical care in diabetes-2016 abridged for primary care providers. Clin Diabetes 2016;34(1):3–21.
29. National Kidney Foundation. KDOQI clinical practice guideline for diabetes and CKD: 2012 update. Am J Kidney Dis 2012;60(5):850–86.
30. Link DK. Management of the chronic kidney disease patient. Physician Assistant Clinics 2016;1(1):43–54.
31. Bennett A, Parto P, Krim SR. Hypertension and ethnicity. Curr Opin Cardiol 2016; 31(4):381–6.
32. Tu W, Pratt JH. A consideration of genetic mechanisms behind the development of hypertension in blacks. Curr Hypertens Rep 2013;15(2):108–13.
33. Chrysant SG, Danisa K, Kem DC, et al. Racial differences in pressure, volume and renin interrelationships in essential hypertension. Hypertension 1979;1(2): 136–41.
34. Wright JT Jr, Dunn JK, Cutler JA, et al. Outcomes in hypertensive black and nonblack patients treated with chlorthalidone, amlodipine, and lisinopril. JAMA 2005;293(13):1595–608.
35. Weinberger MH, Miller JZ, Luft FC, et al. Definitions and characteristics of sodium sensitivity and blood pressure resistance. Hypertension 1986;8(6 Pt 2):II127–134.
36. Weir MR, Ferdinand KC, Flack JM, et al. A noninferiority comparison of valsartan/hydrochlorothiazide combination versus amlodipine in black hypertensives. Hypertension 2005;46(3):508–13.

37. Racial differences in response to low-dose captopril are abolished by the addition of hydrochlorothiazide. Br J Clin Pharmacol 1982;14(Suppl 2):97s–101s.
38. Sica DA, Douglas JG. The African American Study of kidney disease and hypertension (AASK): new findings. J Clin Hypertens (Greenwich) 2001;3(4):244–51.
39. Ruggenenti P, Fassi A, Ilieva AP, et al. Preventing microalbuminuria in type 2 diabetes. N Engl J Med 2004;351(19):1941–51.
40. Haller H, Ito S, Izzo JL Jr, et al. Olmesartan for the delay or prevention of microalbuminuria in type 2 diabetes. N Engl J Med 2011;364(10):907–17.
41. Tight blood pressure control and risk of macrovascular and microvascular complications in type 2 diabetes: UKPDS 38. UK Prospective Diabetes Study Group. BMJ 1998;317(7160):703–13.
42. Writing Group M, Mozaffarian D, Benjamin EJ, et al. Heart disease and stroke statistics-2016 update: a report from the American Heart Association. Circulation 2016;133(4):e38–360.
43. Xie X, Atkins E, Lv J, et al. Effects of intensive blood pressure lowering on cardiovascular and renal outcomes: updated systematic review and meta-analysis. Lancet 2016;387(10017):435–43.
44. Estacio RO, Jeffers BW, Gifford N, et al. Effect of blood pressure control on diabetic microvascular complications in patients with hypertension and type 2 diabetes. Diabetes Care 2000;23(Suppl 2):B54–64.
45. Schrier RW, Estacio RO, Esler A, et al. Effects of aggressive blood pressure control in normotensive type 2 diabetic patients on albuminuria, retinopathy and strokes. Kidney Int 2002;61(3):1086–97.
46. Estacio RO, Coll JR, Tran ZV, et al. Effect of intensive blood pressure control with valsartan on urinary albumin excretion in normotensive patients with type 2 diabetes. Am J Hypertens 2006;19(12):1241–8.
47. Beckett NS, Peters R, Fletcher AE, et al. Treatment of hypertension in patients 80 years of age or older. N Engl J Med 2008;358(18):1887–98.
48. Treatment of hypertension in the elderly. N Engl J Med 2008;359(9):971–4.
49. Williamson JD, Supiano MA, Applegate WB, et al. Intensive vs standard blood pressure control and cardiovascular disease outcomes in adults aged ≥75 years: a randomized clinical trial. JAMA 2016;315(24):2673–82.
50. Karayiannis C, Phan TG, Srikanth V. Intensive vs standard blood pressure control for older adults. JAMA 2016;316(18):1920–1.

Evaluation of Chest Pain in the Primary Care Setting

Daniel T. Thibodeau, MHP, PA-C, DFAAPA[a,b],*

KEYWORDS

- Chest pain • Physician assistant • Physical examination • Laboratory studies
- Nuclear Stress Test • Pharmacologic Stress Test

KEY POINTS

- Chest pain presentations can be extensive depending on etiology.
- A careful history and physical examination aid the practitioner in determining the correct diagnosis.
- Laboratory studies and ancillary testing should be focused on top considerations.
- Treatment varies depending on history, physical, and test results.

INTRODUCTION

The presentation of chest pain in the primary care setting is a challenge for physician assistants (PAs). Because of the extensive nature of a differential diagnosis that includes many systems, accurately diagnosing the etiology of chest pain is key. Several points lead a practitioner to accurately direct their investigation and treatment plans based on sound fundamental practices when the patient presents to their practice. It is important for the PA to start their encounter with the patient in an organized, practical, and directed fashion. Failure to do so may lead the PA to prolong their treatment and not come up with an accurate diagnosis.

STATISTICS AND DEMOGRAPHICS

Heart disease remains the number one cause of death in the United States for individuals age 35 and older. In some regions of the United States the prevalence of heart disease is significant (**Fig. 1**).[1,2] Throughout the United States evaluations for the complaint of chest pain have been consistently high. As it relates to emergency visits, the complaint of chest pain has consistently remained a top complaint of individuals

Author Disclosure: Mr D. T. Thibodeau has no conflicts of interest and no disclosures to report.
[a] Eastern Virginia Medical School, Norfolk, 700 W. Olney Road, Lewis Hall 3168, Norfolk, VA 23505, USA; [b] Cardiovascular Specialists Inc, 5838 Harbour View Boulevard, Suite 270, Suffolk, VA 23435, USA
* Eastern Virginia Medical School, Norfolk, 700 W. Olney Road, Lewis Hall 3168, Norfolk, VA 23505.
E-mail address: thiboddt@evms.edu

Heart Disease Death Rates, 2008–2010
Adults, Ages 35+, by County

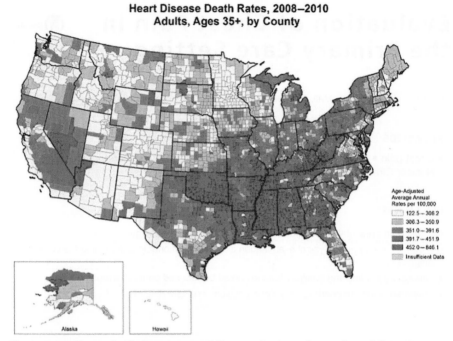

Fig. 1. Heart disease death. Rates are spatially smoothed to enhance the stabilitiy of rates in counties with small populations. (*From* CDC. Available at: https://www.cdc.gov/heartdisease/facts.htm. Accessed on November 22, 2016.)

visiting emergency rooms. This trend does not seem to have let up, and the number of visits has remained consistent (**Figs. 2** and **3**).[3]

CASE EXAMPLE 1

A 56-year-old man who has been followed in the family practice presents with the complaint of chest pain. He states that over the last 3 weeks he has been having a

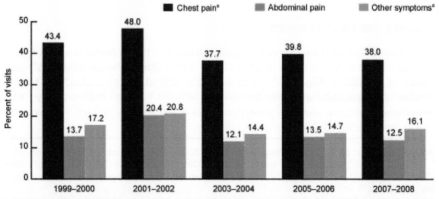

Fig. 2. Immediate and emergent noninjury emergency department visits for persons aged 18 years and older: United States, 1999 to 2008. Notes: Figures are based on 2-year averages. Emergent visits are those in which the patient should be seen within 14 minutes. [a] Trend is significant ($P<.05$). (*From* Emergency department visits for chest pain and abdominal pain: United States, 1999–2008. NCHS Data Brief, No. 43, September 2010. Available at: https://www.cdc.gov/nchs/data/databriefs/db43.pdf. Accessed on November 22, 2016.)

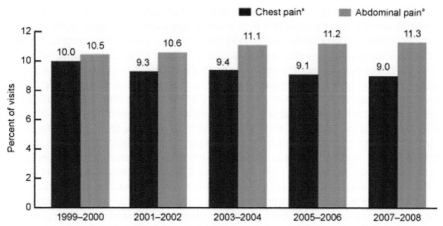

Fig. 3. Noninjury emergency department visits for chest pain and abdominal pain for persons aged 18 years and older: United States, 1999 to 2008. Notes: Figures are based on 2-year averages. [a] Trend is significant (*P*<.05). (*From* Emergency department visits for chest pain and abdominal pain: United States, 1999–2008. NCHS Data Brief, No. 43, September 2010. Available at: https://www.cdc.gov/nchs/data/databriefs/db43.pdf. Accessed on November 22, 2016.)

substernal pain, nonradiating, and at times makes him feel slightly short of breath. Resting helps with the symptoms, and he also has taken acetaminophen during one episode, which relieved his pain. He had another episode, which lasted for about 10 minutes, and was concerned so he asked to be seen in the office. His past medical history is significant for hypertension for 12 years, and borderline dyslipidemia for which he is watching and modifying his diet. His examination has a blood pressure (BP) of 146/90, pulse of 88, and has a normal physical examination.

This tends to be a typical case of a patient who presents to the primary care office with chest pain. By the previous history the patient has two risk factors (hypertension, lipids), and a history that is consistent and concerning for possible coronary artery disease (CAD). His BP is slightly elevated despite taking medications for his hypertension. This type of clinical presentation exemplifies the need for further evaluation and work-up for his chest pain.

HISTORY

A complete, detailed medical history is essential in accurately diagnosing a patient who has chest pain. Several components of the history must be included to ensure every consideration is taken into account for an accurate diagnosis.

It should be noted that early on the PA should determine if the patient is having an acute event, whether it is cardiac in nature, or is another etiology. A quick assessment of the patient's pain level and other factors must initially be taken into account. If the practitioner believes that the patient is having an acute event, measures should be taken to get the patient to an appropriate acute care setting, such as a local emergency room or hospital. In addition, the PA working with his or her medical staff must ensure to properly treat the patient and manage their symptoms before emergency medical services arrives at the practice. At no time should a PA direct a patient to an acute care setting by private vehicle if the PA is concerned that the patient may be having an acute coronary or other life-threatening illness.

The first process to any medical history should start with a basic open-ended question to allow the patient to describe their primary complaint and concerns for the visit. Once the patient has had sufficient time to describe their presenting complaint the PA should follow-up with more detailed questions to round out the history. Onset of symptoms for chest pain allows the practitioner to determine if the patient is having an acute, subacute, or chronic condition that warrants attention. Aspects to the patient's chest pain should also include any activities or other aspects that either cause provocation or palliate their symptoms.[4] In addition other signs of heart disease as it relates to CAD are such symptoms as shortness of breath, weakness, tiredness, reduced exertional capacity, dizziness, palpitations, and in some cases tachycardia and palpitations. Another important feature to obtain when taking a history is determining the quality and nature of the chest pain. An important feature to determine is if the quality of the chest pain is similar to a prior event where the patient has had prior cardiac history. Keep in mind that the symptoms of females as it relates to cardiac disease may not be similar to that of males. Some female patients who present with chest pain may have mild symptoms, and in several cases their complaints are often downplayed. This may cause the practitioner to not consider a cardiac etiology because of the limiting symptoms of the female patient. Radiation of symptoms is also an important feature with chest pain, but also helpful in determining if another etiology may be present. Systemic features, such as sweating, nausea and vomiting, leg pain or claudication symptoms, and abdominal discomfort all can help the clinician in developing a working diagnosis.[5] Some other considerations to round out the history of present illness is if the patient has ever had or experienced this pain before, and what were the circumstances related to that other episode. Any therapies, medications, or other activities that either caused the pain to worsen or improve should also be elicited from the patient during the history.

As with any other patient who presents with symptoms of an acute or subacute diagnosis, a medical history is important. Prior history of all conditions, including those that are treated or untreated, is helpful in understanding the broader picture of addressing the patient's complaint. A complete list of all prescribed and over-the-counter medications, including alternative therapies, should be obtained from the patient or their medical records. A complete family history and social history to include all risk behaviors should also be done. This includes questions related to alcohol, tobacco, and other illicit drugs, but also to explore social setting and possible risks and occupational history and any exposures that may explain the patient's presenting symptoms. Lastly, a review of systems should be taken to ensure that no other complaints are possibly related to the patient's presenting symptoms.[5]

RISK FACTORS

When considering a differential diagnosis for patient who presents with chest pain, the PA must consider the patient with respect to risk. There are several risk factors that pose increased risk with respect to cardiac disease. Careful consideration for these factors helps aid the clinician in properly treating the patient.[6]

The common traditional risk factors for CAD must be considered when making an evaluation for chest pain. The major risk factors for CAD are age (men ≥45 years, women ≥55 years); a family history of CAD, especially in ages less than or equal to 65 years of age and men; hypertension (>140/90); cigarette smoking; diabetes; hypercholesterolemia; low high-density lipoprotein cholesterol (<40 mg/dL); elevated triglycerides (>200 mg/dL); and obesity. There are several other nontraditional risk factors that may also help the practitioner in risk stratifying patients presenting with chest pain (**Box 1**).

Box 1
Major risk factors for CAD

- Age (men ≥45; women ≥55 years)
- Family history of premature CAD
  - CAD in male first-degree relative <65 years
- Hypertension (>140/90 or on medications)
- Tobacco abuse
- Diabetes mellitus
- Hypercholesterolemia
- Low high-density lipoprotein cholesterol (<40 mg/dL)
- Hypertriglyceridemia (>200 mg/dL)
- Obesity

Coronary Artery Calcium Imaging

Coronary artery calcium imaging has gained traction in the last several years and may be used to risk stratify patients for CAD. A 2013 risk assessment guideline for the American College of Cardiology and the American Heart Association helps with the decision-making guideline and consensus on strategies and protocols to evaluate patients in this capacity. This method, which is the process of using computed tomography to calculate the level of coronary artery calcium deposits, is thought to be a good predictor for disease. Although there are supportive data and statements related to this type of assessment, the overall endorsement has been deemed tepid. Practitioners may see this as another tool in working up patients for possible disease. PAs need to be informed of this technology and that it may be used as a way to determine risk and disease.[7]

CASE EXAMPLE 2

A 69-year-old woman with a history of hypertension, diabetes mellitus, and high cholesterol presented to your office in the early morning with chest pressure that woke her up. It was accompanied by shortness of breath, mild sweating, and nausea. It was intense in the morning on waking up, but has almost subsided. She is still having some chest pressure, which is mild. Her physical examination has a BP of 179/94 and pulse of 90. Her examination has evidence of slightly moist skin, clear lungs, and a regular rate and rhythm. No edema was noted on the peripheral examination.

This clinical situation exemplifies a patient who is still having active chest pain. She has multiple risk factors, and her history of chest pressure along with shortness of breath, sweating, and nausea should caution the PA for active ischemia. In this instance, and because the patient is still having active pain, emergency medical service measures should be taken to stabilize the patient's symptoms and she should be brought to an acute care facility for further evaluation.

PHYSICAL EXAMINATION

A detailed and thorough physical examination, including vital signs, must be done. Once again, any patient who is exhibiting signs on the physical examination that indicate an acute and active clinical situation should be considered to be transferred to an acute treatment facility. Advanced cardiac life support measures, if necessary, should be followed until emergency medical support has arrived to assume care.

Beginning with vital signs, the PA should note if the patient has any febrile illness, tachycardia or bradycardia, or whether or not the rate is regular. Accurate BP readings are also important, especially in situations of hypertension out-of-control or hypotensive situations. Understanding if the patient is having active symptoms at the time of physical examination is also helpful. Focus should be concentrated on the clinician's ability to identify potential abnormalities on physical examination in matching with the symptoms and complaints the patient is having with the careful history that was taken. Any positive findings on the physical examination may give clues to the practitioner being able to render a working differential diagnosis.[5] Furthermore, these physical examination findings allow the PA to identify those tests needing to be performed to validate or negate a possible diagnosis.

DIFFERENTIAL DIAGNOSIS

The development of a differential diagnosis should be constructed with the mindset to consider all life-threatening illnesses first and foremost. Once done, the PA should methodically consider the most likely causes of the chest pain based on history and physical examination findings. As this list is developed the clinician then can carefully consider the appropriate approach to determine the correct etiology of the patient's chest pain.

Because chest pain can have so many variations of presentation, and the etiology can be wide and varied, the clinician must have a broad approach to consider all possibilities and then narrow down the differential based on the most probable etiologies that exist. A comprehensive differential diagnosis is listed in **Box 2**.

CASE EXAMPLE 3

A 27-year-old man has been experiencing chest pains for the last month. He also notices that he feels like he gets a faster heart rate any time he exerts himself with mild to moderate activity. He denies any shortness of breath, no lightheadedness or dizziness, and no syncope. He presents with a BP of 132/77, pulse of 64, and his physical examination is essentially normal. His electrocardiogram (ECG) rhythm strip is shown in **Fig. 4**. The patient is not having any chest pain or fast heart rate feelings on history and physical.

This type of clinical presentation is quite common in a primary care office. Although this patient has a lower risk for coronary heart disease, he still may pose a risk for other types of cardiovascular diseases. A more comprehensive history must be taken in the setting, and determination if a cardiovascular etiology is present must still be ruled out. His faster heart rate on exertion should alert the clinician that the patient might be experiencing a possible arrhythmia. His resting rhythm strip shows a normal sinus rhythm without evidence of abnormality. Although traditional stress testing may not be fruitful for a diagnosis, the clinician must consider other types of monitoring to rule out arrhythmia, BP changes, or other types of noncardiac conditions that can cause the feelings of a fast heart rate.

CLINICAL WORK-UP

The clinical work-up for the evaluation of chest pain has three distinct goals. The most important goal is to determine any acute illnesses that may pose a life-threatening illness for the patient. The second goal is to determine any cardiac etiology that

Box 2
Differential diagnosis for chest pain

- Cardiovascular
  - Myocardial ischemia (angina, infarction)
  - Aortic stenosis
  - Aortic dissection
  - Pulmonary embolus
  - Cardiomyopathy
  - Myocarditis
  - Mitral valve prolapse
  - Pulmonary hypertension
  - Hypertrophic obstructive cardiomyopathy
  - Carditis
  - Aortic insufficiency
  - Left ventricular hypertrophy
  - Coronary artery dissection

- Pulmonary
  - Pneumonia
  - Pleuritis
  - Pneumothorax
  - Tumor
  - Pleural effusion

- Gastrointestinal
  - Gastroesophageal reflux disease
  - Biliary disease
  - Esophageal spasm
  - Peptic ulcer syndrome
  - Mallory-Weiss tear
  - Pancreatitis
  - Hepatitis
  - Gastritis

- Musculoskeletal
  - Arthritis
  - Cervical or thoracic disk disease
  - Shoulder disease or arthritis
  - Costochondritis
  - Subacromial bursitis
  - Muscular strain

- Other causes
  - Herpes zoster
  - Breast disorder
  - Cellulitis
  - Anxiety disorder
  - Chest wall tumors
  - Thoracic outlet syndrome

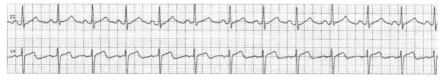

Fig. 4. Normal sinus rhythm.

may be present and needing further investigation by more extensive testing. The final underlying goal is to consider and rule out any other noncardiac reason for the patient's chest pain and consider further work-up to determine its cause. It should be emphasized that if the clinical work-up and results of laboratory studies and other testing point to a noncardiac etiology, the PA should continue with their evaluation and eventual treatment of the patient's pain.

LABORATORY STUDIES

Laboratory testing should be considered when evaluating patients with chest pain. In many instances the laboratory studies not only evaluate the cardiac conditions that tend to be the most concerning, but also create a clinical laboratory work-up to rule out other possible conditions considered within the working differential diagnosis.

Complete Blood Count

The complete blood count has value to evaluate the blood levels that may contribute or point to an alternative diagnosis. The white blood cell count may indicate an inflammatory or possible infectious process. The hemoglobin and hematocrit may indicate an anemic process, which when coupled with a hypoxia condition may cause cardiac demand ischemia events. Depending on the severity, this may contribute to chest pain in a patient. Other abnormalities to the hemoglobin and hematocrit, such as polycythemia, can also point the practitioner in another direction and away from a cardiac source. Certainly, if the patient has any evidence of bruising or bleeding the platelet count is of value.

Comprehensive Metabolic Profile

Practitioners may consider evaluating the blood with a comprehensive metabolic profile. This is of value in several clinical settings and aids the practitioner toward understanding the clinical picture, whether or not a cardiac condition exists. The first consideration within this assay is an evaluation of any electrolyte abnormalities. Sodium, potassium, and chloride levels help with considering other conditions that may impair electrolyte function, medication side effects, and other etiologies. Renal function plays a significant role in several acute, subacute, and chronic conditions. Evaluation of renal function and comparisons of the patient's known baseline can be a useful tool in the clinical work-up. Should the PA suspect hepatic involvement, then liver function testing, such as amylase and lipase, may be helpful. Although they do not always point to a cardiac condition they may be helpful in consideration for hepatic disease, biliary, or pancreatic problems. In some cases these tests help rule out cardiac etiology and assist in considering other problems, such as cholelithiasis, cholecystitis, and pancreatitis.

Troponin

A key blood test for the evaluation of chest pain is troponin. This biomarker is released on damage of cardiac cells and serum assays reveal the level of troponin (specifically troponin I), which can be elevated from the early onset of injury and peaks within a 32-hour window of time (**Fig. 5**).[8] An elevation of this test implies an ischemic condition and indicates further investigation into the patient's chest pain complaints.

There are some conditions that can erroneously elevate troponin levels that may not necessarily indicate cardiac injury. The most common types of erroneous elevations are heart failure, renal disease, thromboembolism, sepsis, infection and inflammatory, arrhythmias, and chemotherapy (**Box 3**).[9]

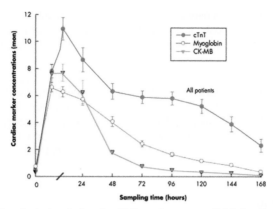

Fig. 5. Troponin levels during ischemia. AMI, acute myocardial infarction; MI, myocardial infarction. CK, creatinine kinase; CKMB- creatinine kinase myocardial band (*From* Korff S, Katus HA, Giannitsis E. Differential diagnosis of elevated troponins. Heart 2006;92(7):987–993; with permission.)

Brain Natriuretic Peptide

The serum testing of brain natriuretic peptide indicates that atrial stretch receptors have caused a release of brain natriuretic peptide. An elevation of this test may indicate the condition of heart failure. Stroke, sepsis, and other inflammatory conditions

---

Box 3
Conditions associated with elevated troponin levels in the absence of ischemic heart disease

- Cardiac contusion
- Cardioinvasive procedures (surgery, ablation, pacing, stenting)
- Acute or chronic congestive heart failure
- Aortic dissection
- Aortic valve disease
- Hypertrophic cardiomyopathy
- Arrhythmias (tachyarrhythmia or bradyarrhythmia)
- Apical ballooning syndrome
- Rhabdomyolysis with cardiac injury
- Severe pulmonary hypertension, including pulmonary embolism
- Acute neurologic disease (eg, stroke, subarachnoid hemorrhage)
- Myocardial infiltrative diseases (amyloid, sarcoid, hemochromatosis, scleroderma)
- Inflammatory cardiac diseases (myocarditis, endocarditis, pericarditis)
- Chronic kidney disease
- Drug toxicity (eg, cocaine)
- Respiratory failure
- Sepsis
- Burns
- Extreme exertion (eg, endurance athletes)

may increase this level, but if elevated it should alert the practitioner to consider heart failure as a possible diagnosis. If elevated without a history of heart failure, the PA should consider a heart failure work-up as a reason for the patient's chest pain.

Other Blood Testing

There may be some other blood testing that the PA could consider during their work-up. However, these tests do not lead to a cardiac etiology, but rather an alternative diagnosis. Some of these tests are blood cultures for possible infectious processes, erythrocyte sedimentation rate for inflammatory disease, and C-reactive protein, which are nonspecific. The PA should develop a differential diagnosis to determine testing.

ANCILLARY TESTING

As the clinician starts his or her consideration and algorithm for ordering ancillary testing several considerations need to be taken into account. The first obvious consideration is whether or not the patient has the ability to perform the test being considered. An evaluation by initiating a resting ECG should be done. The clinician should note if there are any active changes to the ECG, and use this tracing to compare with prior ECG tracings. The clinician should also ensure that no dangerous arrhythmias, ectopy, or QT prolongation is present. Any significant change from a prior ECG should give the clinician cause for concern.

Other considerations for ancillary testing should be to accurately determine the right indications for the test. There are also physical limitations, and the body habitus of the patient or other physical limitations (eg, severe kyphosis or scoliosis, amputee) need to be taken into account. In addition, a history of prior coronary revascularization should be considered especially when performing a stress test where the patient will have exertion.

Electrocardiogram

The ECG is useful when determining the cause of the patient's chest pain. Such factors as rate, rhythm, access changes, and hypertrophy can be found on an ECG. More importantly, any evidence of ongoing active ischemia, prior infarct evidence, or any abnormality different from the patient's prior ECG may suggest a new etiology and a possibility for the patient's complaint.[10] If the patient has presented more than once for the same chest pain, serial ECGs is helpful in determining any changes that may have happened. It is also important to note that if a patient is having current symptoms, the ECG is useful in determining acute versus chronic condition. All ECGs should be done using the standard 12-lead tracing (**Fig. 6**). Single-lead rhythm strips, although helpful, may not necessarily give the clinician the full clinical picture.

Chest Radiograph

The chest radiograph is another valuable test within the clinical work-up. It gives the practitioner several pieces of information to help with several diagnosis possibilities. One of the initial pieces of information is if there are any bony abnormalities present, and if so to determine if these correlate with the patients symptoms. Next, assessment of the airway and lung fields to determine any fluid, infiltrate, evacuated air, effusions, or other lung abnormality should be done. Cardiac size, shape, and any evidence of enlargement of the pulmonary vasculature should also be viewed. Position of the diaphragm and any evidence of gastrointestinal abnormalities should also be considered.

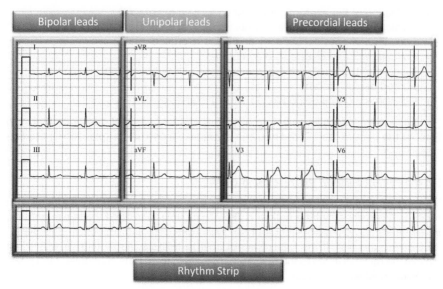

Fig. 6. Representation of a typical 12-lead electrocardiogram. The tracing is broken into the four areas of evaluation: Bipolar leads (I, II, III), unipolar leads (aVR, aVL, aVF), precordial leads (V1-V6), and a baseline rhythm strip below.

Echocardiogram

One valuable noninvasive test that some practitioners may order is the transthoracic echocardiogram. The test provides information related to cardiac size, chamber dimensions, and wall function, and valvular assessment and any evidence of pericardial space abnormalities.[11] It can also give information related to pulmonary pressures, which is helpful especially in patients with a history of smoking, chronic obstructive pulmonary disease, and other pulmonary disorders that can present with chest pain.

NONINVASIVE TESTING

There are several different types of noninvasive testing that can be performed for the evaluation of the patient who presents with chest pain. It is important the PA understand which test is the best test to perform, and which tests are going to yield the best information to render a diagnosis or rule out a cardiac etiology.

One of the first fundamental aspects to consider is to ensure that the PA can give the proper indication for the test. As part of this indication the practitioner must consider several aspects for the proper test. They must indicate that the patient presents with

- Symptoms consistent with angina pectoris
- Chest pain concerning for a cardiac etiology
- Prior history or recent episode of Acute Coronary Syndrome
- Known history of coronary heart disease or valvular disease
- History of heart failure
- History of arrhythmias

The use of exercise testing has several useful tools that can detect the following[12,13]:

- Detection of CAD in patients with chest pain (chest discomfort) syndromes or potential symptom equivalents

- Evaluation of the anatomic and functional severity of CAD
- Prediction of cardiovascular events and all-cause death
- Evaluation of physical capacity and effort tolerance
- Evaluation of exercise-related symptoms
- Assessment of chronotropic competence, arrhythmias, and response to implanted device therapy
- Assessment of the response to medical interventions

In addition the practitioner has to answer some fundamental questions that help direct to the correct test. Some of these questions (along with explanations) are discussed next.

Can the Patient Perform the Test Being Ordered?

Those patients who have the ability to perform an exercise treadmill test should have it ordered. This means that the patient is likely to be able to tolerate the stress portions on the treadmill, achieve peak heart rate during exercise, and limit chest pain symptoms during the test. If the patient is not able to tolerate the testing, or would not achieve the minimal limits to the test, then the patient should be scheduled for a pharmacologic nuclear stress test.[13]

Does the Patient Have Evidence of Abnormal Changes to the Electrocardiogram?

Abnormalities to the ECG should be taken seriously and considerations for acute changes must be addressed to ensure the patient is not having an acute coronary event. If the patient does have changes to the ECG it is necessary to consider that some changes may create a nondiagnostic scenario, reducing the effectiveness of the test.[13] Some of the changes that make the stress testing difficult are

- Left bundle branch block
- ST segment depressions >1 mm to 2 mm
- Prolonged QT segments
- ST-T segment abnormalities
- Ventricular paced rhythms

If these situations exist, the PA must consider if placing the patient in this situation will be of value or potentially negatively impact the patient. Proper consultation with a cardiology group is warranted when there is uncertainty regarding which test should be ordered.

Does the Patient Need an Assessment of Myocardial Viability or Evidence of Disease?

If the patient has a known history of CAD then the practitioner must consider if a noninvasive test is of value. In some cases, and depending on the severity of the known disease, the patient may not benefit with a noninvasive test simply because the disease is too extensive to learn if any new ischemic changes have occurred.[13] This may render this type of testing not very useful. However, if the patient has known, fixed disease and has new symptoms or a new history that may be different from prior disease, or the patient has ongoing symptoms of prior disease, a nuclear stress test may be warranted. In most cases a treadmill exercise test is most likely not a testing option.

Once these questions have been properly vetted the PA can consider the appropriate test. Practitioners should also consider several contraindications for performing stress tests (**Box 4**).

Box 4
Contraindications for performing stress tests

Absolute Contraindications

- Acute myocardial infarction, within 2 days
- Ongoing unstable angina
- Uncontrolled cardiac arrhythmia with hemodynamic compromise
- Active endocarditis
- Symptomatic severe aortic stenosis
- Decompensated heart failure
- Acute pulmonary embolism, pulmonary infarction, or deep vein thrombosis
- Acute myocarditis or pericarditis
- Acute aortic dissection
- Physical disability that precludes safe and adequate testing

Relative Contraindications

- Known obstructive left main coronary artery stenosis
- Moderate to severe aortic stenosis with uncertain relation to symptoms
- Tachyarrhythmias with uncontrolled ventricular rates
- Acquired advanced or complete heart block
- Hypertrophic obstructive cardiomyopathy with severe resting gradient
- Recent stroke or transient ischemic attack
- Mental impairment with limited ability to cooperate
- Resting hypertension with systolic or diastolic BP >200/110 mm Hg
- Uncorrected medical conditions, such as significant anemia, important electrolyte imbalance, and hyperthyroidism

Regular Treadmill Stress Test

Patients who are able to tolerate walking at a normal pace on a flat surface for up to 5 minutes without having symptoms should generally be able to tolerate a regular treadmill stress test. Although there is no scientific proof that certain types of patients are able to perform this test, measures of the patient's heart rate, exercise response recovery, ST segment changes, and hypotension response during exercise may be able to indicate if a patient is at risk for disease. The most universally used assessment tool is the Duke Treadmill Score, which categorizes patients based on risk stratification (**Box 5**).

Box 5
Duke treadmill testing score

- Duke prognostic treadmill score =
  - Exercise time (minutes based on the Bruce protocol) - (5 × maximum ST-segment deviation in mm) - (4 × exercise angina [0 = none, 1 = nonlimiting, and 2 = exercise limiting])
  - Risk levels (based on testing results) =
    - Low risk, score $\geq$ +5
    - Moderate risk, score from −10 to +4
    - High risk, score $\leq$ −11

Other advantages of the stress treadmill testing are its wide availability and low cost. It is indicated for patients who have the ability to tolerate the test and have a normal resting ECG. Patients who have been deemed low risk qualify for this test. However, patients who have abnormalities to the ECG, ongoing symptoms, or intolerance to exercise are not ideal candidates for this test and should be avoided.[12]

Nuclear Stress Testing

Patients who cannot perform an adequate treadmill test and achieve the necessary benchmarks for a successful test should undergo the alternative nuclear stress testing. This testing is done using different modalities to determine any evidence of ischemia or infarcted area.

Pharmacologic

Pharmacologic stress testing can be performed on patients who are not able to tolerate a regular stress test. It is also useful for those patients who have a left bundle branch block or ventricular paced rhythm. However, these rhythms are such that during the testing phase the ECG is not able to be interpreted because of the very nature of their pathology.

Stress Radionuclide Myocardial Perfusion Imaging

Widely used and commonly accepted tests are single-photon emission computed tomography (SPECT) and PET testing. SPECT testing is commonly used, readily available in most clinical areas, and provides information to identify coronary heart disease. There are several different radionuclides that can be used. The most commonly used agents are technetium 99m (Tc-99m sestamibi and Tc-99m tetrofosmin) and thallium 201. Images for these agents can detect defects in resting and stress times. In patients who have a larger body habitus, or for those patients who are obese, the PET scan stress may be more beneficial. PET myocardial perfusion imaging agents include rubidium 82 and N13 ammonia. Similar to SPECT testing, PET testing also uses differences of myocardial perfusion between the stress and resting states.[14]

During this type of testing, two other different types of pharmacologic agents can be used to try to achieve adequate heart rate. These drugs are determined based on patient characteristics and also on the facility preference.

Vasodilator

Among the various vasodilators used in cardiac stress testing, the most commonly used drugs are dipyridamole and adenosine. These agents act by vasodilating the adenosine 2A receptors during stress, thus increasing coronary blood flow. Other agents, such as regodenoson, binodenoson, and apadenoson, also act in the same fashion. Although these drugs are effective in this manner, there are potential side effects that may occur, and some conditions where this medication should be avoided are active bronchospasm, hypotension, sick sinus syndrome or high-grade block without artificial pacing, and active angina or active coronary syndrome. Any of these specific conditions should be automatically avoided and an alternative test should be considered.

Inotrope or Chronotropic

Dobutamine, a synthetic catecholamine that stimulates the β_1-adrenergic receptors to stimulate heart rate, can be used. This is done to increase heart rate for those patients who may not be able to achieve adequate heart rate during testing. It also is helpful in increasing myocardial contractility. This medication is ideal for testing and is the first-

---

Box 6
Sensitivity and specificity of stress test

- Exercise ECG testing, 68% and 77% in 132 studies of more than 24,000 patients
- Planar thallium radionuclide myocardial perfusion imaging, 79% and 73% in six studies of 510 patients
- SPECT radionuclide myocardial perfusion imaging, 88% and 77% in 10 studies of 1174 patients
- Stress echocardiography, 76% and 88% in six studies of 510 patients
- PET scanning, 91% and 82% in three studies of 206 patients

Data from Garber AM, Solomon NA. Cost-effectiveness of alternative test strategies for the diagnosis of coronary artery disease. Ann Intern Med 1999:130(9):719–28.

---

line use for stress echocardiography. It can also be used as a second-line drug in pharmacologic stress radionuclide testing.

Atropine is another medication for use of chronotropic effect and is used sometimes in conjunction with dobutamine to achieve adequate heart rates during testing.

Stress Echocardiography

Stress echocardiography is used to detect any hemodynamic changes that are significant, especially in those patients who have known CAD with decreased wall function from prior infarcted areas. Similar to the radionuclide study, the stress echocardiography also assesses any areas of valvular disease, localized abnormalities, and ejection fraction changes that may be present from changes in perfusion to the myocardium.[15]

In addition to the previously mentioned advantages to stress echocardiography, the testing can also assess global function of the heart before the test and determine any changes that may occur in times of stress. It also measures right ventricular pulmonary pressures and diastolic function and valvular performance.

Stress MRI

Although its use and availability are still growing, stress MRI is another viable testing tool. By use of MRI technology this test can evaluate myocardial viability, ventricular function, location or area of infarct, and perfusion through pharmacologic modalities.

Sensitivity and Specificity of Testing

It is important for the practicing PA to determine which testing is appropriate for their patients. Each testing method has its stronger points and effectiveness. The sensitivity and specificity of each test aids the practitioner in deciding which test to order (**Box 6**). **Table 1** lists testing type and type of modality.

Table 1
Stress tests for chest pain

Type of Test	ECG	Echocardiogram	Nuclear (Technetium or Thallium)
Treadmill	Treadmill ECG	Treadmill echocardiogram	Treadmill nuclear
Chemical (dobutamine, persantine, or adenosine)		Chemical echocardiogram	Chemical nuclear[a]

[a] Most common.

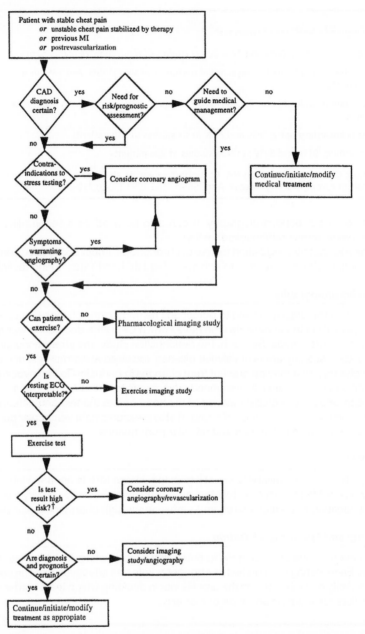

Fig. 7. Clinical context for exercise testing for patients with suspected ischemic heart disease. * Electrocardiogram interpretable unless preexcitation, electronically paced rhythm, left bundle branch block, or resting ST-segment depression >1 mm. † For example, high-risk if Duke treadmill score predicts average annual cardiovascular mortality >3% (see Fig 2⇓ for nomogram). CAD, coronary artery disease; ECG, electrocardiogram MI, myocardial infarction. (*Data from* Gibbons RJ, Balady GJ, Beasley JW, et al. ACC/AHA Guidelines for Exercise Testing: Executive Summary. A Report of the American College of Cardiology/ American Heart Association Task Force on Practice Guidelines (Committee on Exercise Testing). Circulation 1997;96:345–54.)

INVASIVE TESTING
Cardiac Catheterization

Cardiac catheterization is considered when the patient is shown to have a consistent history, physical examination, and risk factors consistent with CAD. In addition, patients who have had other cardiac testing and are shown to be more likely to be positive for coronary disease should be considered for invasive testing.

There are numerous amounts of information that can be gleaned from a cardiac catheterization. The results of this invasive test may determine the appropriate treatment for the root cause of the patient's chest pain.

Fig. 7 aids the PA to consider the most appropriate path and which test to consider.

TREATMENT CONSIDERATIONS

Treatment ultimately depends on the results that are gained from the testing itself. Most testing is able to direct the PA with a better understanding if the patient's chest pain is a potential result of cardiac involvement. However, the type of involvement may vary depending on what the testing has gleaned and if this may be the root cause of the patient's problems. For example, if one had a patient who was evaluated for chest pain and was found to have incidental finding of valvular disease one may have to work the patient up for this in addition to the chest pain, which may or may not relate to the patient's complaint.

In many cases it is best to use the testing results with clinical judgment and treat based on what is known. For those testing results that do not directly point to an etiology that is plausible, it may be necessary to refer the patient to a cardiology group for further evaluation. This is especially the case when the results may indicate that the patient would require additional testing on top of the original work-up. In some cases patients may start with a noninvasive evaluation, and based on findings from this testing may require invasive testing, such as cardiac catheterization or even surgery. In any event, when the PA is unsure as to the next steps, consultation with supervising physician or consultation with a specialist may be warranted.

SUMMARY

Chest pain can be a difficult and involved clinical work-up for the PA. It is imperative that a systematic approach take place, proper testing is done, and follow-up to include possible other key personnel be initiated. Once the etiology has been determined, treatment options can be started.

REFERENCES

1. Kochanek KD, Xu J, Murphy SL, et al. Division of vital statistics. In: Deaths: Final Data for 2009. United States Governmen, Health and Human Services, National Vital Statistics Survey. Washington, DC: United States Government; 2009. p. 1–5.
2. Centers for Disease Control and Prevention. CDC Division for Heart Disease and Stroke. From Centers for Disease Control and Prevention. 2016. Available at: https://www.cdc.gov/dhdsp/data_statistics/fact_sheets/fs_heart_disease.htm. Accessed January 12, 2017.
3. Mozzafarian D, Benjamin EJ, Go AS, et al. Heart disease and stroke statistics—2016 update: a report from the American Heart Association. Circulation 2016; 133(4):e38–360.

4. Bruyninckx R, Aertgeerts B, Bruyninckx P, et al. Signs and symptoms in diagnosing acute myocardial infarction and acute coronary syndrome: a diagnostic meta-analysis. Br J Gen Pract 2008;e1–16.
5. McConaghy JR, Oza Rupal S. Outpatient diagnosis of acute chest pain in adults. Leawood (KS); 2017.
6. Greenland P, Alpert JS, Beller GA, et al. 2010 ACCF/AHA guideline for assessment of cardiovascular risk in asymptomatic adults a report of the American College of Cardiology Foundation/American Heart Association Task Force on Practice Guidelines. J Am Coll Cardiol 2010;56(25):e50–103.
7. McEvoy JW, Martin SS, Blaha MJ. The case for and against a coronary artery calcium trial means, motive, and opportunity. J Am Coll Cardiol 2016;9(8): e995–1002.
8. Law K, Elley R, Tietjens J, et al. Troponin testing for chest pain in primary healthcare: a survey of its use by general practitioners in New Zealand. N Z Med J 2006;119(1238):U2082.
9. Burness CE, Beacock D, Channer KS. Pitfalls and problems of relying on serum troponin. QJM 2005;98:365–71.
10. Mirvis D, Ary Goldberger. Electrocardiography. In: Mann D, editor. Braunwald's heart disease: a textbook of cardiovascular medicine. 10th edition. Philadelphia: Elsevier/Sanders; 2014. p. 126–67.
11. Kimura BJ, Bocchicchio M, Willis CL, et al. Screening cardiac ultrasonographic examination in patients with suspected cardiac disease in the emergency department. J Am Heart Assoc 2001;142:342.
12. Fletcher GF, Ades PA, Kligfield P, et al. Exercise standards for testing and training a scientific statement from the American Heart Association. Circulation 2013;128: 873–934.
13. Gibbons RJ, Balady GJ, Bricker JT, et al. ACC/AHA 2002 guideline update for exercise testing: summary article a report of the American College of Cardiology/ American Heart Association Task Force on Practice Guidelines (Committee to Update the 1997 Exercise Testing Guidelines). Circulation 2002;106(14):1883–92.
14. Bateman TM, Heller GV, McGhie AI, et al. Diagnostic accuracy of rest/stress ECG-gated Rb-82 myocardial perfusion PET: comparison with ECG-gated Tc-99m sestamibi SPECT. J Nucl Cardiol 2006;13(1):24–33.
15. Pellikka PA, Nagueh SF, Elhendy AA, et al. American Society of Echocardiography recommendations for performance, interpretation, and application of stress echocardiography. J Am Soc Echocardiogr 2007;20(9):1021–41.

Cardiac Arrhythmias

Moving to the Beat of a Different Drummer

Nicholas Marshall, MS, PA-C

KEYWORDS

- Atrial fibrillation • Atrioventricular block • Long QT syndrome • Sick sinus syndrome
- Cardiac arrhythmia

KEY POINTS

- Atrial fibrillation is likely the most common arrhythmia, requiring understanding of its symptoms, diagnosis, and therapeutic strategies. Atrial flutter has its own treatment algorithm.
- Atrioventricular block, a major cause of symptomatic bradycardia, and sick sinus syndrome, with age-related changes of the myocardium, may lead to pacemaker placement.
- Long QT syndrome has a strong genetic predisposition. Patients with the diagnosis should have genetic counseling for themselves and their family.
- Wolff-Parkinson-White syndrome can carry a high mortality rate if not intervened on with ablation.
- Sinus arrhythmia is likely a benign, if not adventitious, process that does not require intervention.

INTRODUCTION

Cardiac arrhythmias are represented in large sections of the populations and can be seen in clinical patients routinely. These can range from the benign and latent to the lethal and acutely obvious. They may also be caused by an underlying issue, whether known or not, or by a single event. Knowing the basics of many of these arrhythmias is key to successful diagnosis. Having a deeper understanding of their mechanisms, presenting symptoms, diagnostic properties, and current therapy guideline will enhance the level of care that physician assistants can bring to patients.

ATRIAL FIBRILLATION

Likely the most common arrhythmia that one will encounter, in both inpatient and outpatient presentations, is atrial fibrillation (AF).[1] As of 2014, it was estimated by the American

Author Disclosure: Mr N. Marshall has no conflicts of interest and no disclosures to report.
University of Massachusetts Medical School, 55 North Lake Avenue, Worcester, MA 01655, USA
E-mail address: nmarshallpa@gmail.com

College of Cardiology (ACC) that there are anywhere from 2.7 to 6.1 million Americans with AF, with 750,000 admissions and 130,000 deaths for AF-related problems.[2]

As the population continues to age, this number is expected to increase, thus increasing the demand and interactions with health care providers for monitoring and therapy for AF. Over the past 20 years, starting with the Framingham study publishing epidemiologic data in 1982, the information and understanding related to AF and its causes and subsequent therapeutic options have greatly increased, improving outcomes and changing therapy options.[3] Based on data from the AnTicoagulation and Risk Factors in Atrial Fibrillation (ATRIA) trial, it is expected that over the next 50 years the population will see a 2.5-fold increase in AF prevalence.[4]

Prevalence from AF has a direct and linear relationship to age, outside of specific risk factors and comorbidities, with an incidence of 9.9 per 1000 person-years. For patients ages 55 to 60 years, rates are as low as 0.7%; however, incidence rates were high given lifetime risk at 20.7 per 1000 person-years. This is compared with those 85 years or older in whom the rates are increased to 17.8%, incidence of 1.1 per 1000 person-years, with rates similar between men and women. Risk of AF are 24.8% and 22.9% lifetime for men and female aged 55 years, respectively.[5] These numbers are similar to those published in 1982 from the Framingham study. Older patients are at higher risk of developing AF. About 9% of patients older than the age of 65 years will have issues with AF, compared with just 2% of those younger than 65 years.

Risk Factors

Although age is the largest independent risk factor, it is not alone. Patients with hypertension (HTN), specifically those that are not well controlled, also carry a high risk of developing AF.[6] Overall, HTN can account for 14% to 22% of cases of AF. Direct myocardial damage, most notably due to infarction, and subsequent atrial dilation due to reduced left ventricular (LV) function are significant causes of AF and the risk reduction of these should be targeted for AF prevention.[7,8] Many other medical diagnoses are linked to an increased risk of AF development, including acute pulmonary embolism, acute and chronic alcoholism, pneumonia with or without sepsis, pericarditis, and severe electrolyte abnormalities.[8]

What is Atrial Fibrillation?

Before AF can be effectively understood and treated, it must be defined. A simple definition is a cardiac arrhythmia "characterized by the presence of rapid, irregular, fibrillary waves that vary in size, shape, and timing."[6] Its full definition is a bit more complicated. The typical electrical activity of the heart is rhythmic and repeatable based on the sinoatrial (SA) node. In AF, however, this typical pattern is in chaos. Usually, the pacemaker current and chronicity of normal electrical stimuli of the atria is maintained by potassium (K) movement through inward rectifier K current (I_K) channels in conjunction with the pacemaker current, also known as funny current (I_f) pacemaker with its effects of diastolic depolarization. In AF, this does not happen in a controlled sequence but, instead, with multiple cellular depolarizations with re-entry.[3] This causes elevated atrial contractions with rates as high as 400 to 600 beats per minute (BPM), causing atrial contractions to resemble quivering, rather than controlled, contractions.[9–11]

The initiation of AF usually requires a trigger; typically, either underlying cardiac or noncardiac disease is also present.[6] In addition to the trigger, the driver, or the mechanism causing and maintaining the atrial rate, is caused by 3 distinct means: (1) an ectopic focus, (2) single circuit reentry, or (3) multiple circuit reentry. Once these drivers converge to create a self-sustaining circuit consisting of multiple reentry circuits, a sustained AF rate or rhythm is created.[6]

Diagnosis of AF is made on electrocardiogram (EKG) with findings of normal sinus rhythm (NSR) replaced by irregularly irregular QRS complex intervals.[8] Per the 2012 European guidelines, 3 criteria are needed for the diagnosis of AF: (1) absolutely irregular RR interval without third-degree atrioventricular (AV) block (AVB); (2) absence of discernable P waves; and (3), if visible, a variable atrial cycle.[12] Within the diagnosis, 3 distinct entities of AF can be found based on duration of episodes: paroxysmal, persistent, and permanent.

Symptoms

From latent to shock, AF can present in a myriad of different ways. If symptoms are felt by patients, they is likely to be palpitations with irregular heart rate, chest pain with or without shortness of breath, fatigue, and the lightheadedness of syncope. Signs and symptoms can even escalate as far as overt heart failure with or without pulmonary edema, angina, and ischemia or infarction.[6,13] However, the most common symptoms are more likely to be fatigue and other nonspecific complaints not directly attributed to AF. Patients who present to the clinic with newly diagnosed AF do not require admission to the hospital if asymptomatic and in good control of ventricular rate; however, close follow-up is prudent.[6]

Treatment

The primary reason for treatment of AF is its correlation with thromboembolic events, the greatest concern being risk of stroke. Within patient populations with AF, the risk of stroke is up to 5 times higher than those with NSR, and AF can be directly related to more than 15% of stokes in the United States in those 80 years and older, showing the highest correlation of 36% of strokes related to AF.[14]

Stroke is not the only manifestation of AF pushing for therapy to be undertaken in these patients. Cognitive impairment can be associated with AF, even without a direct correlation to ischemic stroke, with rates as high as 40% increased risk. Thus, there is a suggestion that silent strokes are frequent in patients with AF, irrespective of overt signs and symptoms of acute embolic stroke. Meta-analysis has shown that silent strokes in patients with AF can be found based on MRI data in 40% of subjects studied, and this was not associated with permanent AF compared with paroxysmal.[15] To date, 20% of ischemic stroke is attributed to subclinical AF when no other cause can be found. The asymptomatic atrial fibrillation and stroke evaluation in pacemaker patients and the atrial fibrillation reduction atrial pacing (ASSERT) trial, published in 2016, looked at pacemaker interrogations for findings of subclinical AF. They found that asymptomatic AF was 8 times as common as clinically noted AF based on the subjects studied, highlighting a 2.5-fold increased risk of stroke, whether clinical or subclinical.[16]

Outside of stroke risk, AF can directly lead to reductions in LV systolic function and even to signs of heart failure in patients for whom ventricular rates are not controlled. Tachycardia-induced cardiomyopathy, a syndrome of dilation of the LV with reduction in LV ejection fraction from myocardial stress, has been found to have a direct relationship to uncontrolled heart rates over a long period of time.[8,17] However, once therapy is started with rate-controlling agents and the ventricular rates are controlled, these deteriorations can be reversed to some degree.[17]

AF can carry a dramatic reduction in the quality of life of those it affects. Multiple studies have shown marked improvement in quality of life in postablation patients using multiple different measurement scores.[18]

Different strategies can be initiated based on rate control versus rhythm control. Therapies involving statins and angiotensin-converting enzyme inhibitor (ACEi) or angiotensin receptor blocker (ARB) are being added to the tool bag for reducing the risk of developing AF. AF was initially treated with the hopes of restoration of NSR. However, there have now been multiple studies that have looked at outcomes based on rate control or rhythm controlled strategies. Multiple studies have shown rate control being noninferior to rhythm control. The Pharmacological Intervention in Atrial Fibrillation (PIAF) study and the strategies of treatment of atrial fibrillation (STAF) study both showed noninferiority of rate control, with STAF also not finding any difference in all endpoints between rate control versus rhythm. These studies suggest that, for patients with high risk of recurrence of AF, a rate control therapy strategy can be used successfully to abate the morbidity and mortality associated with AF.[12,19] Most notably, in 2004, the Atrial Fibrillation Follow-up Investigation of Rhythm Management (AFFIRM) trial stated that rate control was an "acceptable, if not preferred, option."[20] This was additionally shown in the How to Treat Chronic Atrial Fibrillation (HOT CAFE) trial.[21] From there, additional studies were completed for guidance in rate control to show an effective heart rate to target. The duel studies rate control efficacy in permanent atrial fibrillation (RACE) and RACE II initially looked at rate versus rhythm control, then followed with established targets for medication-based rate control. The primary RACE study showed that rate control was noninferior to rhythm control while looking at a target heart rate of less than 100 BPM. The follow-up RACE II trial looked to further clarify rate control targets based on 2 arms: a strict versus lenient resting heart rate, with lenient control of heart rate less than 110, with an endpoint of reduction in heart failure admissions. Lenient rate control was shown to be noninferior to strict control based on heart rate less than 110 versus less than 80. Within the lenient arm, due to reduced medication need, secondary endpoints showed a reduction in adverse medication events, such as syncope, and a reduction in need for permanent pacemaker implantation.[22,23]

Statin therapy is now being looked at in terms of reducing risk of AF development. Previously, it was thought that once a patient's cholesterol levels were in check due to statin dosing, the drugs could be discontinued as a means to contain the cost of medical care. Retrospectively, in Taiwan, subjects that had ended their statin dosing had similar rates to those that had not been on a statin, and those that were still on therapy had low incidence of AF.[24]

ACEi or ARB similarly have been shown to reduce the overall incidence of AF and thus can be used as a primary and secondary therapy for AF risk reduction. The risk reduction can be attributed to the ACEi or ARB reduction in myocardial restructuring, reduced atrial fibrosis development, and reduction in cardiac afterload.[25]

Rate Control Strategies

Both the ACC and the European Society of Cardiology have published guidelines for management of AF with multiple recommendations. Per these guidelines for rate control, target resting heart rate should be less than 80 BPM; however, in patients with preserved systolic function and who remain asymptomatic, a goal of less than 110 BPM is advised.[2] Rate control should be achieved with oral medications such as beta-blockers (BBs) or nondihydropyridines calcium channel blockers (CCBs) for patients with multiple duration of AF rate, whether they are paroxysmal, persistent, or permanent AF. Intravenous dosing can be used in the setting of rapid ventricular response (RVR) to control heart rate, unless unstable vital signs present that necessitate electrical cardioversion.[2] In patients who are adherent to the rate control medications, whether it be the BB or CCB, the mortality risk of AF is significantly reduced, particularly in the BB group. Previously, digoxin had been used for rate control but this no longer appears in the 2014 guidelines and studies have pointed out that digoxin can be associated with an increased mortality risk when used for rate control without the addition of a BB or CCB. Rate control was achieved in 70% of patients taking a BB compared with 54% and 58% in those in a CCB or digoxin, respectively.[17,20]

Rhythm Control

The primary end-point of rhythm control is the return and persistence of a NSR. With return of NSR, the risk of stroke related to AF is abated and thus anticoagulation can be avoided. This is particularly important for those patients for whom anticoagulation would be contraindicated or who cannot tolerate the reduction in cardiac output. Dr Rothman[26], in an abstract in the *American Journal of Medicine*, stated that, in surveys of primary care physicians, 25% elect rhythm control so that their patients can avoid anticoagulation.[14] It had also been postulated that those patients with predescribed heart failure would most benefit from rhythm control compared with rate control. This is often based on the loss of atrial kick and thus reduction in cardiac output in AF. In patients with NSR, the controlled and rhythmic contractions, in concert with ventricular contractions, adds to about 20% of LV stroke volume and increased cardiac output based on the Frank-Starling principle.[3,6,8,27] Bedeviling rate control versus rhythm control in heart failure patents is that heart failure itself is a direct cause of AF. Despite this, evidence has shown that rate control strategies are just as effective in these patients' mortality as rhythm control.[28]

Primarily, conversion from an AF rhythm to NSR is produced with electrical cardioversion. AF rates can self-convert to NSR and can be seen in 2 out of 3 of patients who had AF of less than 24 hours. However, should AF persist for a week or more, conversion to NSR without medical intervention is rare.[6] There are 2 main means to elicit return of NSR: electrical shock and chemical cardioversion. Pharmacologic cardioversion can be achieved with a variety of medications, including but not limited to amiodarone, propafenone, flecainide, dofetilide, and ibutilide, per the 2014 guidelines.[2]

Electrical cardioversion is achieved through the use of direct current electrical stimulation. There are, however, risks of inducing stroke with conversion from AF to NSR, thus consideration of anticoagulation, both preconversion and postconversion, should be considered. The one caveat to this is that patients with AF with RVR not improved with medical therapy can be cardioverted in the absence of anticoagulation.[2] This would include those with RVR and signs of new or worsening heart failure, hypotension, or myocardial infarction as related to the loss of atrial kick, and the increased myocardial demand of an elevated heart rate. Of these patients, cardioversion, whether chemical or electrical, should not be held in the absence of anticoagulation given the risk of ongoing RVR.[2]

For patients with stable hemodynamic status who have been known to have AF for less than 48 hours, electrical cardioversion can be initiated without anticoagulation before sinus rhythm conversion. Should the duration of AF be unable to be determined, or is known to be more than 48 hours with stable hemodynamics, anticoagulation should be started and maintained at therapeutic levels for 3 weeks before patient returns for conversion, then for 4 weeks following successful cardioversion. Cardioversion can still be attempted without prior anticoagulation if a transesophageal echocardiogram is obtained. If imaging shows no evidence of clot, cardioversion can be completed. Regardless of anticoagulation leading up to cardioversion, it is still recommended to continue anticoagulation for the next 4 weeks postprocedure.[2]

Surgical options for both directed cardioversion and maintenance of NSR are available. Historically, multiple techniques have been created; however, the first major procedure to have success was the Cox-Maze, primarily the third iteration, developed in the late 1980s.[12] This technique, performed in the operating room, allowed surgeons to redirect the electrical impulse of the SA node by carefully placing incisions to the pulmonary veins, posterior aspects to the left atria, as well as by excision of the left atrial appendence, an area of considerable concern for clot formation.[6] Since that time, catheter ablation via means of radiofrequency, ultrasound, or thermal, by either cold or hot sources, has overcome the surgical procedures of direct AF ablation and have been the predominant means of ablation.[12,29] Ablation has moved into the forefront given the technical difficulty of surgical interventions and high time-investment.[30] Catheter ablation is also not without its differences in technique, time for completion, and dependence on interventionist training. Regardless, either modality of catheter ablation, specifically cryoablation versus radio frequency, has been shown to be similar in terms of therapeutic outcome and procedural risks for those with drug-refractory AF as a means of rhythm control.[29]

Anticoagulation

As mentioned, a major consequence of AF is stroke risk. Given not only the risk but also the potential disastrous outcomes of ischemic or embolic stoke associated with AF, current guidelines implore providers to counsel their patients on the need for anticoagulation and implement a strategy of anticoagulation in those at highest risk of stroke and without significant contraindications. This leads to the question of who is a candidate for anticoagulation and who is not. There are extensive calculations available for clinicians to calculate stroke risk and, therefore, highlight which patient should receive therapeutic anticoagulation versus those who can forgo it. Perhaps the most noted calculator has been the CHAD2 score: assigning a number value to certain risks, and based on those values, determining a strategy for no anticoagulation, aspirin alone, and therapeutic anticoagulation. This system is not without its flaws, therefore other means have been developed, such as the HAS-BLED[31] score, and the CHA_2DS_2-VASc scores, which is the current recommended score per the 2014 ACC guidelines.[2]

It is clear from the recommendations for patients with high scores that anticoagulation should be offered to minimize risk of stroke. In patients with low risk, CHA_2DS_2-VASc of 0 for men and 1 for women, the stroke risk is a slow as 0.49 per 100 person-years at 1 year. Increase the risk by 1 point and the risk markedly increases to 1.55 per 100 person-years, highlighting an increase of 3.01-fold over the lower values. In the European 2012 and ACC 2014 guidelines, low CHA_2DS_2-VASc score can be managed without therapeutic anticoagulation.[32]

Anticoagulation is not without its risks, primarily bleeding. Oral anticoagulation has been linked to both gastrointestinal bleeding and intracranial bleeds, both of which can be fatal. Bleeding risk calculators do currently exist; however, the accuracy of the score is widely variable as no current guidelines outline the use of bleeding risk scores.[33]

Therapeutic anticoagulation has traditionally been implemented using vitamin K antagonist (VKA), most notably warfarin. Overall, oral anticoagulation has good evidence for reduction of risk of stroke when taken as prescribed. Even with strict adherence to their prescription, maintaining therapeutic levels based on the international normalized ratio (INR) with VKAs, is difficult. Therapeutic goals are achieved and/or maintained only 65% to 70% of the time.[33] Newer drugs have since been approved by the US Food and Drug Administration for therapeutic anticoagulation in AF patients, primarily in cases not caused by valvar disease. Within this journal there is an excellent paper describing in detail the multitude of drugs available for anticoagulation. The current 2014 guidelines note that VKAs are the preferred agent for nonvalvular AF, AF in conjunction with mechanical heart valves, and in patients with prior stroke. Newer medications, such as the direct Xa inhibitors or direct thrombin inhibitors, are also indicated in nonvalvular AF, as well as in those patients for whom a therapeutic INR is difficult to maintain.[2]

ATRIAL FLUTTER

Atrial flutter (AFL) was first described in the 1880s with its characteristic EKG findings of a sawtooth pattern, shown only 20 years later.[34] Since that time, extensive study has been conducted on atrial arrhythmias, mostly in AF; however, AFL research has also increased.

Invariably, AFL is compared with AF and with good reason. Studies have often linked the 2 together, looking at epidemiologic data, therapeutic options, mortality, and quality of life. Although there are similarities between AFL and AF, they are distinct entities that should be thought of as separate disease processes with similar outcomes and similarities in therapeutic goals.

There had been a well-described relationship between the 2 processes such that AF is frequently seen in AFL and vice versa.[35] AF is also often shown as being both the cause and effect of AFL with studies showing 56% of solitary or lone AFL will later develop into AF. Patients who undergo chemical cardioversion with class Ic or III for AF can develop AFL at a 15% to 20% rate of risk.[36] Those who undergo catheter ablation for AFL (primarily lone) will show AF at follow-up.[34] Both will require anticoagulation due to risk of thromboembolism; mainly stroke risk. Rhythm control with catheter and surgical ablation techniques in addition to chemical cardioversion techniques are also similar.[37] There are similar epidemiologic patterns between AFL and AF. AF is significantly more common the AFL, with AFL seen as little as one-tenth as frequently, with hospital rates of 34.6% to 4.5%, respectively. These rates are based on discharge diagnosis of arrhythmias in 1990 per the Marshfield Epidemiologic Study Area (MESA) database with an incidence noted to be 88 per 100,000 person years.[36]

As in AF, AFL is more likely to be seen in the elderly, with a similar, linear relationship with 5 per 100,000 at age 50 years, which increases to 587 per 100,000 at age 80 years or older.[34] Similar predictive medical conditions are also present, such as HTN, but patients with chronic obstructive pulmonary disease (25%–12%), patients who smoke (49%–37%), and patients with congestive heart failure (28%–17%) are seen more often in AFL than in AF.[35]

The differences, however, abound. As previously discussed, AF is primarily a consequence of inappropriate pacemaker propagation and electrical discharge within the left atria in a chaotic means without a clear pattern.[35] AFL is a repeatable pattern with a clear, rotating, wave-like, orderly progression. Although AF triggers are usually found in the left atria near the pulmonary veins, AFL is primarily a disease of the right atria, most specifically to the cavotricuspid isthmus (CTI).[34] AFL can be easily discerned versus AF on EKG based on the sawtooth pattern, most likely seen in the inferior leads (II, III, AVF, V_1).[36] Compared with the chaotic appearance of AF, AFL has a specific, orderly appearance with atrial heart rates (the F wave) from 250 to 350.[35]

AFL is typically not a sustained rhythm but rather paroxysmal. Thus, the symptoms at presentation will likely be described by the patient as intermittent. Typically, patients will have complaints of palpitations, chest pressure, and dyspnea; syncope is rarely seen unless a preexisting heart condition is present.[36]

Therapy for AFL is primarily catheter ablation; however, it should be tailored based on the specific type of AFL to target that specific foci. Grossly, AFL and be grouped into 2 groups: CTI or non-CTI. EKG tracings can help to differentiate between different types based on the wave morphology on 12-lead looking at the inferior leads and V1.[37]

A CTI circuit can be diagnosed as the cause of the flutter in 90% of patients if the flutter wave is also seen inferiorly in V1.[36] However, the 2015 guidelines state that EKG interpretation should not be used other than to state whether AFL is related to CTI; distinct mapping is needed to determine other causes.[37]

Although electrical cardioversion and/or ablation is the preferred means of rhythm control, chemical cardioversion is feasible using a similar medication profile as AF, namely ibutilide and dofetilide, with the addition of magnesium for synergy and reduced risk of torsades de pointes.[38] Rate control is not recommended because AFL is well known to be difficult to control; however, there are cases in which heart rates with AFL are amenable to rate control medications; therefore, it is suggested to use BB or CCB. Note that drug doses may need to be higher and there is a likely need for multiple mediations.[38]

ATRIOVENTRICULAR BLOCK

There are 3 types of AVB with 1 type being split in 2. Each of these types can be viewed via either an electrical or anatomic means, with the most recognized means of classification being electrical with first-degree and second-degree (types I and II), and third-degree blocks.[35,36] Each has its own unique EKG findings to differentiate them.

AVB is typically acquired, usually with advancing age, and is thought likely to be caused by fibrous deposits of myocardium. Fibrous deposition in the areas of the aortic and mitral valves, near the AV node and bifurcation, increase the risk for electrical blocking effects.[39] Studies have shown that as humans age there is a natural prolongation of the PR interval, even in the absence of cardiac disease, between the third and ninth decades of life.[40] AVB can also be caused by direct damage to the myocardium due to myocardial infarcts; heart failure; heart valve surgery; infections, such as endocarditis and Lyme disease; toxic exposure, including prescriptions; and disease processes, such as sarcoidosis.[41,42] There are congenital causes of AVB, mainly related to congenital defects in the structure of the heart. These are exceedingly rare, with incidence of 1 in 22,000 live birth. Congenital causes carry a high mortality rate without prompt intervention.[43]

Each type of AVB carries its own unique electrical characteristics and treatment options varying by type and symptoms. Should symptoms be present, they are usually related not to the block itself but to bradycardia or arrhythmias.[39]

First-degree AVB is found on EKG with a prolongation of the PR interval to greater than 0.2 of a second.[38] AVB can be incidentally found on routine testing and is often asymptomatic, especially without associated cardiac disease. In 1986, EKGs of healthy patients in Manitoba showed 20% of subjects in their seventh decade had PR intervals greater than 200 milliseconds but rarely greater than 220 milliseconds.[36]

Therapy for first-degree heart block is usually not required. Should marked PR interval prolongation be noted on EKG (>300 milliseconds), there can be incomplete ventricular filling and a reduced cardiac output, which may lead to patients being symptomatic. In those with symptomatic first-degree AVB, a pacemaker is a reasonable approach to symptom control, otherwise no therapy is needed.[35,36]

Second-degree AVB is broken into 2 types, with nomenclature supporting either notation as type or Mobitz I or II. Each type is distinct in both electrical and anatomic ways.

Type I on EKG will show a progressively elongating PR interval with subsequent loss of QRS complex as the block progresses. Anatomically, it represents a delay of impulses through the AV node, which eventually leads to complete transient block.

Type II also has a prolonged PR interval and eventual loss of QRS complex. Type II can be discerned from type I because it has fixed PR intervals both before and after the lost beat. QRS complex with type II block is frequently wide. Anatomically, type II is often due to a block within the intra-His or infra-His complex. Due to the wide QRS, as well as its anatomic location, type II can be described as advanced block or as high-degree (and grouped with third-degree). Should this block be associated with a wide QRS duration, frequently the patient will be symptomatic. Wide QRS should also raise concern, symptoms aside, because this frequently leads to complete blocks.[38]

Third-degree, or complete, heart block, is complete block of electrical conduction through the AV node, with a dissociated rate of contraction between the atria and the verticals. Heart rates at this degree of block are an escape rhythm and can cause profound bradycardia and subsequent related symptoms.

High-grade heart block, consisting of second-degree type II and third-degree, are grouped together in many of the current guidelines for management that consist of permeant pacemaker (PPM) placement. PPM can be placed for some instances of first-degree block and second-degree type I; however, high-grade most cases will necessitate PPM placement, regardless of current symptoms.

SICK SINUS SYNDROME

Sick sinus syndrome (SSS) is a constellation of diseases of the SA node causing abnormal propagation and conduction of an electrical signal. It is manifested by bradycardia, with and without cardiac pauses, as well as by tachy-brady arrhythmias, with diagnosis being made on EKG during clinic spot checks or on Holter monitor.[44] Of particular interest is the relationship between the tachy-brady syndrome and AF.[45] Symptoms are usually progressive over time and are a result of low cardiac output because the heart rate is insufficient to meet the needs of the tissues, primarily the brain.[44] As is seen in patients without SA node dysfunction, exercise usually produces an increased heart rate and correction of the bradycardia; this is not seen in cases of SSS.[46] Typically, symptoms begin as fatigue, lightheadedness, or dizziness, progressing to syncope and other signs of cerebral hypoperfusion, as well as causing heart failure in some.[44] SSS typically is seen in the elderly, median age noted at 74 years, without difference between sexes. Causes of SSS are typically related to degeneration in the of the SA node itself, usually described by atrial fibrosis. However, multiple diseases have been attributed to SSS, including amyloidosis, ischemic heart disease, and cardiomyopathies, as well as a host of metabolic abnormalities.[45] Treatment more often than not involves placement of a permanent pacemaker unless causative agents are found and mitigated.[44,47,48] Currently, there are no oral medications for treatment and most medications will exacerbate the syndrome.[47] In 2009, of almost 250,000 pacemakers implanted, roughly half were due to SSS. Although the pacemaker can relieve symptoms, it does not affect mortality rates.[44]

LONG QT SYNDROME

Long-QT syndrome (LQTS) is a silent but potentially devastating phenomena. Although easily identifiable on 12-lead EKG, looking for it is often not as clear. LQTS is currently a leading cause of sudden cardiac death (SCD), particularly in younger populations.[49] If not incidentally found on 12-lead, LQTS is typically discovered after an episode of syncope. Mortality rates can be as high as 21% within 1 year after syncopal episode if not properly managed. Those who are managed within the guidelines have a significant drop in mortality to 1% based on studies with 15-year follow-up.[49] Overall risk of death can be further stratified based on the duration of the QT segment with risk by age 40 years as low as 20% if QTc is less than 446 seconds. Conversely, if QTc is greater than 498 seconds, risk of SCD increases to more than 70%. These limits of QT prolongation represent the lowest and the highest quartile for risk stratification.[50]

Cause has been identified within 2 distinct groups: those with a genetic basis and those that are medication-induced. Known mutations to 10 different genes, including Ankyrin-B (ANKB) gene, with hundreds of mutations within that single gene are to blame.[48] Mutations in the genes responsible for ion channel and membrane targeting in cardiac conduction pathways leading to abnormally long QT segments.[50] Elongation in the QT segment attributed to medication also carries a long list of causes and is more common than congenital prolongation.

Diagnosis is found on surface EKG with the QT segment noted to be longer than 450 ms (440 in men, 460 in women) in the absence of QT-prolonging medications or conditions (outpatient approach). Typically, an EKG will be ordered for family history of LQTS, family history of SCD at young age, or for physical childhood sports. However, it is often found during evaluations for symptomatic episodes, such as palpitations, syncope or near syncope, dysrhythmias with ventricular tachycardia (with tendency toward torsades de pointes), and cardiac arrest.[50]

Once the electrical diagnosis is made, genetic testing should be completed. Should mutations within the 10 known genes be found, the specific phenotype and protein deficiency should be identified and typed. There are multiple types, labeled LQTS type 1 to 12, each with their own causes and triggers for arrhythmias. For each type, a specific gene mutation causing an abnormal protein has been identified.[51]

Current therapies can be divided into 3 groups: lifestyle modification therapy, medication requirement, and implanted therapy with implanted cardioverter defibrillator (ICD).[52] Regardless of duration of QTc in patients with known genetic predisposition, lifestyle therapy should be instituted. This consists of abstinence from competitive sports; avoidance of loud noise, such as concerts; and loud alarm clocks or telephones next to the bed, particularly for those with LQTS because loud noises during sleep are associated with SCD. Finally, medications or therapies that are known to prolong the QTc should be avoided.[50] No active therapy outside lifestyle modifications are required if, on routine 12-lead, the QTc is normal in patients with positive genetic mutation screening. However, this should be tailored to specific patients on a case-by-case evaluation.[49] In those who require medication therapy, BBs are first-line therapy, with long-acting medications, such as atenolol and nadolol, preferred.[53] Care is advised because some BBs are themselves associated with QTc prolongation and need to be avoided.[54] ICD is often required and should be strongly considered for QTc greater than 500 milliseconds, for those with symptoms at young age, for those with recurrent syncope despite beta blocker therapy, and for patients who have survived cardiac arrest.[50] BB therapy, despite the presence of an ICD, should continue.[52]

WOLFF-PARKINSON-WHITE SYNDROME

Wolff-Parkinson-White (WPW) syndrome is a supraventricular tachyarrhythmia with elevated ventricular rates due to accessory electrical pathways perpetuating the rhythm. First reported by Dr Wolff and colleagues in 1930,[55] WPW was often described as a bundle branch pattern in patients who were typically young. EKG findings of patients at that time were described as showing a shortened PR segment, with a more recently described finding of a delta wave, or a short PR segment with slurred QRS complex.[48] Later studies found an association between aberrant electrical pathways within the AV node and bundle of His that allowed the electrical stimuli to persist and drive a continued ventricular stimulation. This pathway, known as the bundle of

Kent, mitigated the typical slowing of the AV node and is thus associated with the formation of often malignant tachyarrhythmias, including SCD.[48,55] Patients with WPW can present with palpitation, near syncope, or syncope. SCD, rare as a complication of WPW, is noted to be 0.05% to 0.2% per year.[56] When WPW causes SCD it is usually due to AF leading to ventricular fibrillation. A case study was published of an unfortunate 23-year-old patient with an implanted recorder that showed rapid progression from sinus rhythm, with pre-excitation to AF leading to ventricular fibrillation, which he could not be resuscitated from.[57]

WPW is typically attributed to genetics, with multiple genes being shown in patients with known accessory pathways. Two specific genes have been identified: PRKAG2 and BMP2, both with dominant patterns.[48] Familial pattern of a WPW patient can be described with 3.4% of patients found to have a first-degree relative with similar genetic markers for WPW.[48]

Therapy consists mostly of catheter ablation performed on survivors of SCD and those with noted AF or symptomatic WPW.[55,57] Oral medication therapy is not advised, specifically CCB and digoxin, because these may worsen electrical conduction via accessory pathway.[55]

SINUS ARRHYTHMIA

Sinus arrhythmia is a cyclic slowing of the resting heart rate related to respiratory cycle variation. As patients exhale, a marked slowing of the RR interval with increased RR interval on inhalation may be noted on EKG. This pattern was first described by Ludwing in a paper published in 1847, as well as by Adrian and colleagues[58] in 1932. Two mechanisms have been identified: direct vagal stimulation due to respiration and lung inflation hindering vagal cardiac stimulation. Despite its causes, this phenomenon is nonpathologic and is frequently seen in the young (most predominantly in infants), athletes, and the elderly, and may be beneficial for improved alveoli gas exchange.

REFERENCES

1. Cappato R, Sorgente A. Catheter ablation in atrial fibrillation: a state-of-the-art review. Res Rep Clin Cardiol 2015;6:153–7.
2. January CT, Wann LS, Alpert JS, et al. 2014 AHA/ACC/HRS guideline for the management of patients with atrial fibrillation: executive summary. J Am Coll Cardiol 2014;64(21):2246–80.
3. Iwasaki YK, Nishida K, Kato T, et al. Atrial fibrillation pathophysiology: implications for management. Circulation 2011;124(20):2264–74.
4. Alan S, Go M, Elaine M, et al. Prevalence of diagnosed atrial fibrillation in adults: national implications for rhythm management and stroke preventions: the AnTicoagulation and Risk Factors in Atrial Fibrillation (ATRIA) Study. JAMA 2001; 285(18):2370.
5. Heeringa J, van der Kuip DA, Hofman A, et al. Prevalence, incidence and lifetime risk of atrial fibrillation: the Rotterdam study. Eur Heart J 2006;27(8):949–53.
6. Falk RH. Atrial fibrillation. N Engl J Med 2001;344(14):1067–78.
7. Willam B, Kannel M, Abbott RD, et al. Epidemiological features of chronic atrial fibrillation. The Framingham Study. N Engl J Med 1982;306:1018–22.
8. Dang D, Arimie R, Haywood LJ. A review of atrial fibrillation. J Natl Med Assoc 2002;94(12):1036–48.
9. Atrial fibrillation: current understandings and research imperatives. The National Heart, Lung, and Blood Institute Working Group on Atrial Fibrillation. J Am Coll Cardiol 1993;22(7):1830–4.

10. Hohnloser SH, Kuck K-H, Lilienthal J. Rhythm or rate control in atrial fibrillation—Pharmacological Intervention in Atrial Fibrillation (PIAF): a randomised trial. Lancet 2000;356(9244):1789–94.

11. Nattel S. New ideas about atrial fibrillation 50 years on. Nature 2002;415(6868):219–26.

12. Calkins H, Kuck KH, Cappato R, et al. 2012 HRS/EHRA/ECAS Expert Consensus Statement on Catheter and Surgical Ablation of Atrial Fibrillation: recommendations for patient selection, procedural techniques, patient management and follow-up, definitions, endpoints, and research trial design. Europace 2012;14(4):528–606.

13. American Heart Association. What is Atrial Fibrillation. American Heart Association; 2015. p. 1–2. Available at: http://www.heart.org/idc/groups/heart-public/@wcm/@hcm/documents/downloadable/ucm_300294.pdf.

14. Reiffel JA. Atrial fibrillation and stroke: epidemiology. Am J Med 2014;127(4):e15–6.

15. Kalantarian S, Ay H, Gollub RL, et al. Association between atrial fibrillation and silent cerebral infarctions: a systematic review and meta-analysis. Ann Intern Med 2014;161(9):650–8.

16. Healey JS, Connolly SJ, Gold MR, et al. Subclinical atrial fibrillation and the risk of stroke. N Engl J Med 2012;366:9.

17. Chao TF, Liu CJ, Tuan TC, et al. Rate-control treatment and mortality in atrial fibrillation. Circulation 2015;132(17):1604–12.

18. Mohanty S, Mohanty P, Di Biase L, et al. Results from a single-blind, randomized study comparing the impact of different ablation approaches on long-term procedure outcome in coexistent atrial fibrillation and flutter (APPROVAL). Circulation 2013;127(18):1853–60.

19. Carlsson JÖ, Miketic S, Windeler JÜ, et al. Randomized trial of rate-control versus rhythm-control in persistent atrial fibrillation. J Am Coll Cardiol 2003;41(10):1690–6.

20. Olshansky B, Rosenfeld LE, Warner AL, et al. The Atrial Fibrillation Follow-up Investigation of Rhythm Management (AFFIRM) study: approaches to control rate in atrial fibrillation. J Am Coll Cardiol 2004;43(7):1201–8.

21. Opolski G, Torbicki A, Kosior DA, et al. Rate control vs rhythm control in patients with nonvalvular persistent atrial fibrillation: the results of the Polish How to Treat Chronic Atrial Fibrillation (HOT CAFE) Study. Chest 2004;126:476–86.

22. Van Gelder IC, Hagens VE, Bosker HA, et al. A comparison of rate control and rhythm control in patients with recurrent persistent atrial fibrillation. N Engl J Med 2002;347(23):1834–40.

23. Van Gelder IC, Groenveld HF, Crijns HJ, et al. Lenient versus strict rate control in patients with atrial fibrillation. N Engl J Med 2010;362(15):1363–73.

24. Chang CH, Lee YC, Tsai CT, et al. Continuation of statin therapy and a decreased risk of atrial fibrillation/flutter in patients with and without chronic kidney disease. Atherosclerosis 2014;232(1):224–30.

25. Schneider MP, Hua TA, Bohm M, et al. Prevention of atrial fibrillation by Renin-Angiotensin system inhibition a meta-analysis. J Am Coll Cardiol 2010;55(21):2299–307.

26. Rothman SA. AFib Treatment: General Population. Am J Med 2014;127:e16.

27. Heist EK, Mansour M, Ruskin JN. Rate control in atrial fibrillation: targets, methods, resynchronization considerations. Circulation 2011;124(24):2746–55.

28. Roy D, Talajic M, Nattel S, et al. Rhythm control versus rate control for atrial fibrillation and heart failure. N Engl J Med 2008;358(25):2667–77.

29. Kuck KH, Brugada J, Furnkranz A, et al. Cryoballoon or radiofrequency ablation for paroxysmal atrial fibrillation. N Engl J Med 2016;374(23):2235–45.

30. Wynn GJ, Todd DM, Webber M, et al. The European Heart Rhythm Association symptom classification for atrial fibrillation: validation and improvement through a simple modification. Europace 2014;16(7):965–72.

31. Pisters R, Lane DA, Nieuwlaat R, et al. A novel user-friendly score (HAS-BLED) to assess 1-year risk of major bleeding in patients with atrial fibrillation: the Euro Heart Survey. Chest 2010;138(5):1093–100.

32. Lip GY, Skjoth F, Rasmussen LH, et al. Oral anticoagulation, aspirin, or no therapy in patients with nonvalvular AF with 0 or 1 stroke risk factor based on the CHA2DS2-VASc score. J Am Coll Cardiol 2015;65(14):1385–94.

33. Moss JD, Cifu AS. Management of anticoagulation in patients with atrial fibrillation. JAMA 2015;314(3):291–2.

34. Bun SS, Latcu DG, Marchlinski F, et al. Atrial flutter: more than just one of a kind. Eur Heart J 2015;36(35):2356–63.

35. Mareedu RK, Abdalrahman IB, Dharmashankar KC, et al. Atrial flutter versus atrial fibrillation in a general population: differences in comorbidities associated with their respective onset. Clin Med Res 2010;8(1):1–6.

36. Lee KW, Yang Y, Scheinman MM, University of California-San Francisco SFCAUSA. Atrial flutter: a review of its history, mechanisms, clinical features, and current therapy. Curr Probl Cardiol 2005;30(3):121–67.

37. Page RL, Joglar JA, Caldwell MA, et al. 2015 ACC/AHA/HRS guideline for the management of adult patients with supraventricular tachycardia: a report of the American College of Cardiology/American Heart Association Task Force on Clinical Practice Guidelines and the Heart Rhythm Society. J Am Coll Cardiol 2016; 67(13):e27–115.

38. Epstein AE, DiMarco JP, Ellenbogen KA, et al. 2012 ACCF/AHA/HRS focused update incorporated into the ACCF/AHA/HRS 2008 guidelines for device-based therapy of cardiac rhythm abnormalities: a report of the American College of Cardiology Foundation/American Heart Association Task Force on Practice Guidelines and the Heart Rhythm Society. Circulation 2013;127(3):e283–352.

39. Chow GV, Marine JE, Fleg JL. Epidemiology of Arrhythmias and conduction disorder in older adults. Clin Geriatr Med 2012;28(4):539–53.

40. Masin JW, Ramseth DJ, Chanter DO, et al. Electrocardiographic reference ranges derived from 79,743 ambulatory subjects. J Electrocardiol 2006;40(And 3):228–34.

41. National Heart L, and Blood Institute. What causes heart block? [Website]. 2016. Available at: https://www.nhlbi.nih.gov/health/health-topics/topics/hb/causes. Accessed Novemebr 23, 2016.

42. Society HR. Heart Block. 2016. Available at: http://www.hrsonline.org/Patient-respurces/heart-diseases-disorders/heart-block. Accessed November 23, 2016.

43. Friedman D, Duncanson LJ, Glickstein J, et al. A review of congenital heart block. Images Paediatr Cardiol 2003;5(3):36–48.

44. Semelka M, Gera J, Usman S. Sick sinus syndrome: a review. Am Fam Physician 2013;87(10):691–6.

45. Jensen PN, Gronroos NN, Chen LY, et al. Incidence of and risk factors for sick sinus syndrome in the general population. J Am Coll Cardiol 2014;64(6):531–8.

46. Ewy GA. Sick sinus syndrome: synopsis. J Am Coll Cardiol 2014;64(6):539–40.

47. John RM, Kumar S. Sinus node and atrial arrhythmias. Circulation 2016;133(19): 1892–900.

48. Park DS, Fishman GI. The cardiac conduction system. Circulation 2011;123(8): 904–15.
49. Schwartz PJ, Crotti L, Insolia R. Long-QT syndrome: from genetics to management. Circ Arrhythm Electrophysiol 2012;5(4):868–77.
50. Roden DM. Clinical practice. Long-QT syndrome. N Engl J Med 2008;358(2): 169–76.
51. Hedley PL, Jorgensen P, Schlamowitz S, et al. The genetic basis of long QT and short QT syndromes: a mutation update. Hum Mutat 2009;30(11):1486–511.
52. Douglas P, Zipes M, Camm AJ, et al. ACC/AHA/ESC 2006 Guidelines for Management of Patients With Ventricular Arrhythmias and the Prevention of Sudden Cardiac Death–Executive Summary: A Report of the American College of Cardiology/American Heart Association Task Force and the European Society of Cardiology Committee for Practice Guidelines (Writing Committee to Develop Guidelines for Management of Patients With Ventricular Arrhythmias and the Prevention of Sudden Cardiac Death): Developed in Collaboration With the European Heart Rhythm Association and the Heart Rhythm Society. Circulation 2006; 114(10):1088–132.
53. Shu J, Zhou J, Patel C, et al. Pharmacotherapy of cardiac arrhythmias–basic science for clinicians. Pacing Clin Electrophysiol 2009;32(11):1454–65.
54. Wexler RK, Pleister A, Raman S. Outpatient Approach to Palpitations. Am Fam Physician 2011;84(1):63–9.
55. Pediatric and Congenital Electrophysiology Society (PACES), Heart Rhythm Society (HRS), American College of Cardiology Foundation (ACCF). PACES/HRS expert consensus statement on the management of the asymptomatic young patient with a Wolff-Parkinson-White (WPW, ventricular preexcitation) electrocardiographic pattern: developed in partnership between the Pediatric and Congenital Electrophysiology Society (PACES) and the Heart Rhythm Society (HRS). Endorsed by the governing bodies of PACES, HRS, the American College of Cardiology Foundation (ACCF), the American Heart Association (AHA), the American Academy of Pediatrics (AAP), and the Canadian Heart Rhythm Society (CHRS). Heart Rhythm 2012;9(6):1006–24.
56. Priori SG, Blomstrom-Lundqvist C, Mazzanti A, et al. 2015 ESC Guidelines for the management of patients with ventricular arrhythmias and the prevention of sudden cardiac death: The Task Force for the Management of Patients with Ventricular Arrhythmias and the Prevention of Sudden Cardiac Death of the European Society of Cardiology (ESC). Endorsed by: Association for European Paediatric and Congenital Cardiology (AEPC). Eur Heart J 2015;36(41):2793–867.
57. Olen MM, Baysa SJ, Rossi A, et al. Wolff-Parkinson-White syndrome: a stepwise deterioration to sudden death. Circulation 2016;133(1):105–6.
58. Yasuma F, Hayano J. Respiratory sinus arrhythmia: why does the heartbeat synchronize with respiratory rhythm? Chest 2004;125(2):683–90.

Anticoagulation: The Successes and Pitfalls of Long-Term Management

Eric W. Cucchi, MS, PA-C[a,b,*]

KEYWORDS

- Anticoagulation • Direct oral anticoagulation • Warfarin • Venous thromboembolim
- Atrial fibrillation • Anticoagulation reversal

KEY POINTS

- Direct oral anticoagulation is as effective as warfarin for the management of venous thromboembolism and nonvalvular atrial fibrillation.
- Direct oral anticoagulation is a safe alternative to warfarin.
- An understanding of the differences between direct oral anticoagulation is imperative to choose the correct medication for the individual patient.
- Understanding bleeding risks, which medications are reversible and which agents are available for reversing anticoagulation due to direct oral anticoagulants is critical.

INTRODUCTION

For decades, the mainstay of therapeutic anticoagulation has been vitamin K antagonists (VKAs), with warfarin being the most commonly used. Therapeutic anticoagulation with warfarin therapy is fraught with limitations. Newer classes of medications have emerged, and data have suggested that they are a safe alternative to warfarin.

There is a requirement for frequent laboratory evaluations when using warfarin. With a median number of blood draws in an 18-month period being as many as 20,[1] it can result in discomfort and can be time consuming. The international normalized ratio (INR) can be affected by multiple variables, including age; sex; body weight; smoking; diabetes mellitus (DM); liver failure; congestive heart failure; lung disease; previous anticoagulation; cultural, educational, socioeconomic influences; and food and drug

Disclosure Statement: The author has no conflicts of interest and no disclosures to report.
[a] Affiliate Practitioner Critical Care Residency Program, Critical Care, UMass Memorial Medical Center, The Graduate School of Nursing, University of Massachusetts Medical School, 55 Lake Avenue North, HA318, Worcester, MA 01655, USA; [b] UMass Memorial Medical Center, eICU, 281 Lincoln Street, Worcester, MA 01605, USA
* UMass Memorial Medical Center, 55 Lake Avenue North, HA318, Worcester, MA 01655.
E-mail address: Eric.Cucchi2@umassmemorial.org

Physician Assist Clin 2 (2017) 603–622
http://dx.doi.org/10.1016/j.cpha.2017.06.003
2405-7991/17/© 2017 Elsevier Inc. All rights reserved.

interactions.[2] Subsequently, the variables involved can result in difficulty maintaining patients within a therapeutic range. On average, patients spend approximately 60% of the time in the therapeutic range.[1,3,4] With the difficulties associated with VKAs, there has been a need for alternatives. Recent innovations in anticoagulation therapeutics have dramatically changed the landscape of patient care. Several new classes of medications have emerged, and the all-encompassing terminology is now direct oral anticoagulants (DOACs). DOACs include essentially 2 classes of medications: direct thrombin inhibitors (dabigatran) and Factor Xa antagonists (rivaroxaban, apixaban, and edoxaban). With 4.1 million patient visits for DOACs in 2014,[5] these medications are becoming more and more popular because of the potential benefits of no longer requiring frequent blood checks, fewer food and drug interactions, rapid onset and offset compared with warfarin, and less need for bridging therapy.[6] The potential downside to these medications is that there is a risk of increased plasma concentration with decreased renal function and, in the case of Factor Xa inhibitors, a lack of antidote in severe bleeding.[6]

DOACs are proving themselves as effective and safe as warfarin. In a meta-analysis[7] including 27,023 patients treated DOACs compared with warfarin in the treatment of acute venous thromboembolism (VTE), the overall VTE reoccurrence rate was similar in both groups with a reduction of major bleeding by 39% in the DOAC group. Intracranial and fatal bleeding rates occurred significantly less in the DOAC groups, and all-cause mortality was similar in both groups. Similar results have been found in patients with atrial fibrillation (afib) treated with a DOAC versus a VKA. A meta-analysis of 71,683 patients demonstrated a reduction of stroke and systemic embolism (SSE) by 19%, major bleeding by 14%, and intracranial hemorrhage by 52% by DOACs compared with warfarin; however, there was a higher rate of gastrointestinal bleeds (GIBs).[8] Two *Cochrane Reviews* showed no difference in recurrent VTE, deep vein thrombosis (DVT), nonfatal pulmonary embolism (PE), all-cause mortality, and major bleeding.[9,10]

With similar efficacy and an improved safety profile, DOACs are likely to be used with increased frequency. Although the term DOAC is all encompassing, there are differences between the individual medications in terms of mechanism of actions, dosing, and approvals that are important for the physician assistant to become familiar with so that the proper medication for the individual patient can be prescribed.

ANTICOAGULATION MEDICATIONS

The purpose of anticoagulation is not to directly lyse a previously established thrombus but to prevent propagation of the clot and to allow endogenous anticoagulation factors to reduce the clot burden. Several classes of medications exist that inhibit thrombus formation at different points along the clotting cascade. Because of the risk of bleeding that exists, novel reversal agents had to be developed alongside these newer classes of anticoagulants, because the reversal agents currently used for VKAs are ineffective in reversing the DOACs.

VITAMIN K ANTAGONISTS

In the United States, the mainstay of anticoagulation for years has been warfarin, which is the only vitamin K antagonist on the market. Warfarin acts by blocking the synthesis of the Vitamin K–dependent pathways, which are Factors II, VII, IX, and X as well as proteins C and S. An anticoagulation effect usually occurs within 24 hours, but peak effect may take up to 72 hours. The half-lives of the individual factors are Factor II, 60 hours; VII, 4 to 6 hours; IX, 24 hours; X, 48 to 72 hours; protein C, 8 hours; and protein S, 30 hours. Clinically, the duration of effect of a single dose of warfarin is generally 2 to 5 days[11] (**Table 1**).

DIRECT ORAL ANTICOAGULATION

There are currently 2 major classes of DOACs: direct thrombin inhibitor and factor Xa inhibitors. Each medication within their respective classes carries its own risks and benefits.

DIRECT THROMBIN INHIBITOR
Dabigatran Etexilate Mesylate

Dabigatran etexilate mesylate is a prodrug and is converted to dabigatran and acyl glucuronides, which both then directly inhibit thrombin. Thrombin is involved in the conversion of fibrinogen into fibrin, which allows the thrombus to form[12] (see **Table 1**).

Dabigatran was studied in the RE-LY trial,[13] which evaluated 18,113 patients with nonvalvular afib and one or more of the following: history of stroke or transient ischemic attack (TIA), left ventricular ejection fraction (LVEF) less than 40%, NYHA class ≥ II, age ≥75 or 65 to 74 with DM, hypertension (HTN), or coronary artery disease, were randomly assigned to blinded dabigatran 110 mg or150 mg versus unblinded warfarin with a goal INR of 2 to 3. Dabigatran 150 mg dosing was superior to warfarin in preventing SSE. In terms of safety, there was no difference in major bleeding, but on secondary analysis, there was a higher rate of GIB but less intracranial bleeding in the dabigatran group. Dyspepsia was more common in the dabigatran group as compared with the warfarin group.

Dabigatran's use in VTE treatment was evaluated in the RE-COVER trial,[14] which found that 150 mg of dabigatran was noninferior compared with warfarin dosed for a goal INR of 1 to 2, with similar bleeding rates.

Dabigatran was also evaluated in thromboembolic prevention in patients with mechanical valves in the RE-ALIGN study,[15] which was stopped early because of high rates of thromboembolism and a higher bleeding risk. This effect may be due to the possibility that the clot burden is too extensive for dabigatran to be effective when dosed at clinical concentrations.[16]

FACTOR XA INHIBITORS
Rivaroxaban

Rivaroxaban is a selective Factor Xa inhibitor with prothrombinase activity, resulting in decreased thrombin generation.[17] It was approved for SSE reduction in patients with nonvalvular afib, treatment of DVT and PE, and for prophylaxis of DVT in patients undergoing total knee or total hip replacements.[17]

Use of rivaroxaban was assessed in the ROCKET-AF trial[18]; this trial looked at 14,264 patients who had afib and a history of stroke, TIA, systemic embolism, or 2 or more of the following: heart failure or an LVEF of 35% or less, HTN, age 75 or more, and DM. In this group of patients, rivaroxaban was found to be noninferior to warfarin with a similar risk for both major and nonmajor bleeding. Interestingly, the need for transfusion, a hemoglobin decline of 2 or more g/dL, and major GIB were higher in the rivaroxaban group compared with warfarin. However, critical bleeding, fatal bleeding, and intracranial bleeding were more prevalent in the warfarin group.

A secondary analysis further evaluated the GIB risk of the ROCKET-AF trial and found that 48% had UGIB, 23% had LGIB, and 29% had rectal bleeding. Patients at risk tended to be older, with chronic illness, with higher CHADS scores, with chronic obstructive pulmonary disease, with obstructive sleep apnea, smoked cigarettes,

Table 1
Pharmacodynamics and pharmacokinetics of warfarin and direct oral anticoagulants

Medication	Absorption	Distribution	Elimination	T/12	Metabolism	Renal Impairment	Hepatic Impairment	Drug Interactions
Warfarin	~100% within 4 h	0.14 L/kg 99% protein bound	Mostly urine Some by bile	20–60 h, mean 40 h	Cytochrome P-450	No dosing reduction required	No dosing reduction required, however may decrease metabolism and response of drug may be increased	Many
Dabigatran	3%–7% C_max 1–3 h	50–70 L 35% protein bound	Urine 80% Renal clearance	12–17 h	Esterase catalyzed hydrolysis	Dosing reduction required	No dosing changes required	P-gp inhibitors (rifampin)
Rivaroxaban	10 mg dose: 80%–100% 20 mg dose: 66% fasting 76% 15- and 20-mg dose should be taken with food C_max 2–4 h	50 L 92%–95% Protein bound	Urine 30% Feces 21%	5–9 h	CYP3A4/5 CYP2J2	Dosing reduction required	Unknown beyond Child-Pugh A class	P-gp inhibitors ABCG2 transporters
Apixaban	50% up to 10 mg C_max 3–4 h Food does not affect absorption	21 L 87% Protein bound	Urine 27% Feces	12 h	CYP3A4 CYP1A2, 2C8, 2C9, 2C19, and 2J2	Dosing reduction required	No dosing reduction required	CYP3A4 and P-gp inhibitors
Edoxaban	62% C_max 1–2 h Food does not affect absorption	19.9 L 55% protein bound	Unchanged in the urine 50% Bile/feces 50%	10–14 h	Minimal metabolism via hydrolysis conjugation and oxidation by CYP3A4	Dosing adjustment required	Child-Pugh A or Child-Pugh B no dosing change, no known change for Child-Pugh C	?CYP3A4 and P-gp inhibitors

Data from Refs.[11,12,17,22,28]

used nonsteroidal anti-inflammatory drugs, used proton pump inhibitors or histamine-2 blockers, and had anemia.[19] These findings illustrate the need to identify which patients would benefit from which medication. Rivaroxaban may be used in acute medical conditions for DVT prophylaxis, and although it is noninferior to enoxaparin, it did carry an increased bleeding risk.[20] In patients with PE, rivaroxaban was noninferior to warfarin in preventing recurrent VTE, but was associated with similar bleeding risk.[21]

Apixaban

Apixaban is another selective inhibitor of Factor Xa with a prothombinase activity indicated for risk reduction in SSE in patients with nonvalvular afib, prophylaxis of DVT in patients whom have undergone total hip arthroplasty or total knee arthroplasty, and treatment of DVT/PE and reduction of risk for reoccurrence after initial therapy.[22] For treatment of DVT/PE, there was no difference in efficacy between apixaban and warfarin in regards to recurrence rates; however, there was less bleeding risk.[23] The ARISTOLE trial[24] evaluated apixaban versus warfarin in patients with nonvalvular afib and found that apixaban was superior to warfarin in prevention of SSE. Most of the benefit appeared to be in the prevention of hemorrhagic stroke, rather than system embolism. In this study, there was a lower risk of major bleeding as well as mortality benefits. Importantly, when bleeding did occur, there were similar mortalities and thromboembolic events.[25] A large meta-analysis also found less bleeding risk compared with VKAs.[26] Interestingly, in patients on aspirin alone for SSE prevention in afib patients, apixiban had increased efficacy without any increase in bleeding.[27]

Edoxaban

Edoxaban is another Factor Xa inhibitor with prothrombinase inhibition activity that is approved for reducing the risk of SSE in patients with nonvavular afib and for the treatment of DVT/PE after 5 to 10 days of parenteral anticoagulation.[28]

The Hokusai-VTE[29] group found that enoxaparin/unfractionated heparin (UFH) bridge followed by edoxaban was noninferior compared with bridging before warfarin therapy to prevent VTE. The ENGAGE AF-TIMI 48 study[30] showed that edoxaban 60 mg was superior to warfarin and noninferior at 30 mg daily and was associated with lower bleeding risks. The rate of hemorrhagic stroke was statistically lower in both groups compared with warfarin. The high-dose edoxaban was not statistically better in improving ischemic stroke compared with warfarin, whereas the lower dose had somewhat higher rates than warfarin. All bleeding rates except for GIB were lower in the edoxaban group. In patients with a CrCl greater than 95 mL/min, there was an increased rate of ischemic stroke with edoxaban 60 mg daily compared with warfarin.

Reversal Agents

Bleeding is a serious concern when prescribing any anticoagulation. The effects of warfarin can be easily reversed by several different methods. Vitamin K, prothrombin complex concentrate (PCC), fresh frozen plasma, or Factor VII has been used, although differences in "reversed" versus "nonreversed" patient outcome data are sparse.[2,31] Currently, only dabigatran has a Food and Drug Administration (FDA)-approved reversal agent. Medications are currently being studied for the reversal of the Factor Xa inhibitors. Although there is no clear evidence of increased risk of bleeding of DOACs compared with warfarin, patients who bled while taking dabigatran had better outcomes than those reversed with warfarin.[32] No matter the medication, there is a need for reversing the effects of the medications when patients do suffer a bleed or require an emergent surgery.

PCC comes in 2 forms: 3 factor, which includes Factors II, IX, X, or 4 factor, which contains Factors II, VII, IX, X, Protein C and S.[2] These PCCs have been shown to normalize prothrombin times in warfarin and rivaroxaban but not dabigatran.[33] Edoxaban 60 mg before punch biopsy was given PCC and in the highest concentration of PCC reversed the prothrombin time.[34]

In 2015, idarucizumab received FDA approval for the reversal of dabigatran. It is a humanized mouse monoclonal antibody fragment that binds to dabigatran at 350 times that of its affinity to thrombin. In patients with severe bleeding or need for urgent/emergent surgery, a total of 5 grams (2.5 grams boluses × 2 within 15 minutes of each another) of idarucizumab showed normalization of diluted thrombin time, ecarin clotting times, activated partial thromboplastin, and thrombin time in 88% to 98% of patients within minutes.[35]

There are no currently approved reversal agents for Factor Xa inhibitors. One of the most promising is andexanet alfa, which is a modified recombinant protein derived from human coagulation Factor X. The mechanism of action[36] is high-affinity binding to Factor Xa inhibitors within the vasculature, reducing unbound plasma levels.

ANNEXA-R[36] and ANNEXA-A[36] were randomized controlled trials to evaluate the efficacy of reversal on 20 mg of rivaroxaban and 5 mg of apixaban as well as to access the safety in older healthy volunteers. In both groups, the Factor Xa activity was reduced compared with placebo. The reversal of the anti-Xa activity lasted for 2 hours before returning to levels seen in the placebo groups. When the bolus was followed by a 2-hour infusion, a similar reduction in Factor Xa was found compared with placebo. No serious adverse reactions were noted.

ANNEXA-4[37] was a prospective study that included 67 adults in a safety population versus 47 in an efficacy population who had received Factor XA inhibitors who had acute major bleeding. Adequate hemostasis was achieved in 79% of patients, and thrombotic events occurred in 18% of patients.

What Direct Oral Anticoagulant Should I Choose for My Patient?

The appropriate medication to select for a patient requires careful consideration. In terms of prevention for SSE in afib patients, one should calculate the CHADS-VASC[38] score (**Table 2**), and if greater than 2, patients should be considered for anticoagulation, assuming no contraindications.

The patient's risk of bleeding should also be assessed before administration of an anticoagulant. The HAS-BLED[39] score (**Tables 3** and **4**) is a tool to gauge bleeding risk.

Once the patient's need for anticoagulation and risk of bleeding have been assessed, a medication can be selected.

There are a few considerations regarding the medications that need to be weighed before initiation. The first is that if the patient is currently on warfarin, is it appropriate to switch the patient to a DOAC? Time in therapeutic range (TTR) studies have found that when a patient's warfarin TTR is higher, therapeutic endpoints were similar to those of dabigatran, rivaroxaban, and apixaban.[40–42] Therefore, if a patient is maintaining an appropriate INR level, then no additional therapeutic benefit is gained form a DOAC. Other considerations that may alter the risk/benefit include drug and food interactions or complicated dosing regimens.

All of the Factor Xa inhibitors come with black box warnings that suggest if the medication is stopped prematurely, there could be an increased risk of ischemic events in the absence of an adequate alternative. In addition, there is a risk of spinal/epidural hematoma in patients receiving neuroaxial anesthesia or spinal puncture. Edoxaban carries an additional black box warning for using 60-mg dosing in patients with a

Table 2
Dosing and indications of warfarin and direct oral anticoagulants

Medication	Dosing	Indication
Warfarin	Dosed to maintain a therapeutic INR of 2–3	Prophylaxis and/or treatment of VTE/PE
	Dosed to maintain a therapeutic INR of 2–3	Prophylaxis and/or treatment of thromboembolic complications associated with afib
	Dosed to maintain a therapeutic INR of 2.5–3.5	Prophylaxis and/or treatment of throbmoebmolic complications cardiac valve replacement
	Dosed to maintain a therapeutic INR of 2–3?	To reduce risk of death, recurrent MI, and thromboembolic events after MI
Dabigatran	CrCl >30 mL/min: 150 mg twice a day	Reduction of SSE in afib
	CrCl 15–30 mL/min: 75 mg twice a day	Reduction of SSE in afib
	CrCl <15 mL/min or dialysis: no recommendation	Reduction of SSE in afib
	CrCl 30–50 mL/min with P-gp inhibitor use: 75 mg twice a day	Reduction of SSE in afib
	CrCl <30 mL/min with P-gp inhibitor use: avoid	Reduction of SSE in afib
	CrCl >30 mL/min: 150 mg twice a day	Treatment and reduction of risk of recurrence DVT/PE
	CrCl ≤30 mL/min or dialysis: no recommendation	Treatment and reduction of risk of recurrence DVT/PE
	CrCl <50 mL/min with P-gp inhibitors: avoid	Treatment and reduction of risk of recurrence DVT/PE
Rivaroxaban	CrCl >50 mL/min: 20 mg daily with evening meal	Reduction of SSE risk in nonvalvular afib
	CrCl 15–50 mL/min: 15 mg daily with evening meal	Reduction of SSE risk in nonvalvular afib
	15 mg twice a day with food × 21 d then 20 mg daily with food	Treatment of DVT/PE
	20 mg daily with food	Prevention of recurrence of DVT/PE
	10 mg daily × 35 d	DVT prophylaxis following total hip replacement
	10 mg daily × 12 d	DVT prophylaxis following total knee replacement
Apixaban	5 mg twice daily	Reduction of SSE risk in nonvalvular afib
	2.5 mg twice daily if patient meets at least 2 of the following criteria: Age ≥80 y ≤60 Kg Cr ≥1.5 mg/dL	Reduction of SSE risk in nonvalvular afib
	2.5 mg twice daily with the initial dose 12–24 h after surgery ×35 d ×12 d	DVT prophylaxis following: Total hip replacement Total knee replacement
	10 mg twice a day × 7 d then 5 mg twice a day after 6 mo of treatment then 2.5 mg daily	Treatment of DVT and PE

(continued on next page)

Table 2 (continued)		
Medication	**Dosing**	**Indication**
Edoxaban	60 mg daily	Reduction of SSE risk in nonvalvular afib
	CrCl >95 mL/min: avoid use	Reduction of SSE risk in nonvalvular afib
	CrCl 15–50 mL/min: 30 mg daily	Reduction of SSE risk in nonvalvular afib
	60 mg daily after 5–10 d of parenteral anticoagulation	Treatment of DVT and PE
	CrCl 15–50 mL/min, 60 kg or less, or taking P-gp inhibitor: 30 mg daily	Treatment of DVT and PE

Data from Refs.[11,12,17,22,28]

CrCl greater than 95 mL/min, because of an increased risk of ischemic stroke.[12,17,22,28]

Certain populations may have additional risk factors when considering anticoagulation. If a patient has a history of HTN, then the blood pressure should be controlled, ideally to less than 130/80 mm Hg.[43]

For patients with chronic kidney disease, the DOACs will require careful consideration to dosing.[2] A meta-analysis[44] looked at patients enrolled in the RE-LY, ROCKET AF, ARISTOTLE, and ENGAGE-AF TIMI 48 trials with a growth factor receptor (GFR) greater than 80 and found no difference and perhaps a slight improvement in bleeding risk. In patients with a mild (50–80 mL/min/1.73 m^2) to moderate (<50 mL/min/1.73 m^2) reduction in GFR, there was a reduced risk of SSE as well as major bleeding.

Caution should also be used in elderly patients. Not only does this population often have HTN and renal impairment, but also there is a potential increased risk of gastrointestinal bleeding in patients older than 75 years old on dabigatran. In this same population of patients aged 75 or greater, there is an increased risk of intracranial hemorrhage with dabigatran and apixiban use. Conversely, rivaroxaban may have a decreased risk of bleeding in elderly patients.[45] There are no current data for pregnant or pediatric populations.[2]

Table 3 CHA_2DS_2-VASc	
Age	<65: 0 points 65–74: 1 point ≥75: 2 points
Sex	M: 0 points F: 1 point
Congestive heart failure	1 point
HTN	1 point
Stroke/TIA/thromboembolism	2 points
Vascular disease	1 point
Diabetes	1 point

Data from Lip GY, Nieuwlaat R, Pisters R, et al. Refining clinical risk stratification for predicting stroke and thromboembolism in atrial fibrillation using a novel risk factor-based approach: the Euro Heart Survey on atrial fibrillation. Chest 2010;137(2):263–72.

Table 4 HAS-BLED	
HTN	1 point
Renal diseases	1 point
Liver disease	1 point
Stroke history	1 point
Prior major bleeding or predisposition to bleeding	1 point
Labile INR	1 point
Age >65	1 point
Medication usage predisposing to bleeding	1 point

Data from Pisters R, Lane DA, Nieuwlaat R, et al. A novel user-friendly score (HAS-BLED) to assess 1-year risk of major bleeding in patients with atrial fibrillation: the Euro Heart Survey. Chest 2010;138(5):1093–100.

Knowledge of specific medication variations will also aid in choosing the correct medication for the individual patient. An important consideration is that once-daily dosing can may patient/physician satisfaction.[46] All DOACs used the P-glycoprotein (p-gp) pathways; however, rivaroxaban uses the CYP3A4 pathway in addition to p-gp, whereas warfarin uses cytochrome P450. Patients that are on medications that use one of these pathways may have alterations in the efficacy of the anticoagulant. Patients with concomitant single or dual antiplatelet therapy (aspirin and/or clopidogrel) while using dabigatran have an increased risk of bleeding; however, this did not impact from the efficacy of dabigatran over warfarin (150 mg superior to warfarin) or from its noninferiority (110 mg compared with warfarin).[47] Dabigatran can also cause dyspepsia and may need to be avoided in patients with gastritis, peptic ulcer disease, partial/total gastrectomy, or gastric bypass. Patients that require medications given via a gastric tube may need apixaban or rivaroxaban because these medications can be crushed.

Although there has not yet been a true head-to-head comparison of the DOACs, there are some noted differences in efficacy. Dabigatran 150 mg decreased ischemic stroke, whereas the others improved risk or hemorrhagic strokes. Apixaban had a lower risk of bleeding, whereas other medications/doses were noninferior.

Cost can become burdensome for some patients, and this may require a thoughtful discussion. When comparing patients in the AVERROS study, there was a cost benefit with apixiban versus aspirin alone.[48] When evaluating dabigatran 150 mg twice a day compared with warfarin in patients with Medicare Part D, there is a cost-effectiveness seen both by Medicare and by the patient's out-of-pocket costs. This cost-effectiveness was not translated over to patients without prescription drug coverage.[49] Similarly, edoxaban versus warfarin was found to be cost-effective.[50]

Anticoagulation: Indications and Duration of Therapies

In this new age of a wider array of anticoagulation options, there are several considerations when starting a new oral anticoagulation regimen. Determining who should be treated, when therapy should start, and when therapy should be discontinued should be based on expert opinion, scientific literature, and a frank and shared decision making with the individual patient.

The main indications for therapeutic anticoagulation are DVT and PE; afib and atrial flutter are indications for anticoagulation to prevent SSE. The specifics in treatment of these pathologic entities have been laid out by expert panels and are described in later discussion.

Venous Thromboembolism/Pulmonary Embolism

For DVT or PE, including surgically provoked, the American College of Chest Physicians (ACCP)[51] recommends 3 months of anticoagulation (**Table 5**). DOACs (dabigatran, rivaroxaban, apixabin, or edoxaban) are considered first-line agents for nonvalvular afib and DVT/PE management. VKAs are still the medication of choice for most other anticoagulation needs, such as valvular afib, Factor V Leiden, and so forth. The ACCP suggests that if cancer is present, an extended course of low-molecular-weight heparin (LMWH) should be used. This management regimen is also supported by a 2014 *Cochrane Review* of 10 randomized controlled studies with a total of 1981 patients that found LMWH to be superior to VKAs in patients with cancer. No survival benefit was noted, but there was a reduction in recurrent VTE.[52]

In patients with an unprovoked first proximal leg DVT or PE with a low to moderate bleeding risk, the recommendation by the ACCP is extended anticoagulation, defined as a duration without a scheduled stop date. The need for anticoagulation should be evaluated annually. Conversely, if there is a high bleeding risk, the recommendation is 3 months of anticoagulation. Once the anticoagulation therapy is complete, then the recommendation is for initiation of aspirin in the absence of contraindications.

Isolated distal DVT without symptoms should be reimaged 2 weeks after the initial study, for evaluation of extension into the deep system. If the clot propagates into the deep system, then this would require anticoagulation. In patients with subsegmental

Table 5
2016 American College of Chest Physicians recommendations

Indication	Preferred Medication	Duration
Proximal DVT or PE without cancer	DOAC	3 mo of anticoagulation
Proximal DVT or PE with cancer, low/moderate/high risk of bleeding	LMWH	Unscheduled stop date
Proximal DVT/PE provoked by surgery	DOAC	3 mo
Proximal DVT/PE provoked by transient risk factor	DOAC	3 mo
Isolated Distal DVT provoked by transient risk factor, asymptomatic	Surveillance with serial imaging × 2 wk	NA
Isolated distal DVT provoked by transient risk factor, symptomatic	DOAC	3 mo
First unprovoked VTE, low/moderate risk of bleeding	DOAC	Unscheduled stop date
First unprovoked VTE, high risk of bleeding	DOAC	3 mo
Second unprovoked VTE, low/moderate risk of bleeding	DOAC	Unscheduled stop date
Second unprovoked VTE, high risk of bleeding	DOAC	3 mo
Subsegmental PE without DVT, low risk for recurrence	Surveillance	NA
Subsegmental PE without DVT, high risk for recurrence	DOAC	3 mo

Abbreviation: DOAC, direct oral anticoagulation, specifically dabigatran or rivaroxaban or apixaban or edoxaban.

Data from Kearon C, Akl EA, Ornelas J, et al. Antithrombotic therapy for VTE disease: CHEST guideline and expert panel report. Chest 2016;149(2):315–52.

PE, the current recommendation is to monitor as long as they are low risk for recurrent VTE.

For patients who have had failure of therapeutic anticoagulation, it is recommended that the patient's regimen be transitioned to LMWH for at least 1 month. If there is recurrence of VTE on LMWH, then the recommendation is to increase the dose by 25% to 33%.

Atrial Fibrillation/Atrial Flutter

Afib affects as many as one-third of adults greater than 80 years old[53] and is associated with a 5-fold increase in stroke incidence.[54] In addition, afib at the time of stroke carries a higher risk of mortality at 1 year (49.5% compared with 27.1% in patients without stroke).[55] Traditionally, warfarin has been the mainstay of prevention of stroke in afib/flutter for decades. Compared with placebo, there is a 64% reduction in the risk of stroke and a 39% decrease compared with antiplatelet therapy.[56]

In 2014, the American Heart Association, American College of Cardiology, and the Heart Rhythm Society in collaboration with the Society of Thoracic Surgeons recommended that anticoagulation be a decision between the provider and the patient with consideration of risk factors independent of the pattern of afib (paroxysmal, persistent, or permanent). Atrial flutter carries a similar risk of stroke and should be treated the same way as afib. Risk assessment should be conducted with a validated risk score such as the CHA_2-DS_2-VASc (see **Table 2**). Assessing when to initiate anticoagulation in patients with nonvalvular afib should begin with a CHA_2-DS_2-VASc score; when the score is greater than2, then the recommendation would be to initiate anticoagulation. The regimen in nonvalvular afib may include warfarin, dabigatran, rivaroxaban, or apixaban. If warfarin is used, then the INR must be assessed frequently upon initiation, up to weekly, and once the target INR is achieved and stable, then this may be adjusted. If the INR target cannot be met, then dabigatran, rivaroxaban, or apixaban may be considered in nonvalvular afib. The need for ongoing anticoagulation should be reevaluated at periodic intervals to ensure the risk/benefit ratio remains favorable.

For patients with mechanical heart valves, warfarin continues to be the only approved anticoagulant, with a target INR of 2 to 3 or 2.5 to 3.5 based on the type and position of the valve regardless of the CHA_2-DS_2-VASc score. If interruption in treatment, such as surgery or invasive procedure, is required, patients should be bridged with LMWH.[53]

Prevention of Deep Vein Thrombosis/Pulmonary Embolism Following Joint Surgery

In addition to therapeutic treatment, both rivarboxan and apixaban have been approved by the FDA for VTE prophylaxis in patients after total hip arthroplasty and total knee arthroplasty.[17,22]

Discontinuation

Once initiation of medications has occurred, there are several instances when the medications will need to be withheld or discontinued while undergoing therapy. Generally, any procedure that is associated with major bleeding, such as elective surgery or endoscopic procedures that are associated with major bleeding, will require the medication to be temporarily held.[57] Patients undergoing neuroaxial catheterization are at risk for hematoma and permanent paralysis.[12,17,22,28] Permanent discontinuation should be performed whenever there is hypersensitivity or intolerance to the medication. Other possible indications for discontinuation of anticoagulation include refusal by the patient, medication nonadherence, poor short-term prognosis, and poor functional status with total dependency, and high risk of bleeding. Comorbid conditions whereby caution should be taken and risk/benefit should be analyzed include alcohol abuse, risk of falls, age, previous intracranial bleed, history of bleeding, need for concomitant antiplatelet medications, and use of nonsteroidal anti-inflammatory drugs.[57]

The ACCP[58] recommends bridging for high-risk procedures, such as urologic surgery, cardiac device procedure, colon polypectomy, surgery on highly vascular organs, bowel resection, major surgery with extensive tissue injury, and cardiac, intracranial, or spinal surgeries. No bridging is necessary in low-risk and patient-specific, or moderate or low-risk procedures.

Bridging usually begins in patients whom had been on warfarin when the INR is less than 2; then UFH is stopped 4 to 6 hours before surgery, and LMWH is stopped 24 hours before.

Management of these medications in the perioperative period is unclear. In one study,[59] standard bleeding risk procedures in a patient with a CrCl greater than 80 dabigatran was held for 24 hours before, and in high risk of bleeding patients dabigatran was held for 48 hours. For patients with decreased CrCl, the dabigatran could be held up to 6 days before surgery depending on the risk of bleeding and the severity of renal dysfunction. In this study, most patients were resumed on postoperative day 1, and bleeding risk was limited.[60–136]

SUMMARY

Warfarin has been the mainstay of oral anticoagulation for decades but is limited by several factors, including time in therapeutic window, frequent blood monitoring, complex dosing strategies that can be confusing for some, and bleeding risk. We have now entered an age wherein we can simplify dosing regimens, limit blood testing, and maintain as effective, or in some cases more effective, anticoagulation compared with warfarin. This age does have limitations. The availability of multiple options requires additional consideration to choose the most optimal medication for the patient. Age, kidney function, and bleeding risk all are of concern. Some practitioners may consider that no longer monitoring INR has some disadvantages to consider, including reduced certainty of patient compliance. Bleeding risk is something of deeper concern now that not all of these medications have approved "reversal" antidotes. Further research is needed to ensure that all patients who require anticoagulation remain safe. Despite overall bleeding risk associated with anticoagulants, the efficacy and safety profile of the DOACs are now considered the primary treatment for most thrombotic states or as the primary prevention.

REFERENCES

1. Pokorney SD, Simon DN, Thomas L, et al. Patients' time in therapeutic range on warfarin among US patients with atrial fibrillation: results from ORBIT-AF registry. Am Heart J 2015;170(1):141–8, 148.e1.
2. Schaefer JK, McBane RD, Wysokinski WE. How to choose appropriate direct oral anticoagulant for patient with nonvalvular atrial fibrillation. Ann Hematol 2016;95(3):437–49.
3. Agarwal S, Hachamovitch R, Menon V. Current trial-associated outcomes with warfarin in prevention of stroke in patients with nonvalvular atrial fibrillation: a meta-analysis. Arch Intern Med 2012;172(8):623–31 [discussion: 631–3].
4. Matchar DB, Samsa GP, Cohen SJ, et al. Improving the quality of anticoagulation of patients with atrial fibrillation in managed care organizations: results of the managing anticoagulation services trial. Am J Med 2002;113(1):42–51.

5. Barnes GD, Lucas E, Alexander GC, et al. National trends in ambulatory oral anticoagulant use. Am J Med 2015;128(12):1300–5.e2.

6. Kalabalik J, Rattinger GB, Sullivan J, et al. Use of non-vitamin K antagonist oral anticoagulants in special patient populations with nonvalvular atrial fibrillation: a review of the literature and application to clinical practice. Drugs 2015;75(9): 979–98.

7. van Es N, Coppens M, Schulman S, et al. Direct oral anticoagulants compared with vitamin K antagonists for acute venous thromboembolism: evidence from phase 3 trials. Blood 2014;124(12):1968–75.

8. Ruff CT, Giugliano RP, Braunwald E, et al. Comparison of the efficacy and safety of new oral anticoagulants with warfarin in patients with atrial fibrillation: a meta-analysis of randomised trials. Lancet 2014;383(9921):955–62.

9. Robertson L, Kesteven P, McCaslin JE. Oral direct thrombin inhibitors or oral factor Xa inhibitors for the treatment of deep vein thrombosis. Cochrane Database Syst Rev 2015;(6):CD010956.

10. Robertson L, Kesteven P, McCaslin JE. Oral direct thrombin inhibitors or oral factor Xa inhibitors for the treatment of pulmonary embolism. Cochrane Database Syst Rev 2015;(12):CD010957.

11. Warfarin [package insert]. Taro Pharmaceutical Industries L, Haifa Bay, Israel; 1999.

12. Pradaxa [package insert]. Boehringer Ingelheim Pharmaceuticals I, Ridgefield, CT; 2015.

13. Hijazi Z, Hohnloser SH, Oldgren J, et al. Efficacy and safety of dabigatran compared with warfarin in relation to baseline renal function in patients with atrial fibrillation: a RE-LY (Randomized Evaluation of Long-term Anticoagulation Therapy) trial analysis. Circulation 2014;129(9):961–70.

14. Schulman S, Kearon C, Kakkar AK, et al. Dabigatran versus warfarin in the treatment of acute venous thromboembolism. N Engl J Med 2009;361(24):2342–52.

15. Eikelboom JW, Connolly SJ, Brueckmann M, et al. Dabigatran versus warfarin in patients with mechanical heart valves. N Engl J Med 2013;369(13):1206–14.

16. Jaffer IH, Stafford AR, Fredenburgh JC, et al. Dabigatran is less effective than warfarin at attenuating mechanical heart valve-induced thrombin generation. J Am Heart Assoc 2015;4(8):e002322.

17. Xarelto [package insert]. Janssen Ortho L, Gurabo, PR or Bayer Pharma AG. Leverkusen Germany; 2016.

18. Patel MR, Mahaffey KW, Garg J, et al. Rivaroxaban versus warfarin in nonvalvular atrial fibrillation. N Engl J Med 2011;365(10):883–91.

19. Sherwood MW, Nessel CC, Hellkamp AS, et al. Gastrointestinal bleeding in patients with atrial fibrillation treated with rivaroxaban or warfarin: ROCKET AF Trial. J Am Coll Cardiol 2015;66(21):2271–81.

20. Cohen AT, Spiro TE, Spyropoulos AC. Rivaroxaban for thromboprophylaxis in acutely ill medical patients. N Engl J Med 2013;368(20):1945–6.

21. Buller HR, Prins MH, Lensin AW, et al. Oral rivaroxaban for the treatment of symptomatic pulmonary embolism. N Engl J Med 2012;366(14):1287–97.

22. Eliquis [package insert]. Bristol-Myers Squibb Company P, NJ; 2016.

23. Agnelli G, Buller HR, Cohen A, et al. Oral apixaban for the treatment of acute venous thromboembolism. N Engl J Med 2013;369(9):799–808.

24. Granger CB, Alexander JH, McMurray JJ, et al. Apixaban versus warfarin in patients with atrial fibrillation. N Engl J Med 2011;365(11):981–92.

25. Held C, Hylek EM, Alexander JH, et al. Clinical outcomes and management associated with major bleeding in patients with atrial fibrillation treated with

apixaban or warfarin: insights from the ARISTOTLE trial. Eur Heart J 2015; 36(20):1264–72.

26. Touma L, Filion KB, Atallah R, et al. A meta-analysis of randomized controlled trials of the risk of bleeding with apixaban versus vitamin K antagonists. Am J Cardiol 2015;115(4):533–41.

27. Connolly SJ, Eikelboom J, Joyner C, et al. Apixaban in patients with atrial fibrillation. N Engl J Med 2011;364(9):806–17.

28. Savaysa [package insert]. Daiichi Sankyo Co. L, Tokyo, Japan; 2016.

29. Hokusai VTEI, Buller HR, Decousus H, et al. Edoxaban versus warfarin for the treatment of symptomatic venous thromboembolism. N Engl J Med 2013; 369(15):1406–15.

30. Eisen A, Giugliano RP, Ruff CT, et al. Edoxaban vs warfarin in patients with non-valvular atrial fibrillation in the US Food and Drug Administration approval population: an analysis from the Effective Anticoagulation with Factor Xa Next Generation in Atrial Fibrillation-Thrombolysis in Myocardial Infarction 48 (ENGAGE AF-TIMI 48) trial. Am Heart J 2016;172:144–51.

31. Dowlatshahi D, Butcher KS, Asdaghi N, et al. Poor prognosis in warfarin-associated intracranial hemorrhage despite anticoagulation reversal. Stroke 2012;43(7):1812–7.

32. Hart RG, Diener HC, Yang S, et al. Intracranial hemorrhage in atrial fibrillation patients during anticoagulation with warfarin or dabigatran: the RE-LY trial. Stroke 2012;43(6):1511–7.

33. Eerenberg ES, Kamphuisen PW, Sijpkens MK, et al. Reversal of rivaroxaban and dabigatran by prothrombin complex concentrate: a randomized, placebo-controlled, crossover study in healthy subjects. Circulation 2011;124(14): 1573–9.

34. Zahir H, Brown KS, Vandell AG, et al. Edoxaban effects on bleeding following punch biopsy and reversal by a 4-factor prothrombin complex concentrate. Circulation 2015;131(1):82–90.

35. Pollack CV Jr, Reilly PA, Eikelboom J, et al. Idarucizumab for dabigatran reversal. N Engl J Med 2015;373(6):511–20.

36. Siegal DM, Curnutte JT, Connolly SJ, et al. Andexanet alfa for the reversal of Factor Xa inhibitor activity. N Engl J Med 2015;373(25):2413–24.

37. Connolly SJ, Milling TJ Jr, Eikelboom JW, et al. Andexanet alfa for acute major bleeding associated with factor Xa inhibitors. N Engl J Med 2016;375(12): 1131–41.

38. Lip GY, Nieuwlaat R, Pisters R, et al. Refining clinical risk stratification for predicting stroke and thromboembolism in atrial fibrillation using a novel risk factor-based approach: the Euro Heart Survey on atrial fibrillation. Chest 2010;137(2):263–72.

39. Pisters R, Lane DA, Nieuwlaat R, et al. A novel user-friendly score (HAS-BLED) to assess 1-year risk of major bleeding in patients with atrial fibrillation: the Euro Heart Survey. Chest 2010;138(5):1093–100.

40. Wallentin L, Yusuf S, Ezekowitz MD, et al. Efficacy and safety of dabigatran compared with warfarin at different levels of international normalised ratio control for stroke prevention in atrial fibrillation: an analysis of the RE-LY trial. Lancet 2010;376(9745):975–83.

41. Piccini JP, Hellkamp AS, Lokhnygina Y, et al. Relationship between time in therapeutic range and comparative treatment effect of rivaroxaban and warfarin: results from the ROCKET AF trial. J Am Heart Assoc 2014;3(2):e000521.

42. Wallentin L, Lopes RD, Hanna M, et al. Efficacy and safety of apixaban compared with warfarin at different levels of predicted international normalized ratio control for stroke prevention in atrial fibrillation. Circulation 2013;127(22): 2166–76.

43. Toyoda K, Yasaka M, Uchiyama S, et al. Blood pressure levels and bleeding events during antithrombotic therapy: the Bleeding with Antithrombotic Therapy (BAT) Study. Stroke 2010;41(7):1440–4.

44. Del-Carpio Munoz F, Gharacholou SM, Munger TM, et al. Meta-analysis of renal function on the safety and efficacy of novel oral anticoagulants for atrial fibrillation. Am J Cardiol 2016;117(1):69–75.

45. Sharma M, Cornelius VR, Patel JP, et al. Efficacy and harms of direct oral anticoagulants in the elderly for stroke prevention in atrial fibrillation and secondary prevention of venous thromboembolism: systematic review and meta-analysis. Circulation 2015;132(3):194–204.

46. Engelberger RP, Noll G, Schmidt D, et al. Initiation of rivaroxaban in patients with nonvalvular atrial fibrillation at the primary care level: the Swiss Therapy in Atrial Fibrillation for the Regulation of Coagulation (STAR) Study. Eur J Intern Med 2015;26(7):508–14.

47. Dans AL, Connolly SJ, Wallentin L, et al. Concomitant use of antiplatelet therapy with dabigatran or warfarin in the Randomized Evaluation of Long-Term Anticoagulation Therapy (RE-LY) trial. Circulation 2013;127(5):634–40.

48. Lip GY, Lanitis T, Mardekian J, et al. Clinical and economic implications of apixaban versus aspirin in the low-risk nonvalvular atrial fibrillation patients. Stroke 2015;46(10):2830–7.

49. Salata BM, Hutton DW, Levine DA, et al. Cost-effectiveness of dabigatran (150 mg twice daily) and warfarin in patients >/= 65 years with nonvalvular atrial fibrillation. Am J Cardiol 2016;117(1):54–60.

50. Magnuson EA, Vilain K, Wang K, et al. Cost-effectiveness of edoxaban vs warfarin in patients with atrial fibrillation based on results of the ENGAGE AF-TIMI 48 trial. Am Heart J 2015;170(6):1140–50.

51. Kearon C, Akl EA, Ornelas J, et al. Antithrombotic therapy for VTE disease: CHEST guideline and expert panel report. Chest 2016;149(2):315–52.

52. Akl EA, Kahale L, Barba M, et al. Anticoagulation for the long-term treatment of venous thromboembolism in patients with cancer. Cochrane Database Syst Rev 2014;(7):CD006650.

53. January CT, Wann LS, Alpert JS, et al. 2014 AHA/ACC/HRS guideline for the management of patients with atrial fibrillation: a report of the American College of Cardiology/American Heart Association Task Force on Practice Guidelines and the Heart Rhythm Society. J Am Coll Cardiol 2014;64(21):e1–76.

54. Roger VL, Go AS, Lloyd-Jones DM, et al. Heart disease and stroke statistics–2012 update: a report from the American Heart Association. Circulation 2012; 125(1):e2–220.

55. Marini C, De Santis F, Sacco S, et al. Contribution of atrial fibrillation to incidence and outcome of ischemic stroke: results from a population-based study. Stroke 2005;36(6):1115–9.

56. Hart RG, Pearce LA, Aguilar MI. Meta-analysis: antithrombotic therapy to prevent stroke in patients who have nonvalvular atrial fibrillation. Ann Intern Med 2007;146(12):857–67.

57. Suarez Fernandez C, Formiga F, Camafort M, et al. Antithrombotic treatment in elderly patients with atrial fibrillation: a practical approach. BMC Cardiovasc Disord 2015;15:143.

58. Douketis JD, Spyropoulos AC, Spencer FA, et al. Perioperative management of antithrombotic therapy: Antithrombotic Therapy and Prevention of Thrombosis, 9th ed: American College of Chest Physicians Evidence-Based Clinical Practice Guidelines. Chest 2012;141(2 Suppl):e326S–50S.

59. Schulman S, Carrier M, Lee AY, et al. Perioperative management of dabigatran: a prospective cohort study. Circulation 2015;132(3):167–73.

60. Daniels PR. Peri-procedural management of patients taking oral anticoagulants. BMJ 2015;351:h2391.

61. Agnelli G, Buller HR, Cohen A, et al. Apixaban for extended treatment of venous thromboembolism. N Engl J Med 2013;368(8):699–708.

62. Alexander JH, Lopes RD, James S, et al. Apixaban with antiplatelet therapy after acute coronary syndrome. N Engl J Med 2011;365(8):699–708.

63. Apostolakis S, Guo Y, Lane DA, et al. Renal function and outcomes in anticoagulated patients with non-valvular atrial fibrillation: the AMADEUS trial. Eur Heart J 2013;34(46):3572–9.

64. Avezum A, Lopes RD, Schulte PJ, et al. Apixaban in comparison with warfarin in patients with atrial fibrillation and valvular heart disease: findings from the Apixaban for Reduction in Stroke and Other Thromboembolic Events in Atrial Fibrillation (ARISTOTLE) Trial. Circulation 2015;132(8):624–32.

65. Bansilal S, Bloomgarden Z, Halperin JL, et al. Efficacy and safety of rivaroxaban in patients with diabetes and nonvalvular atrial fibrillation: the Rivaroxaban Once-daily, Oral, Direct Factor Xa Inhibition Compared with Vitamin K Antagonism for Prevention of Stroke and Embolism Trial in Atrial Fibrillation (ROCKET AF Trial). Am Heart J 2015;170(4):675–82.e8.

66. Bertomeu-Gonzalez V, Anguita M, Moreno-Arribas J, et al. Quality of anticoagulation with vitamin K antagonists. Clin Cardiol 2015;38(6):357–64.

67. Blech S, Ebner T, Ludwig-Schwellinger E, et al. The metabolism and disposition of the oral direct thrombin inhibitor, dabigatran, in humans. Drug Metab Dispos 2008;36(2):386–99.

68. Bottger B, Thate-Waschke IM, Bauersachs R, et al. Preferences for anticoagulation therapy in atrial fibrillation: the patients' view. J Thromb Thrombolysis 2015; 40(4):406–15.

69. Botticelli Investigators WC, Buller H, Deitchman D, et al. Efficacy and safety of the oral direct factor Xa inhibitor apixaban for symptomatic deep vein thrombosis. The Botticelli DVT dose-ranging study. J Thromb Haemost 2008;6(8): 1313–8.

70. Bounameaux H, Camm AJ. Edoxaban: an update on the new oral direct factor Xa inhibitor. Drugs 2014;74(11):1209–31.

71. Camm AJ, Lip GY, De Caterina R, et al. 2012 focused update of the ESC Guidelines for the management of atrial fibrillation: an update of the 2010 ESC Guidelines for the management of atrial fibrillation. Developed with the special contribution of the European Heart Rhythm Association. Eur Heart J 2012; 33(21):2719–47.

72. Cohen AT, Spiro TE, Buller HR, et al. Rivaroxaban for thromboprophylaxis in acutely ill medical patients. N Engl J Med 2013;368(6):513–23.

73. Committee R-MW, Ginsberg JS, Davidson BL, et al. Oral thrombin inhibitor dabigatran etexilate vs North American enoxaparin regimen for prevention of venous thromboembolism after knee arthroplasty surgery. J Arthroplasty 2009; 24(1):1–9.

74. Connolly SJ, Ezekowitz MD, Yusuf S, et al. Dabigatran versus warfarin in patients with atrial fibrillation. N Engl J Med 2009;361(12):1139–51.

75. Connolly SJ, Wallentin L, Ezekowitz MD, et al. The long-term multicenter observational study of dabigatran treatment in patients with atrial fibrillation (RELY-ABLE) study. Circulation 2013;128(3):237–43.
76. Dobesh PP, Fanikos J. Direct oral anticoagulants for the prevention of stroke in patients with nonvalvular atrial fibrillation: understanding differences and similarities. Drugs 2015;75(14):1627–44.
77. Douxfils J, Mullier F, Robert S, et al. Impact of dabigatran on a large panel of routine or specific coagulation assays. Laboratory recommendations for monitoring of dabigatran etexilate. Thromb Haemost 2012;107(5):985–97.
78. Eriksson BI, Dahl OE, Rosencher N, et al. Oral dabigatran etexilate vs. subcutaneous enoxaparin for the prevention of venous thromboembolism after total knee replacement: the RE-MODEL randomized trial. J Thromb Haemost 2007; 5(11):2178–85.
79. Eriksson BI, Dahl OE, Rosencher N, et al. Dabigatran etexilate versus enoxaparin for prevention of venous thromboembolism after total hip replacement: a randomised, double-blind, non-inferiority trial. Lancet 2007;370(9591):949–56.
80. Flaker G, Lopes RD, Al-Khatib SM, et al. Efficacy and safety of apixaban in patients after cardioversion for atrial fibrillation: insights from the ARISTOTLE Trial (Apixaban for Reduction in Stroke and Other Thromboembolic Events in Atrial Fibrillation). J Am Coll Cardiol 2014;63(11):1082–7.
81. Friedman RJ, Dahl OE, Rosencher N, et al. Dabigatran versus enoxaparin for prevention of venous thromboembolism after hip or knee arthroplasty: a pooled analysis of three trials. Thromb Res 2010;126(3):175–82.
82. Fuji T, Fujita S, Kawai Y, et al. Efficacy and safety of edoxaban versus enoxaparin for the prevention of venous thromboembolism following total hip arthroplasty: STARS J-V. Thromb J 2015;13:27.
83. Fuji T, Fujita S, Kawai Y, et al. Safety and efficacy of edoxaban in patients undergoing hip fracture surgery. Thromb Res 2014;133(6):1016–22.
84. Fuji T, Fujita S, Tachibana S, et al. A dose-ranging study evaluating the oral factor Xa inhibitor edoxaban for the prevention of venous thromboembolism in patients undergoing total knee arthroplasty. J Thromb Haemost 2010;8(11): 2458–68.
85. Fuji T, Wang CJ, Fujita S, et al. Safety and efficacy of edoxaban, an oral factor Xa inhibitor, versus enoxaparin for thromboprophylaxis after total knee arthroplasty: the STARS E-3 trial. Thromb Res 2014;134(6):1198–204.
86. Ganetsky VS, Hadley DE, Thomas TF. Role of novel and emerging oral anticoagulants for secondary prevention of acute coronary syndromes. Pharmacotherapy 2014;34(6):590–604.
87. Geller BJ, Giugliano RP, Braunwald E, et al. Systemic, noncerebral, arterial embolism in 21,105 patients with atrial fibrillation randomized to edoxaban or warfarin: results from the Effective Anticoagulation with Factor Xa Next Generation in Atrial Fibrillation-Thrombolysis in Myocardial Infarction Study 48 trial. Am Heart J 2015;170(4):669–74.
88. Heidbuchel H, Verhamme P, Alings M, et al. Updated European Heart Rhythm Association Practical Guide on the use of non-vitamin K antagonist anticoagulants in patients with non-valvular atrial fibrillation. Europace 2015;17(10): 1467–507.
89. Hernandez I, Zhang Y. Risk of bleeding with dabigatran in 2010-2011 Medicare data. JAMA Intern Med 2015;175(7):1245–7.
90. Holbrook A, Schulman S, Witt DM, et al. Evidence-based management of anticoagulant therapy: Antithrombotic Therapy and Prevention of Thrombosis,

9th ed: American College of Chest Physicians Evidence-Based Clinical Practice Guidelines. Chest 2012;141(2 Suppl):e152S–84S.

91. Hori M, Matsumoto M, Tanahashi N, et al. Rivaroxaban versus warfarin in Japanese patients with nonvalvular atrial fibrillation in relation to the CHADS2 score: a subgroup analysis of the J-ROCKET AF trial. J Stroke Cerebrovasc Dis 2014; 23(2):379–83.

92. Hylek EM, Skates SJ, Sheehan MA, et al. An analysis of the lowest effective intensity of prophylactic anticoagulation for patients with nonrheumatic atrial fibrillation. N Engl J Med 1996;335(8):540–6.

93. Iung B, Rodes-Cabau J. The optimal management of anti-thrombotic therapy after valve replacement: certainties and uncertainties. Eur Heart J 2014;35(42): 2942–9.

94. Kubitza D, Becka M, Voith B, et al. Safety, pharmacodynamics, and pharmacokinetics of single doses of BAY 59-7939, an oral, direct factor Xa inhibitor. Clin Pharmacol Ther 2005;78(4):412–21.

95. Lassen MR, Davidson BL, Gallus A, et al. The efficacy and safety of apixaban, an oral, direct factor Xa inhibitor, as thromboprophylaxis in patients following total knee replacement. J Thromb Haemost 2007;5(12):2368–75.

96. Limdi NA, Nolin TD, Booth SL, et al. Influence of kidney function on risk of supratherapeutic international normalized ratio-related hemorrhage in warfarin users: a prospective cohort study. Am J Kidney Dis 2015;65(5):701–9.

97. Lindahl TL, Baghaei F, Blixter IF, et al. Effects of the oral, direct thrombin inhibitor dabigatran on five common coagulation assays. Thromb Haemost 2011;105(2): 371–8.

98. Lip GY, Agnelli G. Edoxaban: a focused review of its clinical pharmacology. Eur Heart J 2014;35(28):1844–55.

99. Lip GY, Clemens A, Noack H, et al. Patient outcomes using the European label for dabigatran. A post-hoc analysis from the RE-LY database. Thromb Haemost 2014;111(5):933–42.

100. Lip GY, Lane DA. Matching the NOAC to the patient: remember the modifiable bleeding risk factors. J Am Coll Cardiol 2015;66(21):2282–4.

101. Lopes LC, Eikelboom J, Spencer FA, et al. Shorter or longer anticoagulation to prevent recurrent venous thromboembolism: systematic review and meta-analysis. BMJ Open 2014;4(7):e005674.

102. Lutz J, Menke J, Sollinger D, et al. Haemostasis in chronic kidney disease. Nephrol Dial Transplant 2014;29(1):29–40.

103. Lyman GH, Khorana AA, Kuderer NM, et al. Venous thromboembolism prophylaxis and treatment in patients with cancer: American Society of Clinical Oncology clinical practice guideline update. J Clin Oncol 2013;31(17): 2189–204.

104. Mant J, Hobbs FD, Fletcher K, et al. Warfarin versus aspirin for stroke prevention in an elderly community population with atrial fibrillation (the Birmingham Atrial Fibrillation Treatment of the Aged Study, BAFTA): a randomised controlled trial. Lancet 2007;370(9586):493–503.

105. Marcy TR, Truong T, Rai A. Comparing direct oral anticoagulants and warfarin for atrial fibrillation, venous thromboembolism, and mechanical heart valves. Consult Pharm 2015;30(11):644–56.

106. Masson P, Webster AC, Hong M, et al. Chronic kidney disease and the risk of stroke: a systematic review and meta-analysis. Nephrol Dial Transplant 2015; 30(7):1162–9.

107. Maura G, Blotiere PO, Bouillon K, et al. Comparison of the short-term risk of bleeding and arterial thromboembolic events in nonvalvular atrial fibrillation patients newly treated with dabigatran or rivaroxaban versus vitamin K antagonists: a French nationwide propensity-matched cohort study. Circulation 2015; 132(13):1252–60.
108. McCormack PL. Edoxaban: a review in nonvalvular atrial fibrillation. Am J Cardiovasc Drugs 2015;15(5):351–61.
109. Mega JL, Braunwald E, Wiviott SD, et al. Rivaroxaban in patients with a recent acute coronary syndrome. N Engl J Med 2012;366(1):9–19.
110. Mendell J, Tachibana M, Shi M, et al. Effects of food on the pharmacokinetics of edoxaban, an oral direct factor Xa inhibitor, in healthy volunteers. J Clin Pharmacol 2011;51(5):687–94.
111. Minor C, Tellor KB, Armbruster AL. Edoxaban, a novel oral Factor Xa inhibitor. Ann Pharmacother 2015;49(7):843–50.
112. Mookadam M, Shamoun FE, Mookadam F. Novel anticoagulants in atrial fibrillation: a primer for the primary physician. J Am Board Fam Med 2015;28(4): 510–22.
113. Mueck W, Stampfuss J, Kubitza D, et al. Clinical pharmacokinetic and pharmacodynamic profile of rivaroxaban. Clin Pharmacokinet 2014;53(1):1–16.
114. Nagarakanti R, Ezekowitz MD, Oldgren J, et al. Dabigatran versus warfarin in patients with atrial fibrillation: an analysis of patients undergoing cardioversion. Circulation 2011;123(2):131–6.
115. Ogawa S, Shinohara Y, Kanmuri K. Safety and efficacy of the oral direct Factor Xa inhibitor apixaban in Japanese patients with non-valvular atrial fibrillation. The ARISTOTLE-J study. Circ J 2011;75(8):1852–9.
116. Oldgren J, Budaj A, Granger CB, et al. Dabigatran vs. placebo in patients with acute coronary syndromes on dual antiplatelet therapy: a randomized, double-blind, phase II trial. Eur Heart J 2011;32(22):2781–9.
117. Omran H, Bauersachs R, Rubenacker S, et al. The HAS-BLED score predicts bleedings during bridging of chronic oral anticoagulation. Results from the national multicentre BNK Online bRiDging REgistRy (BORDER). Thromb Haemost 2012;108(1):65–73.
118. Piccini JP, Stevens SR, Lokhnygina Y, et al. Outcomes after cardioversion and atrial fibrillation ablation in patients treated with rivaroxaban and warfarin in the ROCKET AF trial. J Am Coll Cardiol 2013;61(19):1998–2006.
119. Pollack CV Jr, Reilly PA, Bernstein R, et al. Design and rationale for RE-VERSE AD: a phase 3 study of idarucizumab, a specific reversal agent for dabigatran. Thromb Haemost 2015;114(1):198–205.
120. Raghavan N, Frost CE, Yu Z, et al. Apixaban metabolism and pharmacokinetics after oral administration to humans. Drug Metab Dispos 2009;37(1):74–81.
121. Raschi E, Poluzzi E, Koci A, et al. Liver injury with novel oral anticoagulants: assessing post-marketing reports in the US Food and Drug Administration adverse event reporting system. Br J Clin Pharmacol 2015;80(2):285–93.
122. Raskob G, Cohen AT, Eriksson BI, et al. Oral direct factor Xa inhibition with edoxaban for thromboprophylaxis after elective total hip replacement. A randomised double-blind dose-response study. Thromb Haemost 2010;104(3):642–9.
123. Redondo S, Martinez MP, Ramajo M, et al. Pharmacological basis and clinical evidence of dabigatran therapy. J Hematol Oncol 2011;4:53.
124. Schwartzenberg S, Lev EI, Sagie A, et al. The quandary of oral anticoagulation in patients with atrial fibrillation and chronic kidney disease. Am J Cardiol 2016; 117(3):477–82.

125. Sennesael AL, Dogne JM, Spinewine A. Optimizing the safe use of direct oral anticoagulants in older patients: a teachable moment. JAMA Intern Med 2015; 175(10):1608–9.

126. Senoo K, Lip GY. Relationship of age with stroke and death in anticoagulated patients with nonvalvular atrial fibrillation: AMADEUS trial. Stroke 2015;46(11): 3202–7.

127. Skanes AC, Healey JS, Cairns JA, et al. Focused 2012 update of the Canadian Cardiovascular Society atrial fibrillation guidelines: recommendations for stroke prevention and rate/rhythm control. Can J Cardiol 2012;28(2):125–36.

128. Song Y, Wang X, Perlstein I, et al. Relative bioavailability of apixaban solution or crushed tablet formulations administered by mouth or nasogastric tube in healthy subjects. Clin Ther 2015;37(8):1703–12.

129. Stangier J. Clinical pharmacokinetics and pharmacodynamics of the oral direct thrombin inhibitor dabigatran etexilate. Clin Pharmacokinet 2008;47(5):285–95.

130. Tendera M, Syzdol M, Parma Z. ARISTOTLE RE-LYs on the ROCKET. What's new in stroke prevention in patients with atrial fibrillation? Cardiol J 2012;19(1):4–10.

131. Tullett J, Murray E, Nichols L, et al. Trial Protocol: a randomised controlled trial of extended anticoagulation treatment versus routine anticoagulation treatment for the prevention of recurrent VTE and post thrombotic syndrome in patients being treated for a first episode of unprovoked VTE (The ExACT Study). BMC Cardiovasc Disord 2013;13:16.

132. Tummala R, Kavtaradze A, Gupta A, et al. Specific antidotes against direct oral anticoagulants: a comprehensive review of clinical trials data. Int J Cardiol 2016; 214:292–8.

133. van Ryn J, Stangier J, Haertter S, et al. Dabigatran etexilate–a novel, reversible, oral direct thrombin inhibitor: interpretation of coagulation assays and reversal of anticoagulant activity. Thromb Haemost 2010;103(6):1116–27.

134. Vedovati MC, Germini F, Agnelli G, et al. Direct oral anticoagulants in patients with VTE and cancer: a systematic review and meta-analysis. Chest 2015; 147(2):475–83.

135. Verheugt FW, Granger CB. Oral anticoagulants for stroke prevention in atrial fibrillation: current status, special situations, and unmet needs. Lancet 2015; 386(9990):303–10.

136. You JJ, Singer DE, Howard PA, et al. Antithrombotic therapy for atrial fibrillation: Antithrombotic Therapy and Prevention of Thrombosis, 9th ed: American College of Chest Physicians Evidence-Based Clinical Practice Guidelines. Chest 2012;141(2 Suppl):e531S–75S.

Acute Coronary Syndrome

Care After a Patient Event and Strategies to Improve Adherence

Craig Hricz, MPAS, PA-C[a,b,*]

KEYWORDS

- Ischemic heart disease • Acute coronary syndrome • Myocardial infarction
- Adherence • Compliance

KEY POINTS

- Appropriate and timely medical management of a patient after an ischemic event has occurred is paramount.
- Following current guidelines and recommendations for appropriate testing increases greater accuracy for diagnosis, and appropriate office follow-up is key.
- Methods to improve patient adherence to medical and lifestyle change recommendations greatly impact overall success and improvement in wellness.

A 62-year-old man presents to you as his primary care provider 1 month after requiring 2 stents in his left anterior descending coronary artery. His history is significant for hypertension and hypercholesterolemia, both of which have been somewhat poorly controlled because of the patient's admitted noncompliance with strictly adhering to his medication regimen and routine office visits. He also continues to smoke a pack of cigarettes daily. This scenario is relatively common, and it is vital that the provider understand the current recommendations for managing a patient after a myocardial infarction (MI). Equal importance should also be placed on understanding the barriers to treatment adherence and to the methods that can be used to overcome these barriers and improve long-term outcomes.

MEDICATION THERAPY IN THE POST–MYOCARDIAL INFARCTION OR POSTINTERVENTION PATIENT

Antiplatelet therapy is crucial to the successful outcome of a patient after a recent event. If the patient had not previously been on aspirin, it should be started immediately

Disclosure Statement: Nothing to disclose.
[a] School of Physician Assistant Studies, Massachusetts College of Pharmacy and Health Sciences, 1260 Elm Street, Manchester, NH 03101, USA; [b] Emergency Department, Wentworth-Douglass Hospital, 789 Central Avenue, Dover, NH 03820, USA
* School of Physician Assistant Studies, Massachusetts College of Pharmacy and Health Sciences, 1260 Elm Street, Manchester, NH 03101.
E-mail address: craig.hricz@mcphs.edu

Physician Assist Clin 2 (2017) 623–631
http://dx.doi.org/10.1016/j.cpha.2017.06.005
2405-7991/17/© 2017 Elsevier Inc. All rights reserved.

and continued indefinitely, assuming there are no allergy or bleeding complications. A dose of 75 to 81 mg daily can be as effective as 325 mg in secondary prevention without the increased risk of gastrointestinal bleeding associated with the higher dose. In addition to aspirin, either clopidogrel, 75 mg daily, or ticagrelor, 90 mg twice daily, should be started and ideally maintained for 12 months. These recommendations are the same regardless of whether the patient is male or female or whether the event was managed medically or a stent was placed. Patients undergoing a coronary artery bypass graft (CABG) should have clopidogrel or ticagrelor restarted if they had been on it before the procedure; however, there is less convincing evidence for initiating one of these agents after CABG. Currently, clopidogrel has a class IIb (may be reasonable) recommendation, and ticagrelor has no recommendation. The preferred agent for patients with chronic kidney disease is ticagrelor. Patients with atrial fibrillation or heart valve replacements that require anticoagulation therapy should be prescribed a proton pump inhibitor, and a reduction in the 12-month timeframe for clopidogrel or ticagrelor should be considered. If there is an allergy or gastrointestinal intolerability to aspirin, clopidogrel or ticagrelor at the same dosing is recommended.[1–3]

Antihypertensive medication selection requires careful consideration. The most recent recommendations from the Joint National Committee, Detection, Evaluation, and Treatment of High Blood Pressure (JNC7) advises a systolic blood pressure of less than 140/90 mm Hg for most patients with the exception of those who also have diabetes or chronic kidney disease, in which case, the target should be lowered to less than 130/80 mm Hg. More intensive lowering has not been found to improve outcomes.

- A β-blocker (carvedilol, metoprolol succinate, or bisoprolol) is recommended for all patients unless contraindicated. The choice of additional agents is largely based on what additional medical history a patient has.
- An angiotensin-converting enzyme inhibitor should be added in patients with a recent MI who also have underlying hypertension, diabetes, heart failure, or a left ventricular ejection fraction of less than 40%.
- An angiotensin receptor blocker is an adequate substitute if an angiotensin-converting enzyme inhibitor is not tolerated.
- A calcium channel blocker other than verapamil or diltiazem, added to a regimen, may be beneficial for patients with angina.

In many cases, more than one medication may be required to adequately control blood pressure or angina symptoms. When a dosage adjustment is required, the β-blocker dose should be maximized before adjustment of any other medication.[1,3]

Diabetes should be managed with a target hemoglobin A1c of less than 7%, but a range of 7% to 9% is acceptable in some cases. The results of one study showed that metformin was superior to insulin plus a sulfonylurea with regard to complications related to diabetes, MI, and death. Patients whose blood sugars were well controlled before a cardiac event, should be maintained on their original medications with the possible exception of those taking rosiglitazone. Studies have found an increase in cardiovascular complications associated with this thiazolidinedione, and it is therefore advised against starting it in patients with ischemic heart disease. Those whose conditions were well controlled with the medication before a cardiac event might be maintained on it, but a discussion with the patient regarding potential adverse effects should be had, and it is advised to strongly consider use of a different medication.[1]

Nitroglycerine sublingual tablets or spray should be prescribed for all patients who have had an event to be used for angina episode relief or preactivity prevention of angina as needed. The patient should be aware that the tablets need to be kept in the original manufacture's bottle in a cool, dry place, and the expiration date should be noted so that the medication has its desired effect when needed. Requiring frequent use of short-acting nitroglycerine is an indication that the disease state has advanced or that adjustments in the current medication regiment need to be made.[1]

Both stress and depression should be managed to improve outcomes. The importance and recommendations regarding smoking cessation, diet, exercise, and lipid management are discussed elsewhere in this issue (see Craig Hricz's article, "Ischemic Heart Disease: Evaluating for Potential Disease in the Previously Undiagnosed, Those Experiencing Angina, and in Those with Stable Disease") and should receive equal importance to medication selection.

FOLLOW-UP SCHEDULE IN THE POST–MYOCARDIAL INFARCTION OR POSTINTERVENTION PATIENT

Patients should be scheduled for an office visit within 2 to 6 weeks of an event; higher-risk patients need to be seen by the end of week 2. Subsequent office visits should be scheduled every 4 to 6 months during the first year and every 6 to 12 months thereafter, assuming the patient's symptoms are stable and they are reliable enough to contact the provider immediately upon any changes in symptoms.[1,3]

These office visits should focus on a high-quality history and physical examination related to the cardiovascular system. Important elements of the history that should be discussed include:

- Interval changes in physical activity
- Development and frequency of new symptoms
- Problems related to the prescribed medications, such as intolerance or inconvenient dosing
- Barriers in adhering to lifestyle recommendations[1]

The physical examination component should always include a complete set of vital signs and a body mass index and waist circumference. Other important physical examination elements include:

- Assessment for fluid retention (increased jugular venous pressure, pulmonary rales/crackles, peripheral edema)
- Auscultation of the heart for new murmurs or rhythm irregularities
- Auscultation of the carotid, aortic, and renal arteries for new bruits, which could signify progressing atherosclerotic disease or aneurysm[1]

An annual electrocardiogram (ECG) is recommended as well as an urgent ECG with any changes in the patient's symptoms. Routine ECGs can provide a baseline, which can be referred to at the time new symptoms arise. The annual ECG will also provide an opportunity to assess for interval changes possibly caused by a silent event or uncover an unknown arrhythmia, which may alter treatment.[1]

Annual laboratory testing should include:

- Hemoglobin/hematocrit
- Thyroid-stimulating hormone
- Lipid panel
- Basic metabolic panel
- Hemoglobin A1c (known diabetics)

Patients who were not diagnosed previously with diabetes should have a fasting blood sugar every 3 years.[1]

Diagnostic testing should be limited to when any changes in the patient's condition occur or when any concerning elements of the history are obtained. An echocardiogram or radionuclide imaging study should be performed if angina symptoms or new or worsening heart failure occur. Appropriate stress testing modalities are discussed in detail elsewhere in this issue (see Craig Hricz's article, "Ischemic Heart Disease: Evaluating for Potential Disease in the Previously Undiagnosed, Those Experiencing Angina, and in Those with Stable Disease"); however, in general, using the same modality as had been previously used is advised for the most accurate determination of any interval disease development.[1]

Resumption of activities should be considered based on both the severity of the patient's event and the specific activity. Adequately managing a patient's anxiety or depression has been found to lessen the degree of long-term disability.

- Resumption of driving can usually occur within 1 week (2–3 weeks for a complicated MI) of discharge assuming the patient's symptoms are well controlled and any state-specific Department of Motor Vehicles criteria have been met.
- Air travel can be resumed within the first 2 weeks after an event assuming the patient is not having anginal symptoms or hypoxia or has not experienced anxiety with prior air travel. If air travel is necessary during the first few weeks after an event, the patient should have a companion accompany them, have nitroglycerine readily available, and use airport wheelchair assistance to avoid excess stress or cardiac demand.
- Sexual activity and other strenuous activities can be resumed gradually once the patient's symptoms are well controlled.

A graded exercise stress test can be helpful when determining the patient's capabilities. The results can be converted using standardized references into common activities that a patient should be able to perform.[3]

STRATEGIES TO IMPROVE PATIENT ADHERENCE

It is estimated that only 50% of patients in developed countries adhere to the medication plan they are prescribed, and even fewer will follow through with the plan or the recommended lifestyle changes after 2 years.[4,5] These statistics provide the primary care provider not only an opportunity but also a significant challenge when it comes to impacting a patient's quality of life, morbidity, and ultimately, mortality. The most successful approach to improving adherence requires education and considering and addressing every modifiable factor that a particular patient might have. Every patient has a different set of factors that prevents him or her from sticking to the plan, requiring a customized approach for each person.

Educating the patient and the patient's family support group is the first step once a diagnosis of coronary artery disease has been established. The provider should explain not only the diagnosis but also the implications of the disease in a manner that is understandable. Providing important statistics found throughout this article may help emphasize the impact that the diagnosis and lack of adherence can have on the patient's quality of life. Another important aspect to education is providing the patient with information on how to recognize when symptoms have changed from baseline and what steps to take if that occurs. All information should be delivered in a way that is easily understood based on the patient's or family member's level of education. It is also recommended that this information be delivered in the language that the patient is most comfortable with. If the language is not one in which the provider is fluent, a qualified translator should be used rather than relying on a family member or friend. In addition to individualized counseling, use of group counseling sessions or formal support groups are also methods that can be used in patient education.[1]

Once the patient comprehends the diagnosis, a thorough discussion of the current recommendations and the proposed treatment plan is warranted. By involving the patient in the early stages of plan preparation, the hope is to develop a higher rate of patient buy-in and responsibility resulting in an increased likelihood of adherence. This buy-in has been referred to as *medication concordance*. The plan should take into consideration:

- The patient's other current medical conditions
- Potential medication side effects, interactions, and dosing frequency
- Insurance coverage
- Cultural beliefs
- Access to resources such as transportation, exercise facilities, and even internet access or comfort level with smartphone applications
- Affordability and access to the recommended dietary plan

The plan should focus on minimizing complexity and potential for confusion, which will greatly impact adherence.[1,5]

Several techniques that a provider can use to facilitate a change in patient behavior have been described.

- Motivational Interviewing requires the practitioner to elicit from the patient reasons they feel change is important, demonstrate empathy, and foster the patient's desire to change. This activity can be facilitated by interviewing using open-ended questions, being an active listener, and affirming the patient's desires to make positive improvements to their lives.
- The Self-efficacy Theory involves setting patient goals that are obtainable, resulting in improved self-confidence and the likelihood that future goals will be met.
- The Transtheoretical Model is centered around the 5 stages of change, identified as phases that an individual will experience while attempting behavioral change. The stages are: precontemplation, contemplation, preparation, action, and maintenance. If the provider can remain cognizant of which stage a particular patient is presently in, it may lead to a more effective approach in moving the individual along this continuum in a positive direction.[4,5]

Care must be taken to avoid the patient perception that change is being forced on them by the provider, as this can lead to a lack of trust and motivation and a reluctance to discuss issues openly. Many of these concepts can be summarized using the acronym SIMPLE. SIMPLE stands for:

- Simplifying the patient's medication regimen
- Informing the patient about the purpose of his or her medications
- Modifying behaviors and beliefs using the techniques mentioned above
- Providing patient-provider communication that builds trust
- Leaving biases and customizing education to the patient's health literacy level
- Evaluating medication adherence in a consistent and recurring manner[4,6]

Patients should be encouraged to perform regular self-monitoring and documentation including:

- Blood pressure
- Blood sugar (when appropriate)

- Physical activity
- Dietary efforts

Benefits of self-monitoring include keeping a patient engaged in their treatment plan, providing the practitioner with some evidence of the treatment plan effectiveness, and assist in generating a patient-provider discussion, which should consist of encouragement and areas for improvement. Another form of self-monitoring is the use of a smartphone app to improve medication adherence. The Web site www.medappfinder.com is a database of apps, which the patient and provider can query based on certain desirable features to decide on one that seems to provide the best fit. Many of these apps allow for the provider to make changes to dosages or regimens through a Web site, and these changes are automatically synced to the patient's app. Other features include the ability to set dosing reminders, record when doses are taken, document why a dose is not taken, and the ability to view a log of adherence over a given period. Many patients will find this type of visual tracking and feedback appealing. Ongoing encouragement at regular intervals is especially important if a patient has been symptom free for some time, as this can lead to the patient thinking their condition has been cured or at least that the medications and lifestyle changes are less of a necessity. Studies find that patients with stable coronary artery disease who do not maintain regular adherence to the medication regiment have a:

- 10% to 40% increased risk of hospital admissions owing to cardiovascular etiologies
- 10% to 30% increase in the need for coronary interventions
- 50% to 80% increase in overall cardiovascular-related mortality

Obviously, these complications are costly not only to the patient but to the health care system in general and could be significantly minimized by improved adherence.[1,5,6]

Because of the excess costs associated with a lack of medication adherence, numerous approaches have been studied and many show some promise.

- Sending out regular mailings as reminders of the importance of adherence has led to some improvement, but frequent face-to-face interactions between the patient and a provider, nurse, or even a pharmacist have repeatedly been found to significantly improve medication adherence.
- Insurance companies have looked into decreasing or removing copays for post-MI medications. Although removing this fee may cost the insurance provider in the short term, the savings related to improved adherence over the long-term would be extremely significant.
- Involvement in formal cardiac rehabilitation programs has shown improved adherence rates.[7,8]

POSTINTERVENTION COMPLICATIONS

Complications after an intervention are divided into 2 categories: poststenting and post-CABG. Each of these can then be further divided into 2 subcategories consisting of restenosis or thrombosis. The process of restenosis involves a gradual renarrowing and generally results in a recurrence of the patient's anginal symptoms. A thrombotic event is a sudden occlusion and generally results in immediate death or a large infarction area associated with a poor prognosis. The timeframe for these complications depends on multiple factors, but the type of stent and the origin of the vessel used for the CABG are the primary factors.

Patients who have undergone a percutaneous intervention with drug-eluting stenting have up to a 20% chance of having a restenosis of the area within 3 to 12 months; whereas an in-stent thrombosis can occur in up to 2% of patients at 30 days with a lower percentage in those who had a drug-eluting stent placed. The primary risk factor that contributes to stent restenosis is diabetes. Other risks include:

- Female sex
- Hypertension
- Elevated body mass index
- Multivessel disease or requiring multiple stents

The primary risk factor for a thrombotic event is the absence of dual platelet therapy, specifically a $P2Y_{12}$ inhibitor, reinforcing the importance of medication adherence. Most stent occlusions are managed with a new-generation drug-eluting stent, but angioplasty using a drug-coated balloon or CABG is also an option.[9–11]

Patients who have undergone a CABG are also at risk for occlusive thrombotic or restenosis events.

- Up to 12% of these patients can have an event within the first 30 days; those receiving a saphenous vein graft are more likely to have an event than those receiving an internal mammary artery graft.
- Up to 40% will have atherosclerotic restenosis within 10 years.

Recommendations lean toward stenting of the occluded area. Low-pressure balloon angioplasty and repeat vessel grafting are also options. To reduce this risk of early thrombosis, aspirin should be started within 6 hours of the CABG. If post-CABG stenting is required, a $P2Y_{12}$ inhibitor should be started. Other complications include low cardiac output syndrome, arrhythmias (primarily tachyarrhythmias), pericarditis, and pericardial effusion with the possibility of developing tamponade or chronic constrictive pericarditis.

- Low cardiac output syndrome generally responds well to fluid resuscitation.
- The risk of arrhythmias can generally be lowered by ensuring that preoperative and postoperative potassium levels are within the normal range, and many cases of atrial fibrillation will spontaneously convert to a normal sinus rhythm if the patient had no prior history of the arrhythmia.
- Pericarditis presents as chest pain, generally increased with lying supine, and usually occurs within the first few weeks after CABG.
- Pericardial effusions occur in many patients at some point within the first 30 days; however, most are asymptomatic and resolve spontaneously. Tamponade is classically identified using Beck's triad, which consists of hypotension, distended neck veins, and muffled heart sounds. Tamponade is a medical emergency.[8,12,13]

SUMMARY

Minimizing myocardial damage and future recurrence should be the goals of patient care after an MI or even after detection of coronary artery disease. For the provider to successfully intervene and positively impact patient outcomes, he or she must know what the most current guidelines recommend and be able to create a medication regimen and recommend lifestyle modifications tailored to the patient's needs with special attention given to each patient's specific barriers. Every effort should be made to use resources and techniques that will assist the patient in adhering to the plan. Providers, or their staff, need to maintain regular contact with these high-risk patients and provide encouragement and positive reinforcement to achieve high adherence rates. Patient education, simplified plans with an attention to specific patient barriers, and regular contact is a formula for improved long-term outcomes.

REFERENCES

1. Fihn SD, Gardin JM, Abrams J, et al. 2012 ACCF/AHA/ACP/AATS/PCNA/SCAI/STS guideline for the diagnosis and management of patients with stable ischemic heart disease. J Am Coll Cardiol 2012;60(24):e44–164.

2. Amsterdam EA, Wenger NK, Brindis RG, et al. 2014 AHA/ACC guideline for the management of patients with non-ST-elevation acute coronary syndromes: executive summary: a report of the American College of Cardiology/American Heart Association Task Force on practice guidelines. Circulation 2014;130(25): 2354–94.

3. Anderson JL, Adams CD, Antman EM, et al. 2012 ACCF/AHA focused update incorporated into the ACCF/AHA 2007 guidelines for the management of patients with unstable angina/non–ST-elevation myocardial infarction. J Am Coll Cardiol 2013;61(23):e179–347.

4. Miller DM, Rose T, Van Amburgh JA. Behavioral interviewing: techniques to improve patients' medication adherence. Consultant 2016;702–5.

5. Cardiovascular disease: risk assessment and reduction, including lipid modification. NICE. Available at: https://www.nice.org.uk/guidance/cg181. Accessed September 26, 2016.

6. Thakkar JB, Chow CK. Adherence to secondary prevention therapies in acute coronary syndrome. Med J Aust 2014;201(10):106–9.

7. Desai NR, Choudhry NK. Impediments to adherence to post myocardial infarction medications. Curr Cardiol Rep 2012;15(1):322.

8. Sengstock D, Vaitkevicius P, Salama A, et al. Under-prescribing and non-adherence to medications after coronary bypass surgery in older adults: strategies to improve adherence. Drugs Aging 2012;29(2):93–103.

9. Levin T, Cutlip D. Intracoronary stent restenosis. In: Post TW, editor. UpToDate. Waltham (MA): UpToDate. Available at: https://www.uptodate.com/contents/intracoronary-stent-restenosis?source=search_result&search=intracoronary%20stent%20restenosis&selectedTitle=1~21. Accessed September 26, 2016.

10. Giacoppo D, Gargiulo G, Aruta P, et al. Treatment strategies for coronary in-stent restenosis: systematic review and hierarchical bayesian network meta-analysis of 24 randomised trials and 4880 patients. BMJ 2015;351:h5392.

11. Cutlip D, Abbott JD. Coronary artery stent thrombosis: incidence and risk factors. In: Post TW, editor. UpToDate. Waltham (MA): UpToDate. Available at: https://www.uptodate.com/contents/coronary-artery-stent-thrombosis-incidence-and-risk-factors?source=search_result&search=coronary%20artery%20stent%20thrombosis&selectedTitle=2~150. Accessed September 26, 2016.

12. Aranki S, Cutlip D, Aroesty J. Early cardiac complications of coronary artery bypass graft surgery. In: Post TW, editor. UpToDate. Waltham (MA): UpToDate. Available at: https://www.uptodate.com/contents/early-cardiac-complications-of-coronary-artery-bypass-graft-surgery?source=search_result&search=early%20cardiac%20complications&selectedTitle=1~150. Accessed September 26, 2016.

13. Aranki S, Aroesty J. Medical therapy to prevent complications after coronary artery bypass graft surgery. In: Post TW, editor. UpToDate. Waltham (MA): UpToDate. Available at: https://www.uptodate.com/contents/medical-therapy-to-prevent-complications-after-coronary-artery-bypass-graft-surgery?source=search_result&search=medical%20therapy%20to%20prevent%20complications&selectedTitle=1~150. Accessed September 26, 2016.

Dyslipidemia
How Low Should We Go? A Review of Current Lipid Guidelines

Harvey A. Feldman, MD[a], Kim Zuber, PA-C[b,c],*, Jane Davis, DNP[c,d]

KEYWORDS

- Hypercholesterolemia • Dyslipidemia • Lipid guidelines
- Statin and nonstatin therapy • Atherosclerotic cardiovascular disease

KEY POINTS

- Though most guidelines recommend fasting lipid panels, a nonfasting test is appropriate for many patients and its convenience may increase compliance with testing.
- The 2013 the American College of Cardiology (ACC) and American Heart Association cholesterol management guideline represents a paradigm shift away from the treat-to-target approach for lowering low-density lipoprotein cholesterol embodied in the 2001 Adult Treatment Panel III guideline to a cardiac risk–based approach.
- Four groups of patients are now identified as being appropriate for statin therapy and the intensity of dosing is based on an assessment of medication benefit versus risk using a global cardiovascular risk calculator.
- The 2016 ACC expert consensus document filled a gap in the 2013 guideline by providing guidance for the use of nonstatin lipid-lowering drugs in patients whose response to statins is suboptimal or who do not tolerate statins.
- Gaps in the 2013 guideline relating to lipid management in children and patients with chronic kidney disease are covered in other recent guidelines, but evidence-based guidance for treating the very elderly is limited.

INTRODUCTION

Despite advances in treatment, atherosclerotic cardiovascular disease (ASCVD) remains the leading cause of death in the United States[1] **(Fig. 1)**.

The management of hypercholesterolemia has been a cornerstone in the fight against ASCVD. For more than a decade before 2013, clinicians relied on the National

Disclosures: None.
[a] Physician Assistant Program, Nova Southeastern University, 3200 South University Drive, Terry Building 1258, Fort Lauderdale, FL 33328-2018, USA; [b] American Academy of Nephrology PAs, 707 Foxwood Street, Oceanside, CA 92057, USA; [c] National Kidney Foundation of Advanced Practitioners; [d] Division of Nephrology, UAB Hospital, 1720 2nd Avenue So, Birmingham, AL 35294, USA
* Corresponding author. American Academy of Nephrology PAs, 707 Foxwood Street, Oceanside, CA 92057.
E-mail address: zuberkim@yahoo.com

Physician Assist Clin 2 (2017) 633–650
http://dx.doi.org/10.1016/j.cpha.2017.06.004
2405-7991/17/© 2017 Elsevier Inc. All rights reserved.

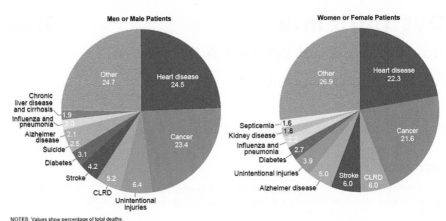

Fig. 1. Percent distribution of the 10 leading causes of death, by sex: United States, 2014. CLRD, chronic lower respiratory disease. (*From* CDC/National Center for Health Statistics 2016. leading causes of death. Available at: http://www.cdc.gov/nchs/fastats/leading-causes-of-death.htm. Accessed May 24, 2017; and *Courtesy of* NCHS, National Vital Statistics System, Mortality.)

Cholesterol Education Program Adult Treatment Panel III (ATP III) guideline for the management of hypercholesterolemia. This guideline was introduced in 2001, fully reported in 2002, and updated in 2004.[2,3]

In 2013, an expert panel from the American College of Cardiology (ACC) and the American Heart Association (AHA) created a new guideline on the treatment of blood cholesterol to reduce atherosclerotic cardiovascular (CV) risk in adults (2013 ACC/AHA guideline).[4,5] This guideline, based on a rigorous analysis of evidence, mainly from randomized clinical trials, is focused on using statins to reduce global ASCVD risk. However, because of its focus on statin therapy, it created uncertainty over the role of nonstatin drugs for high-risk patients who either have a less-than-anticipated response to statins or who have statin intolerance. This gap was filled in 2016 by an ACC expert consensus document.[6]

Disconcerting, however, is the gap between the 2013 ACC/AHA guideline and its implementation. A recent survey of primary care (family practice, internal medicine) and specialty (cardiology, endocrinology) practices revealed that "most clinicians do not completely understand the guideline" and are "moving away from lipid testing to document response and adherence to statin therapy."[7] A recent analysis of 204 cardiology practices showed that a statin was prescribed for only 62% of patients with diabetes and that prescribing patterns varied widely. Moreover, only 58% of patients had a low-density lipoprotein cholesterol (LDL-C) lower than 100 mg/dL.[8] These observations indicate a need for improved understanding of current lipid.

This article highlights the laboratory assessment of hyperlipidemia, the salient features of the 2013 ACC/AHA guideline and the 2016 ACC consensus document, and lipid management in special populations not fully addressed in these guidelines. Additional resources of information are provided to assist practitioners and patients in achieving optimal ASCVD risk reduction through lipid control.

Although lifestyle modifications, including diet, physical activity, smoking cessation, and weight and blood pressure control, are necessary adjuncts to pharmacologic therapy in reducing ASCVD risk, these measures are covered in detail in companion 2013 ACC/AHA guidelines and are not discussed in this article.[9,10]

LABORATORY ASSESSMENT OF HYPERLIPIDEMIA

The 2013 ACC/AHA guideline recommends an initial fasting lipid panel followed by a second fasting panel 4 to 12 weeks after starting statin therapy to determine patient adherence and response. Thereafter, a lipid panel should be obtained every 3 to 12 months as clinically indicated for the same reasons.[5] The lipid panel (CPT code 80061) consists of total cholesterol (TC), high-density lipoprotein cholesterol (HDL-C), triglycerides (TGs), and calculated LDL-C using the Friedewald equation:

$$LDL\text{-}C = TC - HDL\text{-}C - TG/5$$

This calculation is preferred because the direct measurement of LDL-C is time-consuming, expensive, and requires special equipment not universally available. The ratio TG/5 is used as an estimate of very LDL (VLDL) cholesterol; it assumes that the TG to cholesterol ratio of VLDL is 5:1; however, this holds true only in the fasting state.

The Friedewald equation underestimates LDL-C in the presence of

- Postprandial chylomicronemia (ie, after a high-fat meal)
- TG level greater than 400 mg/dL
- Low LDL-C (<70–100 mg/dL), even with TG equal to or greater than 150 mg/dL.

The direct assay for LDL-C also has shortcomings:

- Assay is not standardized
- Accuracy across all LDL-C values is uncertain
- Assay is expensive and not universally available.

Non-HDL-C (TC minus HDL-C), which includes LDL-C and other atherogenic lipid moieties, has been recommended as an alternative, but is not included in the 2013 ACC/AHA guideline.

HDL-C tracks inversely with ASCVD risk and is, therefore, referred to as the good cholesterol. However, there is no evidence that raising HDL-C levels reduces CV risk in statin-treated patients.[5] Likewise, a high HDL-C level should not preclude statin therapy in patients whose LDL-C level and/or other risk factors for ASCVD warrant treatment. The value of including HDL-C in the lipid panel is that it enables one to calculate the TC/HDL-C ratio and non-HDL-C, both of which predict ASCVD better than LDL-C alone.[11]

All current and past guidelines, except for the 2014 Veterans Affairs and Department of Defense (VA/DOT) guideline, recommend that lipid profiles should be obtained in the fasting state (9–12 hours after last meal).[2,4,12] However, recent studies have challenged this practice on several grounds:

- The 2013 ACC/AHA risk calculator incorporates TC and HDL-C rather than LDL-C. These tests are only minimally affected by eating.[13–15]
- In a community-based study, nonfasting LDL-C levels were only 10% lower than in the fasting state.[16] For most patients, this small difference in LDL-C is unlikely to affect CV risk scores, prognosis, or therapeutic decision-making.[17]
- The 2013 ACC/AHA guideline does not target specific LDL-C levels, making precise measurement less critical.
- Routine fasting lipid testing is inconvenient for patients who may have to make a separate trip to the clinic or laboratory, which increases the likelihood that the test will not be done.

So, how does one reconcile the conflicting data? Driver and colleagues[15] provide a practical approach for clinicians to use. They identify patients for whom either a fasting or nonfasting lipid panel is acceptable and others for whom only a fasting sample should be obtained. Their recommendations are listed in **Box 1**.

Besides a lipid panel, liver enzyme tests should also be performed before starting statin therapy.[4] Since 2012, the US Food and Drug Administration (FDA) no longer recommends routine periodic monitoring of liver enzymes after starting therapy because liver injury is rare and testing does not effectively detect or prevent this complication. These tests should only be obtained as clinically indicated. Though not mandated, it is reasonable to also obtain a baseline creatine phosphokinase because statin therapy is contraindicated in patients with very high levels. Routine monitoring during therapy is not recommended and performed only if a patient develops muscle-related symptoms.[4]

DIFFERENCES BETWEEN THE GUIDELINES

The 2013 ACC/AHA guideline represents a paradigm shift from the ATP III guideline in several respects. The most notable differences from the previous guideline relate to the focus and target of therapeutic intervention and the method of risk assessment.

Focus

Whereas the ATP III guideline was focused on reducing only coronary heart disease (CHD), the 2013 ACC/AHA guideline aims to reduce all manifestations of ASCVD (acute coronary syndrome, stable or unstable angina, prior myocardial infarction, coronary or other arterial revascularization, stroke or transient ischemic attack, and atherosclerotic peripheral arterial disease), that is, global risk.

Therapeutic Target

The ATP III guideline recommended achieving specific LDL-C levels based on 10-year risk for CHD derived from the Framingham (CHD) Risk Score. The writers of the 2013 ACC/AHA guideline could find no evidence from randomized controlled trials to support this approach. Although these trials clearly showed risk reduction with statins,

---

Box 1
Selection factors for deciding between fasting versus nonfasting lipid panels

Fasting or nonfasting acceptable

- Assessing an untreated primary prevention patient
- Screening patients for suspected metabolic syndrome[a]

Fasting recommended

- Patients with a family history of genetic hyperlipidemia or premature ASCVD
- Estimating residual risk for a treated patient because response to therapy is better gauged with a fasting lipid panel.
- Assessing patients with or at risk for pancreatitis due to hypertriglyceridemia 500 mg/dL or greater[b]
- Diagnosing hypertriglyceridemia

  [a] If nonfasting, use a triglyceride threshold of 200 mg/dL instead of 150 mg/dL. If it is ≥200 mg/dL, follow with a fasting lipid panel.
  [b] Nonfasting is acceptable in emergency assessment of suspected pancreatitis.
  Adapted from Driver SL, Martin SS, Gluckman TJ, et al. Fasting or nonfasting lipid measurements: it depends on the question. J Am Coll Cardiol 2016;67:1227–34.

they were not designed to determine specific optimal LDL-C targets. Therefore, the new guideline shifts from LDL-C targets to intensity of statin therapy based on the level of global ASCVD risk.

Risk Assessment

Because of the shift from CHD to ASCVD reduction, the new guideline could not use the Framingham CHD Risk Score that assesses only CHD risk. Therefore, the panel developed a new risk assessment tool for ASCVD known as the pooled cohort equations, derived from large community-based cohorts of white and African American populations in the United States. This risk score quickly became the most controversial component of the new guideline and the target of much criticism.

Key differences between the ATP III guideline and the 2013 ACC/AHA guideline are summarized in **Table 1**.

SPECIFIC PROVISIONS OF THE 2013 GUIDELINE

The crux of the 2013 ACC/AHA guideline is the identification of 4 population groups that are at risk for ASCVD and for whom the benefit from statin therapy well exceeds any potential harm[4] (**Box 2**).

Table 1
Key differences between guidelines

	ATP III Guideline	AHA/ACC 2013 Guideline
Methodology	Evidence-based: includes RCTs and other sources of moderate to high strength. Precedes the more rigorous IOM model for state-of-the-guidelines.	Evidence-based: relies on RCTs and meta-analyses of RCTs. Adheres to the IOM model for state-of-the-art guidelines.
Scope or focus	Comprehensive: includes sections on classification of lipids, modifiable and nonmodifiable CHD risk factors, lifestyle interventions, especially dietary, as well as cost-effectiveness issues and drug therapy for both hypercholesterolemia and hypertriglyceridemia.	Narrow (46 pages): Addresses 3 critical questions relevant to clinical care. Two questions relate to use of LDL-C and/or non–HDL-C levels as targets. The third examines the reduction in ASCVD events and adverse effects for each cholesterol-lowering drug class.
Risk assessment	Uses Framingham risk score to determine CHD risk in non-Hispanic whites.	Uses a new risk calculator (pooled cohort equations) to determine ASCVD risk in African Americans and non-Hispanic whites.
Recommendations	Based on specific LDL-C targets for patients at different levels of CHD risk per the Framingham risk score. Recommends using non-HDL-C as a secondary target in patients with hypertriglyceridemia. Recommends use of nonstatin drugs as adjunctive treatment of patients with hypercholesterolemia and/or for hypertriglyceridemia.	Based on intensity of statin therapy for 4 specific groups of patients at increased risk for ASCVD. Makes no recommendation regarding non-HDL-C. Recommends nonstatin drugs only for high-risk patients with statin intolerance or less than anticipated LDL-C reduction. No recommendations for patients with hypertriglyceridemia.

Abbreviations: IOM, Institute of Medicine; RCTs, randomized clinical trials.

Box 2
Always treat these 4 groups of patients with statins

Clinical atherosclerotic disease

LDL-C levels 190 mg/dL or higher, age older than 21 years

Patients with diabetes, ages 40 to 75 years with LDL-C 70 to 189 mg/dL but without ASCVD

Patients ages 40 to 75 years with LDL-C 70 to 189 mg/dL without ASCVD or diabetes but with a 10-year risk of ASCVD 7.5% or more per the pooled cohort equations risk score

Data from Stone NJ, Robinson JG, Lichtenstein AH, et al. 2013 ACC/AHA Cholesterol Guideline Panel. Treatment of blood cholesterol to reduce atherosclerotic cardiovascular disease risk in adults: synopsis of the 2013 American College of Cardiology/American Heart Association cholesterol guideline. Ann Intern Med 2014;160:339–43.

Statins are secondary preventive therapy for the first group (those with known ASCVD), whereas they are for primary prevention in the remaining 3 groups. Because evidence of benefit is lacking, the guideline recommends against treating patients with New York Heart Association class II to IV heart failure and patients on hemodialysis, even though these groups are at increased ASCVD risk.

The guideline defines the intensity of statin therapy appropriate for each of the 4 groups. High-intensity therapy would be expected to lower LDL-C by greater than 50% and moderate-intensity by 30% to 49%. An important difference from the previous guideline is that periodic monitoring of LDL-C is done only to determine adherence and response to therapy, not to achieve a specific LDL-C level. The intensity of statin therapy recommended for each of the 4 groups is shown in **Fig. 2** and relative potency

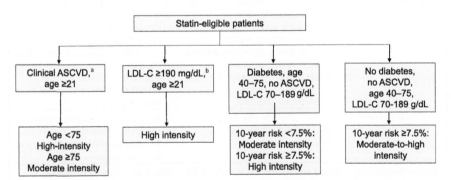

Fig. 2. Intensity of statin therapy for each of the 4 patient groups requiring treatment, ACA/AHA guidelines. [a] 10-year risk not required for patients with clinical ASCVD. [b] 10-year risk not required; evaluate for secondary cause for patients with LDL-C ≥190 mg/dL. (*Data from* Stone NJ, Robinson JG, Lichtenstein AH, et al. 2013 ACC/AHA Cholesterol Guideline Panel. Treatment of blood cholesterol to reduce atherosclerotic cardiovascular disease risk in adults: synopsis of the 2013 American College of Cardiology/American Heart Association cholesterol guideline. Ann Intern Med 2014;160:339–43; and Stone NJ, Robinson JG, Lichtenstein AH, et al. American College of Cardiology/American Heart Association Task Force on Practice Guidelines. 2013 ACC/AHA guideline on the treatment of blood cholesterol to reduce atherosclerotic cardiovascular risk in adults: a report of the American College of Cardiology/American Heart Association Task Force on Practice Guidelines. J Am Coll Cardiol 2014;63(25 Pt B):2889–934.)

of statin drugs corresponding to high and moderate-intensity therapy is shown in **Table 2**.

Not as clearly defined is how to treat patients who belong outside of the 4 groups but who may still be at increased risk of ASCVD. The guideline lists several risk factors that might favor statin therapy in these patients but emphasizes the importance of shared decision-making between patient and clinician because the evidence of benefit from statin therapy is not as strong in these patients (**Box 3**).

Since its release, the 2013 ACC/AHA guideline has been subjected to extensive analysis and controversy. Critical assessment of the guideline has uncovered several gaps in information and lack of solid evidence for some of its recommendations.[18,19] Critics have argued that because the guideline's risk-prediction algorithm (the pooled cohort equations) was derived from decades-old cohorts of whites and African Americans, it may not accurately predict risk in more contemporary populations or in other ethnic groups. The strongest criticism has been that it overestimates 10-year ASCVD risk, especially in people without diabetes or CV disease.[18,20] One study, using data from the National Health and Nutrition Examination Surveys of 2005 to 2010, estimated that the new guideline would increase the number of adults receiving or eligible for statins from 43 million to 56 million.[21] In an analysis of people enrolled in the prospective epidemiologic Multi-Ethnic Study of Atherosclerosis (MESA) who were free of CV disease and diabetes at baseline, the risk calculator grossly overestimated the 10-year rate of developing ASCVD. Whereas the actual rate was 5%, the risk calculator predicted a rate of 9%.[22]

For these reasons, 2 more recently published guidelines have taken a more conservative approach to treatment. The 2014 VA/DOT guideline recommends a risk threshold of greater than 12% (rather than the 7.5% recommended by ACC/AHA) for initiating statin therapy and starting with moderate, rather than high-intensity, therapy for both primary and secondary prevention of ASCVD.[12] Titrating to high-intensity therapy is indicated for secondary prevention only when appropriate, for example, acute coronary syndrome, recurrent cardiovascular disease (CVD) events, or multiple uncontrolled risk factors. In 2016, the US Preventive Services Task Force (USPSTF) issued recommendations on the use of statins for primary prevention.[23] This guideline does not pertain to adults at very high risk of CVD (eg, familial hypercholesterolemia [FH]), and those with established CVD or LDL-C higher than 190 mg/dL because they were excluded from primary prevention trials. Based on its systematic review of evidence of benefit versus harm, the USPSTF advises low-to moderate-dose statins for adults 40 to 75 years of age with no history of CVD but with at least 1 CVD risk factor (dyslipidemia, diabetes, hypertension, or smoking) and a 10-year event risk of 10%

Table 2
Relative potency of statin drugs

Drug	High-Intensity (Daily Dose)	Moderate-Intensity (Daily Dose)
Rosuvastatin	20–40 mg	5–10 mg
Atorvastatin	40–80 mg	10–20 mg
Simvastatin[a]	—	20–40 mg
Pravastatin	—	40–80 mg
Lovastatin	—	40 mg
Fluvastatin	—	80 mg

[a] Caution should be taken with higher doses due to multiple drug interactions.

Box 3
Risk factors favoring statin therapy in patients with indefinite risk for atherosclerotic cardiovascular disease

Family history of premature ASCVD

High-sensitivity C-reactive protein 2 or more

Coronary artery calcium scan score 300 or higher

Ankle-brachial index less than 0.9

LDL-C 160 mg/dL or more, or other evidence of genetic hyperlipidemias

Elevated lifetime risk of ASCVD per pooled cohort equations or 10-year risk between 5.0% to 7.5%

Taking into consideration the risk/benefit ratio of treatment and patient preferences, shared decision-making between patient and clinician is essential.

---

or more using the ACC/AHA pooled cohort equations (grade B recommendation) as well as for those with a calculated risk of 7.5% to 10% (grade C recommendation).[23]

Based on data from the 2009 to 2014 National Health and Nutrition Examination Survey, Pagidipati and colleagues[24] determined that about 9 million more adults, mostly between 40 and 59 years old, would receive statins using ACC/AHA rather than USPSTF guidelines. Although these individuals would have a low 10-year risk for CVD, their mean 30-year risk would exceed 30%, and 28% would develop diabetes. The investigators concluded that reliance on 10-year CVD risk alone might exclude many younger individuals who over their lifetime might benefit from long-term statin therapy.[24] Two other recent studies also found that the 7.5% risk threshold specified in the ACC/AHA guideline is not only reasonable and cost-effective but that an even lower threshold of 3% to 4% would avoid more than 160,000 additional CV events.[25,26] In a review of these newer observations, Pender and colleagues[27] recommend considering the use of statins for asymptomatic individuals ages 40 to 75 with less than a 7.5% 10-year ASCVD risk, as well as for those younger and older than this range, especially those with high coronary artery calcium scores.

Although the guidelines differ from one another in the initiation threshold and intensity of statin therapy, they agree that everyone at age 40 years or older should be considered for possible statin therapy. They all also emphasize the importance of lifestyle modification and, especially, the need for joint decision-making between clinician and patient concerning the benefits and risks of starting statin therapy. Most importantly, however, no guideline is of any value if it is not followed. Unfortunately, such is the case. A recent comparison of statin use before and after the publication of the ACC/AHA guideline showed that use of statins overall, and specifically within each of the 4 guideline-defined at-risk groups, increased only marginally or not at all among 161 cardiology practices.[28] In an accompanying editorial, Blumenthal and colleagues[29] cite several studies that reported significant underuse of statins for both primary and secondary prevention in a variety of other clinical settings.

NONSTATIN DRUG THERAPY

The 2013 ACC/AHA guideline falls short of providing specific recommendations for using nonstatin cholesterol-lowering drugs in statin-intolerant patients and those who do not achieve the expected reduction in LDL-C. It is known that the response of patients to statin therapy is variable, and that not all patients achieve 50% or greater reduction in LDL-C on high-intensity therapy.[30] When the guideline was published, there was no evidence of benefit of adding nonstatin drugs to optimal statin therapy. However, the Improved Reduction of Outcomes: Vytorin Efficacy International Trial (IMPROVE-IT) has demonstrated improved CV outcomes in simvastatin-treated patients receiving ezetimibe versus simvastatin therapy alone.[31,32] Also, a new class of potent cholesterol-lowering drugs, the proprotein convertase subtilisin/kexin type 9 (PCSK9) inhibitors (alirocumab and evolocumab), has appeared. PCSK9 inhibitors decrease LDL-C by up to 60%. Currently, they are indicated as add-on therapy to statins for patients with FH or clinical ASCVD who require additional lowering of LDL-C. Early randomized trials with these 2 PCSK9 inhibitors, primarily designed to demonstrate safety and efficacy of LDL-C lowering, also suggested benefit in reducing CV events.[33,34] However, the recent Further Cardiovascular Outcomes Research With PCSK9 Inhibition in Subjects With Elevated Risk trial rigorously assessed CV outcomes with evolocumab added to statin therapy over a 2-year period in subjects with ASCVD. Evolocumab not only reduced LDL-C to a median value of 30 mg/dL, it also reduced the primary and secondary CV end points by 15% to 20%.[35] These developments prompted the Expert Consensus Panel (ECP) of the American College of Cardiology to recently issue more detailed recommendations for the use of nonstatin drugs in specific patient scenarios.[6] **Fig. 3** is a condensed representation of the ECP recommendations with respect to nonstatin drug therapy.

At this time, only ezetimibe, bile acid sequestrates (BAS) such as colesevelam, and PCSK9 inhibitors are recommended. Because of evidence of nonefficacy and potential harms, niacin is not recommended.[36] The ECP did not recommend omega-3 fatty acids or fibric acid derivatives for treating hypertriglyceridemia because clinical trials have failed to show CV benefit from targeting TGs with these drugs in subjects optimally treated with statins.[6] These recommendations are consistent with the recent

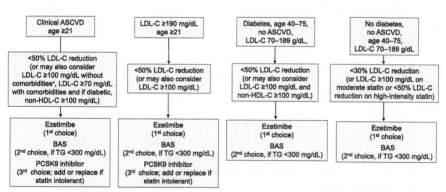

Fig. 3. Indications for adding nonstatin therapy to maximally tolerated statin therapy. In each group, the following steps should be taken before adding nonstatin therapy: address adherence to statin therapy, intensify lifestyle modification, evaluate statin intolerance, refer to specialist if intolerant to even moderate-intensity statins, control other risk factors, discuss risk versus benefits of nonstatin therapy, and ascertain patient's preferences for additional therapy. [a] Comorbidities: diabetes, recent (<3 months) acute ASCVD event, ASCVD while on a statin, baseline LDL-C 190 mg/dL or higher, poorly controlled major ASCVD risk factors, elevated lipoprotein(a), and chronic kidney disease. (*Adapted from* Lloyd-Jones DM, Morris PB, Ballantyne CM, et al. 2016 ACC expert consensus decision pathway on the role of non-statin therapies for LDL-cholesterol lowering in the management of atherosclerotic cardiovascular disease risk: a report of the American College of Cardiology Task Force on Clinical Expert Consensus Documents. J Am Coll Cardiol 2016;68:92–125. Fig. 1.)

FDA withdrawal of approval for niacin and fibrates in combination with statins.[37] However, treatment of severe hypertriglyceridemia (≥500 mg/dL) is still indicated to reduce the risk of acute pancreatitis.

A noteworthy feature of the EPC document is that it resurrects interest in returning, at least partially, to a treat-to-target approach for LDL-C, a viewpoint shared by other experts.[38] It also suggests the use of non-HDL-C as an additional target for patients with diabetes (see **Fig. 3**). Both of these concepts are fully endorsed in the 2014 National Lipid Association recommendations for management of dyslipidemia.[39] Further support for targeting specific LDL-C and non-HDL-C targets comes from the recently published American Association of Clinical Endocrinologists and American College of Endocrinology guidelines for management of dyslipidemia and prevention of CV disease. The guidelines define 5 ASCVD risk categories with corresponding targets for LDL-C, non-HDL-C, and apolipoprotein B.[40] Thus, only a few years since the publication of the ACC/AHA guideline, the pendulum may be swinging back toward a treat-to-target approach.

LIPID MANAGEMENT IN SPECIAL POPULATIONS

The ACC/AHA guideline does not address children, adolescents, the very elderly (>75 year old), patients with chronic kidney disease (CKD), and patients taking drugs that can adversely affect or interact with statins.

Children and Adolescents

Atherosclerosis starts at a young age as evidenced by pathologic changes in the vessels of children and adolescents who died of injury.[41,42] Additional evidence of early-onset atherosclerosis comes from noninvasive clinical tests, such as carotid intima-media thickness (CIMT) assessed with ultrasound and coronary artery calcification seen on computed tomography scans.[43] As in adults, dyslipidemia contributes to CV risk in children.

The most common hereditary dyslipidemia in childhood and adolescence is familial combined hyperlipidemia, present in 20% to 30% of obese children.[41] Untreated patients manifest a pseudodiabetes lipid pattern consisting of elevated LDL-C, TC, and TG levels, along with low HDL-C and a preponderance of small dense atherogenic LDL-C particles. The next most common hereditary dyslipidemia is the heterozygous form of FH, which is seen in 1:200 to 1:500 ratios and associated with LDL-C greater than 160 mg/dL in children.[44] Without treatment, a CV event will occur by age 50 years in 25% of affected women and 50% of affected men.[45] In the much rarer homozygous form of FH, CV events begin in the first decade of life.[45] Dyslipidemia in childhood can also be acquired (**Box 4**).

Lipid screening in childhood and adolescence has been recommended in guidelines from the National Heart, Lung, and Blood Institute (NHLBI) and the American Academy of Pediatrics (AAP), and the National Lipid Association (NLA).[39,41] Both recommend selective screening starting at age 2 years for children likely to have FH (based on family history of FH or premature ASCVD), and universal screening at age 10 years. However, after carefully reviewing evidence on screening for FH and multifactorial dyslipidemia in children, the USPSTF recently concluded that "current evidence is insufficient to assess the balance of benefits and harms of screening for lipid disorders in children and adolescents 20 years or younger".[47] The USPSTF recognizes the association of dyslipidemia with ASCVD. However, it based its conclusions on the following considerations:

Box 4
Secondary causes of childhood dyslipidemia and early atherosclerosis

High risk

- Diabetes mellitus, types 1 and 2
- Chronic kidney disease
- Following organ transplant (heart, kidney)
- Kawasaki disease with persistent coronary artery aneurysms

Moderate risk

- Kawasaki disease with regressed coronary artery aneurysms
- Chronic inflammatory disease (eg, rheumatoid arthritis, systemic lupus)
- Human immunodeficiency virus
- Nephrotic syndrome
- Adolescent depressive and bipolar disorders[46]

Adapted from Zappalla FR, Gidding SS. Lipid management in children. Endocrinol Metab Clin North Am 2009;38:171–83.

- For FH: Although short-term pharmacologic interventions have shown reduction in LDL-C and CIMT, there are no long-term randomized clinical trials (RCTs) showing that this reduces the incidence of or mortality from ASCVD in adulthood.
- For multifactorial dyslipidemia: Screening has not been evaluated in RCTs. Evidence of benefit from lifestyle modification or pharmacologic intervention is inadequate. Elevated levels of LDL-C in adolescents predict abnormal levels 15 to 20 years later with a positive predictive value of only 33% to 37%. Because most children with multifactorial dyslipidemia will not develop premature ASCVD, screening can result in over-diagnosis, unnecessary treatment, and anxiety.

Therefore, pending more definitive data, it is up to the clinician's discretion and judgment to decide who and when to screen and what to recommend or prescribe. The USPSTF acknowledges that "clinical decisions involve more considerations than evidence alone." For now, it would seem prudent to screen children with multiple risk factors, including obesity, metabolic syndrome, secondary causes of dyslipidemia (see **Box 4**) or a strong family history of risk factors, recognizing that only universal screening can identify all children or adolescents with dyslipidemia. However, a recently published AAP survey revealed that screening practices among pediatricians varied widely due to a combination of lack of knowledge, conflicts between the guidelines, and concern about benefit versus harm from treatment.[48]

Treatment should start with lifestyle modifications, which are explained in detail in the pediatric guidelines from the NHLBI/AAP and the NLA.[41] Both guidelines recommend starting pharmacologic therapy at age 10 for patients who fail lifestyle intervention after 6 months and who either have severe dyslipidemia or other comorbid conditions. The guidelines contain algorithms defining the threshold and target levels of LDL-C for treatment; however, these are debatable, as is the appropriate age for starting medication, because of insufficient supporting evidence.[41,47]

Statins are the preferred first-line drugs and are started at the lowest dose. However, because they are contraindicated in pregnancy, adolescent females should be counseled about using effective contraception. Short-term clinical trials have shown no significant adverse side effects, including impairment of growth or sexual maturation.[41] Bile acid sequestrants and ezetimibe are also approved, but the former is poorly tolerated and experience with the latter is limited. Moreover, the long-term benefits versus risks of therapy are unknown.[47]

For hypertriglyceridemia, diet modification with reduced intake of saturated fat and simple sugars, and increased intake of fish or omega-3 fatty acid supplements, along with weight loss and increased physical activity are the primary treatments. Niacin is rarely used because of side effects. Fibrates are used to treat severe TG elevations (>500 mg/dL) to prevent pancreatitis, and referral to a lipid specialist is recommended.[47]

The Elderly

None of the guidelines discussed in this article contain recommendations for patients older than 75 years, yet this growing segment of the population has the highest prevalence of ASCVD.[4,48] Despite the exclusion of the elderly from many clinical trials, there is evidence that these patients do derive benefit from statin therapy for both primary and secondary prevention of adverse CV outcomes.[49] However, data on treatment for patients older than 80 to 85 years are especially limited.

Because elderly patients often have comorbidities, are on multiple medications that increase the risk for drug interactions and side effects, and have altered pharmacokinetics and pharmacodynamics, clinical judgment should guide the decision to initiate statin therapy in this population. Moderate intensity therapy, if initiated, should be started at a low dose to avoid adverse events, and then titrated upward as tolerated.

Despite the evidence of benefit, elderly patients are undertreated and adherence is poor.[48] Medication nonadherence is complex, but improved clinician and patient understanding of the potential benefits of persistence with statin therapy may enhance compliance.

Chronic Kidney Disease

Patients with CKD pose a special challenge to the clinician. Dyslipidemia is very common in this population, which also has a high risk for ASCVD. Yet, at the same time, LDL-C, a potent risk factor for ASCVD in the general population, does not correlate as well with CV outcomes in CKD patients, especially those on chronic dialysis.[50] In end-stage renal disease, other factors such as inflammation, malnutrition, and disorders of mineral metabolism, are more potent determinants of CV morbidity and mortality. In the remaining CKD population, a decreasing benefit from statin therapy is seen as CKD progresses from stage 2 through stage 5 (ie, glomerular filtration rates [GFRs] from <60 to <15 mL/min).[51] This relationship was borne out in a recent meta-analysis of 28 clinical trials in which progressively smaller reductions in major vascular events per each mmol/L reduction in LDL-C were observed as GFR declined; no benefit was seen in dialysis patients.[52] Thus, LDL-C cannot be used for identifying CKD patients who should receive pharmacologic cholesterol-lowering treatment.[51]

The ACC/AHA guideline advises against starting statin therapy in dialysis patients but does not specifically address patients CKD by stage. However, recommendations for these patients were published in the 2013 Kidney Disease: Improving Global Outcomes (KDIGO) clinical practice guideline for lipid management in CKD.[53] Like the ACC/AHA guideline, the KDIGO committee recommends obtaining a baseline lipid panel but advises against routine follow-up tests after therapy is initiated, except when the results would alter management or assess adherence.[53,54]

Due to the paucity of conclusive evidence, most of the KDIGO recommendations for pharmacologic treatment in CKD are weak and, therefore, are designated as suggestions (**Table 3**).

Table 3
Kidney Disease: Improving Global Outcomes recommendations for pharmacologic therapy in chronic kidney disease

Patient Category	Advice	Quality of Evidence
Treatment favored[a]		
Adults, age $\geq$50 y, GFR 30–59 mL/min/1.73 m^2 (stage G3–G5)[b]	Recommend	High
Adults, age $\geq$50 y, GFR $\geq$60 mL/min/1.73 m^2 (stage G1–G2)[b]	Recommend	Moderate
Adults, age <50 y, with comorbidities (stage G1–G5)[b,c]	Suggest	High
Transplant patients, any age	Suggest	Moderate
Dialysis patients already being treated before starting dialysis	Suggest	Low
Treatment not favored		
Adults already on dialysis	Suggest	Low
Children, age <18 y[d]	Suggest	High

[a] Treatment: Statin or statin-ezetimibe combination.
[b] Excludes chronic dialysis and transplant patients.
[c] Must also have known CVD, diabetes, or 10-year risk greater than 10%.
[d] Includes chronic dialysis and transplant patients.
  Data from Wanner C, Tonelli M. Kidney Disease: Improving Global Outcomes Lipid Guideline Development Work Group Members. KDIGO clinical practice guideline for lipid management in CKD: summary of recommendation statements and clinical approach to the patient. Kidney Int 2014;85:1303–9.

For all weak recommendations, clinicians should consider the patient's comorbidities, age, preferences, and risk for ASCVD events versus benefits of treatment before initiating pharmacologic therapy.

Comorbid Conditions Affecting Statin Therapy

Two conditions associated with dyslipidemia worth noting are organ transplantation and human immunodeficiency virus (HIV) because drugs used to treat these conditions can adversely affect statin effectiveness and/or safety.

Dyslipidemia and increased risk for CV morbidity and mortality are both common in cardiac and renal transplant patients.[48,54] Unfortunately, immunosuppressive therapy with corticosteroids, calcineurin inhibitors (cyclosporine more than tacrolimus), and rapamycin (sirolimus) contribute significantly to the pathogenesis of dyslipidemia. KDIGO recommends statin therapy for transplant patients, though the recommendation is weak because it is based on only 1 clinical trial with fluvastatin.[54] However, because several statins, including simvastatin, atorvastatin, and lovastatin, are metabolized by the same hepatic cytochrome P450 isoenzyme (CYP3A4) as the calcineurin inhibitors and rapamycin, the statin level is raised with concurrent therapy, which can cause myopathy and rhabdomyolysis.[48] Although pravastatin, fluvastatin, and rosuvastatin do not rely on CYP3A4, increased levels of all these drugs have been reported with coadministration of cyclosporine in kidney and/or heart transplant recipients. Therefore, consulting with the patient's transplant center is advised before prescribing a statin.

Human Immunodeficiency Virus Patients

The advent of highly active antiretroviral therapy (HAART) has improved and extended the life spans of patients with HIV. However, with increasing age there has been an increasing rate of CV mortality over the past 15 years due to a combination of traditional CVD risk factors, residual virally mediated inflammation despite HIV treatment, and side effects of HAART.[55] CVD is now the second-most common cause of death in the HIV-positive population (after cancer) in countries where HAART is widely used.[56]

Dyslipidemia is common in patients with HIV. Patients manifest the same pseudo-diabetes lipid pattern seen in children and adolescents with familial combined hyperlipidemia. HAART contributes further to the dyslipidemia, especially to the high TG and low HDL-C levels.[56]

Treatment of dyslipidemia in HIV-infected patients follows the same strategies as for uninfected patients, with a key difference. Several types of HAART drugs, especially protease inhibitors, inhibit CYP3A4 and can increase statin levels and toxicity. Therefore, for patients receiving HAART medications, appropriate options are atorvastatin, pravastatin, and rosuvastatin but simvastatin and lovastatin are contraindicated. Ezetimibe can also be used; it is not metabolized through the CYP450 system. For severe hypertriglyceridemia, fibrates are favored; fish oil and niacin can be used, but the latter is less tolerated. Because patients with HIV take many other drugs that are metabolized by the CYP450 system, there is the potential for a range of complex drug interactions. These patients may be best managed in a specialty practice.

SUMMARY

The 2013 ACC/AHA guideline provides evidence-based advice to clinicians regarding lipid management. It clearly establishes statins as the first-line pharmacologic treatment of hypercholesterolemia. Together with the 2016 ACC consensus document that provides guidance for the use of nonstatin drugs, clinicians can now engage in meaningful discussion and shared decision-making with their patients to reduce ASCVD risk. However, both documents leave some uncertainties and gaps in knowledge that only future randomized clinical trials can answer. Guidelines are not edicts; they are fluid documents that require individualized application and periodic revision. They are not a substitute for clinical judgment but, if understood and appropriately applied, can enhance patient care.

ADDITIONAL RESOURCES

For clinicians

2013 ACC/AHA guideline interactive risk calculator (per pooled cohort equations). Available at: http://clincalc.com/cardiology/ascvd/pooledcohort.aspx

Mayo Statin Decision Aid (includes 3 interactive risk calculators: 2013 ACC/AHA, Framingham, and Reynolds). Available at: http://statindecisionaid.mayoclinic.org/index.php/site/index

VA/DOT Management of Dyslipidemia guideline and frequently asked questions. Available at: http://www.healthquality.va.gov/guidelines/CD/lipids/ and http://www.healthquality.va.gov/guidelines/CD/lipids/VADoDLipidsFAQsTable2014.pdf

For patient education

Foundation of the National Lipid Association. Available at: http://www.learnyourlipids.com

CDC. Available at: http://www.cdc.gov/cholesterol/materials_for_patients.htm

REFERENCES

1. CDC/National Center for Health Statistics 2016. Leading causes of death. Available at: http://www.cdc.gov/nchs/fastats/leading-causes-of-death.htm. Accessed May 24, 2017.

2. National Cholesterol Education Program (NCEP) Expert Panel on Detection, Evaluation, and Treatment of High Blood Cholesterol in Adults (Adult Treatment Panel III). Third Report of the National Cholesterol Education Program (NCEP) Expert Panel on Detection, Evaluation, and Treatment of High Blood Cholesterol in Adults (Adult Treatment Panel III) final report. Circulation 2002;106:3143–421.

3. Grundy SM, Cleeman JI, Merz CN, et al, Coordinating Committee of the National Cholesterol Education Program. Implications of recent clinical trials for the National Cholesterol Education Program Adult Treatment Panel III Guidelines. J Am Coll Cardiol 2004;44:720–32.

4. Stone NJ, Robinson JG, Lichtenstein AH, et al. 2013 ACC/AHA Cholesterol Guideline Panel. Treatment of blood cholesterol to reduce atherosclerotic cardiovascular disease risk in adults: synopsis of the 2013 American College of Cardiology/American Heart Association cholesterol guideline. Ann Intern Med 2014; 160:339–43.

5. Stone NJ, Robinson JG, Lichtenstein AH, et al, American College of Cardiology/American Heart Association Task Force on Practice Guidelines. 2013 ACC/AHA guideline on the treatment of blood cholesterol to reduce atherosclerotic cardiovascular risk in adults: a report of the American College of Cardiology/American Heart Association Task Force on Practice Guidelines. J Am Coll Cardiol 2014; 63(25 Pt B):2889–934.

6. Lloyd-Jones DM, Morris PB, Ballantyne CM, et al. 2016 ACC expert consensus decision pathway on the role of non-statin therapies for LDL-cholesterol lowering in the management of atherosclerotic cardiovascular disease risk: a report of the American College of Cardiology Task Force on Clinical Expert Consensus Documents. J Am Coll Cardiol 2016;68:92–125.

7. Virani SS, Pokharel Y, Steinberg L, et al. Provider understanding of the 2013 ACC/AHA cholesterol guideline. J Clin Lipidol 2016;10:497–504.

8. Pokharel Y, Gosch K, Nambi V, et al. Practice-level variation in statin use among patients with diabetes: insights from the PINNACLE registry. J Am Coll Cardiol 2016;68:1368–9.

9. Eckel RH, Jakicic JM, Ard JD, et al, American College of Cardiology/American Heart Association Task Force on Practice Guidelines. 2013 AHA/ACC guideline on lifestyle management to reduce cardiovascular risk: a report of the American College of Cardiology/American Heart Association Task Force on Practice Guidelines. J Am Coll Cardiol 2014;63(25 Pt B):2960–84.

10. Jensen MD, Ryan DH, Apovian CM, et al, American College of Cardiology/American Heart Association Task Force on Practice Guidelines, Obesity Society. 2013 AHA/ACC/TOS guideline for the management of overweight and obesity in adults: a report of the American College of Cardiology/American Heart Association Task Force on Practice Guidelines and The Obesity Society. J Am Coll Cardiol 2014;63(25 Pt B):2985–3023.

11. Arsenault BJ, Boekholdt SM, Kastelein JJ. Lipid parameters for measuring risk of cardiovascular disease. Nat Rev Cardiol 2011;8:197–206.

12. Downs JR, O'Malley PG. Management of dyslipidemia for cardiovascular disease risk reduction: synopsis of the 2014 U.S. Department of Veterans Affairs and U.S. Department of Defense clinical practice guideline. Ann Intern Med 2015;163: 291–7.

13. Craig SR, Amin RV, Russell DW, et al. Blood cholesterol screening influence of fasting state on cholesterol results and management decisions. J Gen Intern Med 2000;15:395–9.

14. Di Angelantonio E, Sarwar N, Perry P, et al. Emerging Risk Factors Collaboration. Major lipids, apolipoproteins, and risk of vascular disease. JAMA 2009;302: 1993–2000.

15. Driver SL, Martin SS, Gluckman TJ, et al. Fasting or nonfasting lipid measurements: it depends on the question. J Am Coll Cardiol 2016;67:1227–34.

16. Sidhu D, Naugler C. Fasting time and lipid levels in a community-based population: a cross-sectional study. Arch Intern Med 2012;172:1707–10.

17. Doran B, Guo Y, Xu J, et al. Prognostic value of fasting versus nonfasting low-density lipoprotein cholesterol levels on long-term mortality: insight from the National Health and Nutrition Examination Survey III (NHANES-III). Circulation 2014; 130:546–53.

18. Ridker PM, Cook NR. Statins: new American guidelines for prevention of cardiovascular disease. Lancet 2013;382(9907):1762–5.

19. Lopez-Jimenez F, Simha V, Thomas RJ, et al. A summary and critical assessment of the 2013 ACC/AHA guideline on the treatment of blood cholesterol to reduce atherosclerotic cardiovascular disease risk in adults: filling the gaps. Mayo Clin Proc 2014;89:1257–78.

20. Cook NR, Ridker PM. Further insight into the cardiovascular risk calculator: the roles of statins, revascularizations, and underascertainment in the Women's Health Study. JAMA Intern Med 2014;174:1964–71.

21. Pencina MJ, Navar-Boggan AM, D'Agostino RB Sr, et al. Application of new cholesterol guidelines to a population-based sample. N Engl J Med 2014;370: 1422–31.

22. DeFilippis AP, Young R, Carrubba CJ, et al. An analysis of calibration and discrimination among multiple cardiovascular risk scores in a modern multiethnic cohort. Ann Intern Med 2015;162:266–75.

23. Bibbins-Domingo K, Grossman DC, Curry SJ, et al, U.S. Preventive Services Task Force. Statin use for the primary prevention of cardiovascular disease in adults: U.S. Preventive Services Task force recommendation statement. JAMA 2016; 316:1997–2007.

24. Pagidipati NJ, Navar AM, Mulder H, et al. Comparison of recommended eligibility for primary prevention statin therapy based on the US Preventive Services Task Force recommendations vs the ACC/AHA guidelines. JAMA 2017;317:1563.

25. Pursnani A, Massario JM, D'Agostino RB Sr, et al. Guideline-based statin eligibility, coronary artery calcification, and cardiovascular events. JAMA 2015;314: 134–41.

26. Pandya A, Weinstein MC, Gaziano TA. Cost-effectiveness of statin therapy for ASCVD–reply. JAMA 2015;314(20):2191–2.

27. Pender A, Lloyd-Jones DM, Stone NJ, et al. Refining statin prescribing in lower-risk individuals: informing risk/benefit decisions. J Am Coll Cardiol 2016;68: 1690–7.

28. Pokharel Y, Tang F, Jones PG, et al. Adoption of the 2013 American College of Cardiology/American Heart Association cholesterol management guideline in cardiology practices nationwide. JAMA Cardiol 2017;2:361–9.

29. Blumenthal RS, Gluckman TJ, Martin SS. Trends in the use of moderate-intensity to high-intensity statin and nonstatin lipid-lowering therapy: turning off the faucet is much more valuable than mopping up the floor. JAMA Cardiol 2017;2:355–6.

30. Karlson BW, Palmer MK, Nicholls SJ, et al. To what extent do high-intensity statins reduce low-density lipoprotein cholesterol in each of the four statin benefit groups identified by the 2013 American College of Cardiology/American Heart Association guidelines? A VOYAGER meta-analysis. Atherosclerosis 2015;241:450–4.

31. Cannon CP, Blazing MA, Giugliano RP, et al, for IMPROVE-IT Investigators. Eze-timibe Added to Statin Therapy after Acute Coronary Syndromes. N Engl J Med 2015;372:2387–97.

32. Bohula EA, Giugliano RP, Cannon CP, et al. Achievement of dual low-density lipo-protein cholesterol and high-sensitivity C-reactive protein targets more frequent with the addition of ezetimibe to simvastatin and associated with better outcomes in IMPROVE-IT. Circulation 2015;132:1224–33.

33. Robinson JG, Farnier M, Krempf M, et al, ODYSSEY LONG TERM Investigators. Efficacy and safety of alirocumab in reducing lipids and cardiovascular events. N Engl J Med 2015;372:1489–99.

34. Sabatine MS, Giugliano RP, Wiviott SD, et al, for OSLER Investigators. Efficacy and safety of evolocumab in reducing lipids and cardiovascular events. N Engl J Med 2015;372:1500–9.

35. Sabatine MS, Giugliano RP, Keech AC, et al. Evolocumab and clinical outcomes in patients with cardiovascular disease. N Engl J Med 2017;376:1713–22.

36. AIM-HIGH Investigators, Boden WE, Probstfield JL, Anderson T, et al. Niacin in patients with low HDL cholesterol levels receiving intensive statin therapy. N Engl J Med 2011;365:2255–67.

37. FDA Federal Register. 2016. Available at: https://www.federalregister.gov/documents/2016/04/18/2016-08887/abbvie-inc-et-al-withdrawal-of-approval-of-indications-related-to-the-coadministration-with-statins. Accessed May 24, 2017.

38. Shrank WH, Barlow JF, Brenan TA. New therapies in the treatment of high choles-terol: an argument to return to goal-based lipid guidelines. JAMA 2015;314:1443–4.

39. Jacobson TA, Maki KC, Orringer CE, et al. NLA expert panel. National Lipid As-sociation recommendations for patient-centered management of dyslipidemia: part 2. J Clin Lipidol 2015;9(Issue 6, Suppl S):S1–122.e1.

40. Jellinger PS, Handelsman Y, Rosenblit PD, et al. American Association of Clinical Endocrinologists and American College of Endocrinology guidelines for manage-ment of dyslipidemia and prevention of cardiovascular disease. Endocr Pract 2017;23(Suppl 2):1–87.

41. Expert panel on integrated guidelines for cardiovascular health and risk reduction in children and adolescents, National Heart, Lung, and Blood Institute. Expert panel on integrated guidelines for cardiovascular health and risk reduction in chil-dren and adolescents: summary report. Pediatrics 2011;128(Suppl 5):S213–56.

42. Zappalla FR, Gidding SS. Lipid management in children. Endocrinol Metab Clin North Am 2009;38:171–83.

43. Daniels SR, Benuck I, Christakis DA, et al. Expert panel on integrated guidelines for cardiovascular health and risk reduction in children and adolescents: full report, 2011. Natl Heart Lung Blood Inst. Available at: https://www.nhlbi.nih.gov/files/docs/peds_guidelines_sum.pdf. Accessed May 24, 2017.

44. Gidding SS, Champagne MA, de Ferranti SD, et al, American Heart Association Atherosclerosis, Hypertension, and Obesity in Young, Committee of Council on Cardiovascular Disease in Young, Council on Cardiovascular and Stroke Nursing, Council on Functional Genomics and Translational Biology, and Council on Life-style and Cardiometabolic Health. The Agenda for Familial Hypercholesterolemia: a Scientific Statement from the American Heart Association. Circulation 2015;132:2167–92.

45. Daniels SR. Familial hypercholesterolemia: the reason to screen children for cholesterol abnormalities. J Pediatr 2016;170:7–8.

46. Goldstein BI, Lotrich F, Axelson DA, et al. Inflammatory markers among adolescents and young adults with bipolar spectrum disorders. J Clin Psychiatry 2015;76:1556–63.

47. Lozano P, Henrikson NB, Dunn J, et al. Lipid screening in childhood and adolescence for detection of familial hypercholesterolemia: a systematic evidence review for the U.S. Preventive Services Task Force. JAMA 2016;316:645–55.

48. Corsini A. The safety of HMG-CoA reductase inhibitors in special populations at high cardiovascular risk. Cardiovasc Drugs Ther 2003;17:265–85.

49. Catapano AL, Graham I, De Backer G, et al, Authors/Task Force Members. ESC/EAS Guidelines for the management of dyslipidaemias: The Task Force for the management of dyslipidaemias of the European Society of Cardiology (ESC) the European Atherosclerosis Society (EAS). Developed with the special contribution of the European Association for Cardiovascular Prevention & Rehabilitation (EASCPR). Eur Heart J 2011;32:1769–818.

50. Tsimihodimos V, Mitrogianni A, Elisaf M. Dyslipidemia associated with chronic kidney disease. Open Cardiovasc Med J 2011;5:41–8.

51. Tonelli M, Wanner C, Kidney Disease: Improving Global Outcomes Lipid Guideline Development Work Group Members. Lipid management in chronic kidney disease: synopsis of the kidney disease: improving global outcomes 2013 clinic practice guideline. Ann Intern Med 2014;160(3):182.

52. Cholesterol Treatment Trialists' (CTT) Collaboration, Herrington WG, Emberson J, Mihaylova B, et al. Impact of renal function on the effects of LDL cholesterol lowering with statin-based regimens: a meta-analysis of individual participant data from 28 randomised trials. Lancet Diabetes Endocrinol 2016;4:829–39.

53. Kidney Disease: Improving Global Outcomes (KDIGO) Lipid Work Group. KDIGO Clinical Practice Guideline for Lipid Management in Chronic Kidney Disease. Kidney Int Suppl 2013;3(Issue 3):259–305.

54. Wanner C, Tonelli M, Kidney disease: Improving Global Outcomes Lipid Guideline Development Work Group Members. KDIGO Clinical Practice Guideline for Lipid Management in CKD: summary of recommendation statements and clinical approach to the patient. Kidney Int 2014;85:1303–9.

55. Feinstein MJ, Bahiru E, Achenbach C, et al. Patterns of cardiovascular mortality for HIV-infected adults in the United States: 1999 to 2013. Am J Cardiol 2016;117:214–20.

56. Giannarelli C, Klein RS, Badimon JJ. Cardiovascular implications of HIV-induced dyslipidemia. Atherosclerosis 2011;219:384–9.

Heart Failure

Daniel T. Thibodeau, MHP, PA-C, DFAAPA[a,b,*]

KEYWORDS

- Heart failure • Management • Classifications • Risk factors

KEY POINTS

- Heart failure is a complex syndrome that results in significant impairment of normal heart pumping function.
- Several factors and risk can significantly reduce patients' survival rate, which is 50% at 5 years.
- A team approach to managing this syndrome includes all members of the health care team and, most importantly, the patients themselves.
- New therapies have improved symptoms and reduction in morbidity.

INTRODUCTION
Definition of Heart Failure

Heart failure is a complex syndrome in which the heart cannot pump blood at a rate commensurate with the metabolic needs of tissues and organs or can do so only with high pressures within the cardiovascular system.[1] This syndrome results from either a structural or functional impairment of the ventricles' ability to fill appropriately or an impairment of the ejection of blood. It should be noticed that the term *heart failure* is preferred over *congestive heart failure* because some patients present without signs or symptoms of volume overload.

Because the heart's inability to either fail or eject a proper amount of volume of blood, heart failure can be broken down into 2 major components of dysfunction. The first condition has to do with the heart's inability to fully relax, thus, causing a passive stiffness throughout the heart and its inability to adequately fill. This passive stiffness has been referred to diastolic heart failure or heart failure with a preserved ejection fraction (HFpEF). In an opposite function, the heart's inability to properly squeeze enough volume out of the heart causes a reduction in the hearts ejection fraction. This condition is commonly referred to as systolic heart failure or heart failure with a reduced ejection fraction (HFrEF).[1]

Author disclosure: Mr D. T. Thibodeau has no conflicts of interest and no disclosures to report.
[a] Eastern Virginia Medical School, Norfolk, 700 W. Olney Road, Lewis Hall 3168, Norfolk, VA 23505, USA; [b] Cardiovascular Specialists Inc, 5838 Harbour View Boulevard, Suite 270, Suffolk, VA 23435, USA
* Eastern Virginia Medical School, Norfolk, 700 W. Olney Road, Lewis Hall 3168, Norfolk, VA 23505.
E-mail address: thiboddt@evms.edu

Physician Assist Clin 2 (2017) 651–670
http://dx.doi.org/10.1016/j.cpha.2017.06.007
2405-7991/17/© 2017 Elsevier Inc. All rights reserved.
physicianassistant.theclinics.com

Clinical case

A 56-year-old female accountant presents to her primary care clinic with the complaint of a 6-week history of increasing shortness of breath, fatigue, and difficulty lying flat. She states that she does not have dyspnea at rest; but anytime she exerts herself upstairs or long walks, she will start feeling short winded. She also notices tightness in all of her shoes. Her past medical history includes hypertension that has been difficult to manage, dyslipidemia, arthritis, and a prior history of a chest pain evaluation that resulted in a normal nuclear stress test. She denies any alcohol use but has a 40 pack-year history of tobacco and quit 2 years ago.

Epidemiology

It is estimated that about 5.7 million adults in the United States have been diagnosed with heart failure. In all deaths, nationally 1 in 9 deaths included heart failure as a contributing cause. Each year greater than 870,000 new cases of heart failure are diagnosed, and it is estimated that by the year 2030 greater than 8 million people will have been diagnosed with the disease. Before 75 years of age, rates are markedly higher in black populations than in whites.[2,3]

Epidemiology results show that heart failure is more common in some areas of the United States than others (**Fig. 1**). What is most alarming with this disease is that the mortality rate of those patients with heart failure dies within 5 years of developing the disease. Despite advances in medications and therapies, this statistic has remained

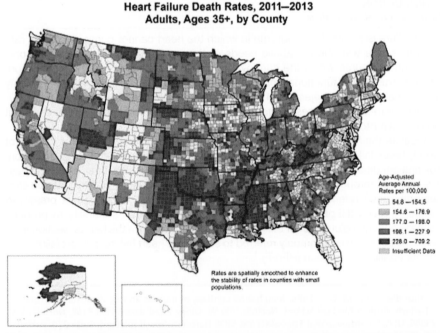

Fig. 1. Interactive atlas of heart disease and stroke. Rates are spatially smoothed to enhance the stability of rates in counties with small populations. (*From* Prevention, C. f. Interactive atlas of heart disease and stroke. Centers for Disease Control and Prevention. 2016. Available at: https://www.cdc.gov/DHDSP/data_statistics/fact_sheets/fs_heart_failure.htm. Accessed August 28, 2016.; and *Courtesy of* National Vital Statistics System; National Counter for Health Statistics, Atlanta, GA.)

relatively flat for greater than a decade. As in the aforementioned case, early detection of the disease is critical to mitigate any harmful damage that can occur when it is not properly found.

Impact on Health Care System

Since 1980, the number of hospitalizations for heart failure–related disease has been increasing.[4] This increase is especially true in the adult female population whereby statistics show the adult female sex outnumbering the number of adult males who are hospitalized each year. About 1 million hospitalizations per year are attributed to heart failure, and these are usually patients who were previously hospitalized for the same problem. New measures to prevent hospitalizations have been underway over the last several years, and aggressive management as an outpatient is key. Because of its significant impact on the health care system, practitioners have been working hard to reduce the number of rehospitalizations that tend to occur over a short period of time. It is estimated that approximately $30.7 billion each year has been contributed by heart failure. This number includes the cost of all health care services, medications, and missed days of work for patients with heart failure.[2]

Pathophysiology of Heart Failure

There are several different mechanisms that cause heart failure. In each of these different instances, an excessive amount of workload is placed on the heart causing its impairment. The 3 most common mechanisms that cause heart failure to occur are by an imposed increased in systolic blood pressure, an increase in diastolic volume, or loss of structural myocardium and substrate. What ensue are electrophysiologic contractility and biochemical changes, which directly alter the structure of the heart and its function. As time continues and the disease remains present, this condition ultimately results in cell death. This cell death eventually leads to alterations in the ability of the heart to function normally. Hypertrophy of the ventricles continues as well as the atria, and this leads to alterations of increased volume loads on the ventricles. This increase in ventricular volume as well as a weakness in the ventricular wall ultimately cause a decrease in the ventricles' ability to eject enough volume and perfuse the body's tissues and organs. These changes and stressors to the myocardium activate neurohormonal mechanisms. The most common mechanism is the renin-angiotensin-aldosterone system (RAAS). The RAAS system causes a reduction in sodium and hypo per through the glomerular filtration system, which causes increased renin release. There is also activation of the sympathetic nervous system (SNS) and cytokines that contribute to growth and remodeling and the ischemic and energy depletion effects that lead to cell death.[5]

An overall analysis of heart failure shows that most individuals with the diagnosis have as many as 5 other major comorbidities.[6] One of the most common causes and disease risk factors for systolic heart failure is coronary artery disease. This disease accounts for up to 50% of all causes of heart failure in the United States. It is also thought that approximately 20% of all other contributors to heart failure have a component of coronary artery disease.[1,4] These ischemic events cause ongoing systolic dysfunction; in some instances of acute smaller attacks, ischemic conditions still persist after the myocardium has been insulted. This persistence leads to a reduction of blood flow and tissue hypoperfusion, which ultimately can lead to apoptosis and cell death. As this mechanism occurs, it causes a fixed defect in the heart's ability to normally function. Multiple structural damages will result in ultimate pump failure in the body's ability to adequately perfuse its tissues.

In addition to the RAAS system hormonal activation, other factors also contribute to the slow progression of pump failure. Multiple chemical receptors throughout the cardiovascular system, including the carotid sinus and aortic arch baroreceptors, cause an increase in sympathetic activity, which in turn causes an increase in sympathetic tone. This mechanism causes an increase of norepinephrine within the system, which increases heart rate and contractility to try to support cardiac function. Because of the increased demands placed on the cardiovascular system, such as hypertension, valvular disease, and pressure overload, the natural response with norepinephrine will not be as great and dysfunction will start to occur. This dysfunction also has an impact throughout the alpha, beta-1, and beta-2 receptors of cardiac cells, which impact the cells ability to contract effectively. This ultimately creates a chronic level of increase in blood pressure as well as an increase in afterload and vasoconstriction of the renal system, which in turn causes a backflow and preservation of sodium and water within the cardiovascular system. In the early stages of this cardiac dysfunction, the body is able to compensate and still function at a relatively adequate level. As time progresses, and the disease continues, this sodium and water retention increases whereby patients start having symptoms. As increased pressures place demand on the heart vasodilators, such as atrial natriuretic peptide and beta natriuretic peptide, these stressors result in the heart's inability to lower atrial, pulmonary, and pulmonary artery wedge pressures. This inability causes a reduction in cardiac output, systemic vascular resistance, and a decrease in the renal system's ability to infiltrate. The activation of the RAAS attempts to increase the excretion of sodium and water to rid the body of volume overload.[7]

Classifications of Heart Failure

There are 2 major classifications of heart failure and they are based on alterations or preservation of the hearts normal ejection fraction. Although there are several less common causes for heart failure, the author focuses on the 2 primary areas of dysfunction.

Systolic heart failure

Systolic heart failure or what is now referred to as HFrEF. This heart disease is a condition whereby the heart has dilated informed large chambers, particularly in the ventricles. The abnormal contractility grossly impairs the heart's ability to adequately perfuse organs and tissues, thus, leading to peripheral disease. These individuals tend to have normal to low blood pressures, and it is more common in men but vary in age groups. The ejection fraction has been reduced (<50%), and this causes a systolic and diastolic impairment that is seen on echocardiogram. Because of this dysfunction, the impairment of the ejection fraction causes a backflow of pressure, which causes stress onto the pulmonary system, organs, and peripheral tissue. The overall prognosis is poor, and ischemic conditions are a contributing factor in more than 50% of all cases.[1,7]

Diastolic heart failure

Diastolic heart failure can also be referred to as HFpEF. This condition is a result of passive stiffness along with a smaller left ventricular cavity that also has concentric hypertrophy. Many individuals with this type of heart failure also have long-standing hypertension, which has a direct impact on the disease. The disease is more common in women, and most of the time it is often caused by other diseases not central to the cardiovascular system. Overall prognosis is poor, especially after hospitalizations. Myocardial ischemia conditions can be commonly seen in this type of heart failure.[1]

Combined systolic and diastolic heart failure

There are some instances whereby patients may have a component of both systolic and diastolic dysfunction. This mixed cardiomyopathy results in multiple comorbidities that greatly impact the ability to manage heart failure.

It should be noted that medical therapies have only been proven to be effective in the treatment of heart failure in patients who have HFrEF. In cases of diastolic heart failure, the underlying cause must be addressed to decrease the load on the heart impacting the heart failure.

Clinical case

A 62-year-old man with a long-standing history of hypertension, diabetes mellitus type II, dyslipidemia, and coronary artery disease as well as an ejection fraction of 40% presents with 4 days of increasing edema to his lower extremities, dyspnea on exertion, and sweating with mild chest pressure as he walks across the room of his house. He has had this before, and the last time he had the symptoms of chest pressure he had his myocardial infarction. He has been unable to sleep lying flat, so he has resorted to sleeping in his reclining chair.

In this clinical example, this patient is exhibiting signs of worsening HFrEF. In many clinical cases that physician assistants evaluate, patients present with a short history of worsening heart failure that is usually caused by a wide variety of reasons. In this instance, the patient's chest pressure may indicate signs of an ischemic condition. Proper clinical evaluation is pertinent in this instance.

Risk Factors and Comorbidities

Because heart failure is a syndrome and not just related to one cause, there are several contributing risk factors, cardiac comorbidities, noncardiac comorbidities, and patient-related factors that contribute to the disease and how it responds to therapy.[6] It is important for the practitioners to not only evaluate the heart failure but also the contributing factors that lead to disease and ultimately to multiple complications because of its complexity. **Table 1** illustrates the more common risk factors that contribute to heart failure. It also lists comorbidities and patient-related factors that must be considered on initial evaluation as well as treatment plans.

The Heart Failure Continuum

Multiple mechanisms over the course of a patient's life with heart failure lead to worsening of the disease. In the early stages, patients may only have evidence of

Table 1
Risk factors and other comorbidities related to heart failure

Risk factors	CAD, hypertension, valvular heart disease, diabetes, cigarette smoking, high/low hematocrit
Cardiac comorbidities	ACS, tachycardia or bradycardia syndromes, hypertension, myocarditis, cardiomyopathy, acute pulmonary embolus, acute valvular regurgitation, acute aortic dissection, cardiac tamponade
Noncardiac comorbidities	Renal dysfunction, respiratory diseases, anemia, arthritis, cognitive dysfunction, depression, COPD, thyroid disorder, polypharmacy, infection, inflammatory markers, sleep apnea
Patient-related factors	Aging, nonadherence, high salt or fluid intake, alcohol use/abuse

Abbreviations: ACS, acute coronary syndrome; CAD, coronary artery disease; COPD, chronic obstructive pulmonary disease.
Data from Refs.[4,8,9]

atherosclerosis or mild coronary artery disease. As new events occur, such as myocardial ischemia in coronary thrombosis events, the worsening of heart failure ensues. This chronic insult to the myocardium and systemic cardiovascular system leads to more chronic issues for patients' elevated filling pressures, which cause remodeling of the ventricles as well as dilatation and leads to increased pressures to the vascular system particularly within the pulmonary vasculature. This chronic condition will cause increased vascular resistance, an increase in the right ventricular afterload, which ultimately leads to worsening of disease and a reduction of ejection fraction. This results in a hypo-perfusion of organs and tissue. As time progresses patient's experience more symptoms of the disease, the potential for arrhythmia activity increases, and more exacerbations of heart failure can occur. This dilatation and remodeling of the myocardium throughout the continuum of heart failure causes patients to have increased symptoms worsening quality of life as it leads to the end stage of the heart disease itself. The number of hospitalizations increases, and eventually patients worsen to the point of needing palliative measures so that exacerbations are limited. End-of-life care occurs when all measures have been exhausted, which ultimately leads to the eventual death of patients[10] (**Fig. 2**).

History and Physical Examination

A careful evaluation of all patients suspected of heart failure must include a thorough history and physical examination. Because heart failure is a syndrome, and not a disease, no single test or physical examination characteristic is diagnostic of heart failure.[1] Early detection is most hindered by patients presenting with nonspecific symptoms and presence of comorbidities. In many cases, presentations change and vary from some patients having no symptoms at all to significant symptoms for people who have advanced stages. In some cases, the rate of the initial misdiagnosis can be up to 50% in primary care practices. Misdiagnoses is especially true for elderly patients with heart failure of a preserved ejection fraction where symptoms may be mild, absent or attributed to other causes.

A careful history must be taken in order to accurately diagnose heart failure. Dyspnea has the highest sensitivity of any of the symptoms for patients. If dyspnea is absent, this makes heart failure less likely; all other symptoms have a much lower sensitivity as it relates to heart failure.[11] There is a progression of patients' dyspnea. Dyspnea on exertion first occurs followed by a progression of paroxysmal nocturnal dyspnea. As the disease worsens, patients become orthopneic and eventually leading

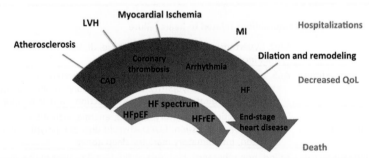

Fig. 2. The heart failure continuum. CAD, coronary artery disease; HF, heart failure; LVH, left ventricular hypertrophy. (*From* Dzau V, Braunwald E. Resolved and unresolved issues in the prevention and treatment of coronary artery disease: a workshop consensus statement. Am Heart J 1991;121:1244–1263.)

to a condition whereby dyspnea occurs at rest. Other common symptoms are fatigue, weakness, exercise intolerance, nocturia, cough, and weight gain. Less common symptoms include cognitive impairment, delirium, and nausea. As the disease progresses, gastrointestinal symptoms, which can be misleading, occur in this patient population. The physical examination will help differentiate patients who have conditions of heart failure or other causes. Evaluation of patients with either cardiac or noncardiac risk factors will show that coronary artery disease is responsible for roughly 50% of patients with heart failure who have decreased left ventricular dysfunction.[12]

A thorough physical examination is required. The overall general appearance of patients will show any signs of resting dyspnea, cyanosis, or cachexia. Vital signs are extremely important as they can determine if patients have been compensated. Blood pressure evaluation along with heart rate and any evidence of arrhythmia is pertinent. Jugular venous distention and elevation of pressures on physical examination have a very high specificity for left intricate or dysfunction. Also with a high specificity is displacement of the point of maximal impact (PMI), implying enlargement of the heart. Patients who have volume overload that the stand the ventricles may have an S3 gallop. In addition, the pulmonary examination can have a variety of adventitious lung sounds. This can range from normal, crackles, rhonchi, or rales. While patients with heart failure can also have lower extremity edema, this proves to be of limited diagnostic value overall. A hepatojugular reflux is also a consideration on examination that has a high specificity. It should be noted that not all patients on physical examination would have abnormal lung sounds while they are in heart failure. Some patients who are well compensated my not have any congestive components as it relates to their pulmonary examination. While evaluating patients, practitioners should be keen on not disregarding those who have normal lung examinations[13] (**Box 1**).

Box 1
Physical examination findings in heart failure

General appearance
Resting dyspnea, cyanosis, cachexia

Vital signs
Blood pressures, heart rate (compensation, arrhythmia)

Head and neck
Jugular venous pressure elevation (very high specificity)

Cardiovascular
Displacement of PMI, S3 heart sounds

Pulmonary
Various adventitious lung sounds (normal, wheezing, crackles, rales); decreased or absent sounds may imply pleural effusion (transudate)

Abdominal
Hepatojugular reflux (high specificity)

Extremity
Lower extremity edema (pitting) (limited diagnostic value)

Differential Diagnosis

Because heart failure is a syndrome and is not composed of one sign, symptom, or physical examination finding, making the diagnosis can sometimes prove difficult. This difficulty is especially true in the early stages of the disease. It is imperative that the practitioner considers other causes that may present as heart failure and evaluate patients to ensure other causes are considered. The brief list of a differential diagnosis for heart failure is shown in **Box 2**.

Testing and Diagnostic Studies

Laboratory testing for heart failure is limited to a few specific assays. Other laboratory testing is performed to evaluate other comorbidities and clinical conditions that can attribute to worsening heart failure. A basic metabolic profile (BMP) to assess electrolyte abnormalities, renal function, and acid-base imbalance is commonly performed. Cardiac biomarkers and enzymes are also drawn for those practitioners concerned with ischemic conditions that may be presenting with heart failure. A variety of other laboratory tests are performed at the same time as these but not necessarily directed toward the assessment of heart failure.[1]

Noninvasive imaging for heart failure can prove to be helpful when making the diagnosis. There are a couple of key diagnostic tests that aid in providing the practitioner a better understanding of the extent of disease. Because heart failure is a syndrome, other noninvasive tests are performed to rule out other causes that may be aiding in the progression of heart failure or ruling out heart failure as the primary reason for patients' symptoms. The diagnostic workup for disease is especially true in conditions whereby suspected ischemic involvement has occurred.

Box 2
Differential diagnosis of heart failure

- Myocardial ischemia
- Pulmonary diseases[a]
- Sleep and breathing disorders
- Obesity-related disease
- Deconditioning
- Malnutrition
- Anemia
- Hepatic failure
- Chronic kidney disease
- Hypoalbuminuria
- Venous stasis
- Depression
- Anxiety and hyperventilation syndrome
- Hyperthyroid and hypothyroid disease

[a]Asthma, chronic obstructive pulmonary disease, pulmonary embolism, pneumonia, primary pulmonary hypertension.
From Heart Failure Society of America, Lindenfeld J, Albert NM, et al. HFSA 2010 comprehensive heart failure practice guideline. J Card Fail 2010;16(6):e1–194. Available at: http://www.hfsa.org/heart-failure-guldelines-2/. Accessed November 11, 2016.

Natriuretic peptides

Initially discovered in brain tissue of laboratory pigs, brain natriuretic peptide was also found to be present in cardiac tissue, specifically ventricular tissue. This poly-peptide is excreted in response to overload of the ventricles that results in myocar-dial stretch. This activation causes a release of the peptide, which has a diuretic, antihypertensive effect and directly inhibits the reading and angiotensin aldosterone system. A serum assay can be obtained to evaluate the level of heart failure patients may be in. This tool can be very helpful in determining the extent of heart failure, and a negative result gives a low probability of heart failure being present. The two more common assays are B-type natriuretic peptide (BNP) and N-terminal prohormone BNP (NT-proBNP), both of which are tests that can be seen in different clinical set-tings. These different assays that can evaluate heart failure have a relative perfor-mance that has shown no significant difference, and their predictive sensitivities seem to be close to equal.

One aspect of note as it relates to BNP is that the test, although positive in heart fail-ure, is not able to differentiate those patients who have HFrEF versus HFpEF. Other factors and stressors may lower BNP levels, such as obesity in those patients with in-sulin resistance. Higher levels of BMP lack specificity, so it is incumbent on the prac-titioner to clinically correlate in those situations. Although this test has been shown to be very helpful in evaluating the disease, only 40% a primary care practices use BMPs for the diagnosis of heart failure.[14–16]

Table 2 outlines recommendations for the use of biomarkers and their level of evi-dence. **Table 3** shows that other clinical conditions and stressors may cause abnormal elevations of natriuretic peptide levels.

Echocardiography

Of all the testing that is performed on patients with heart failure, none of them is more valuable than a 2-dimensional (2D) echo with Doppler. This essential tool is helpful when practitioners suspect heart failure; it is a diagnostic standard for evaluating pa-tients for heart failure of both a reduced and preserved ejection fraction. This helpful

---

Table 2
Biomarkers and recommendations

Biomarker, Application	Setting	LOE
Natriuretic peptides (BNP, NT-proBNP)		
Diagnosis or exclusion of HF	Ambulatory, acute	A
Prognosis of HF	Ambulatory, acute	A
Achieve GDMT	Ambulatory	B
Guidance of acutely decompensated HF therapy	Acute	C
Biomarkers of myocardial injury (troponins, creatine phosphokinase)		
Additive risk stratification	Acute, ambulatory	A
Biomarkers of myocardial fibrosis (ST2, galectin-3)		
Additive risk stratification	Ambulatory	B
	Acute	A

Abbreviations: GDMT, guideline-directed medical therapy; HF, heart failure; LOE, level of evidence.
From Yancy CW, Jessup M, Bozkurt B, et al. 2013 ACCF/AHA guideline for the management of heart failure: a report of the American College of Cardiology Foundation/American Heart Associ-ation Task Force on Practice Guidelines. Circulation 2013;128(16):1810–52.

Table 3
Other causes of elevated BNP

Cardiac	Noncardiac
HF, including RV syndromes	Advancing age
ACS	Anemia
Heart muscle disease, including LVH	Renal failure
Valvular heart disease	Pulmonary causes: obstructive sleep apnea, severe pneumonia, pulmonary hypertension
Pericardial disease	Critical illness
AF	Bacterial sepsis
Myocarditis	Severe burns
Cardiac surgery Cardioversion	Toxic-metabolic insults, including cancer chemotherapy and envenomation

Abbreviation: ACS, acute coronary syndrome; AF, atrial fibrillation; HF, heart failure; LVH, left ventricular hypertrophy; RV, right ventricular.

From Yancy CW, Jessup M, Bozkurt B, et al. 2013 ACCF/AHA guideline for the management of heart failure: a report of the American College of Cardiology Foundation/American Heart Association Task Force on Practice Guidelines. Circulation 2013;128(16):1810–52.

tool assesses the ejection fraction, filling pressures, wall thickness and wall motion, as well as valvular function. The value in this test is due to its low rates of false-positive and false-negative readings. Most patients are able to tolerate the test, and it gives practitioners a wealth of information to either confirm the diagnosis or rule it out. In addition, this test is helpful when a known diagnosis of heart failure exists and the clinical situation warrants an understanding of any changes of the disease that may have taken place from the last time an echocardiogram was performed.[13,17]

Chest radiography
Radiography of the chest is commonly performed in patients with suspected heart failure. Although it is not a good independent predictor for heart failure as a whole, a chest radiograph may show evidence of heart failure signs, such as cardiomegaly, intravascular congestion, and pleural effusions. What is most helpful with the chest radiograph is the evaluation to rule out other causes of why patients may have symptoms consistent with heart failure. It may also aid the practitioner in evaluating other comorbidities, which may also be present during a heart failure exacerbation (ie, pneumonia with heart failure, chronic obstructive pulmonary disease [COPD] with heart failure). It should be noted that, although treatment of heart failure is progressing, a chest radiograph may lag behind in showing clinical improvement. Although this is only one test that can be performed, it should be noted that physical examination and history are key components in determining the progression of either improvement of symptoms or worsening conditions.[18]

Electrocardiogram
The electrocardiogram (EKG) is another essential tool that can be used in heart failure. This assessment allows for evaluation of assessing rate, rhythm, and any structural changes that would suggest an alteration in its function. An examination of the EKG can reveal hypertrophy of atria and ventricles, any evidence of ischemic conditions present or evolving, and any evidence of an arrhythmia that could coincide with heart failure (ie, atrial fibrillation, ventricular arrhythmia)[19] (**Table 4**).

Table 4
Noninvasive imaging: American College of Cardiology Foundation/American Heart Association guidelines

Recommendation	LOE
Acute, new-onset HF suspected: chest radiograph	C
2D echo with Doppler for initial evaluation	C
Repeat EF measurement in patients with HF with significant change in clinical status or who have had treatment that might affect cardiac function or for consideration of device therapy (ICD or biventricular pacemaker)	C
Noninvasive imaging to detect myocardial ischemia and viability reasonable in HF and CAD	C
Viability assessment reasonable before revascularization in patients with HF with CAD	B
Radionuclide ventriculography or MRI useful for assessing LVEF and volume	C
MRI reasonable when assessing myocardial infiltration or scar	B
LV function not routinely reassessed	B

Abbreviations: CAD, coronary artery disease; ICD, implantable cardioverter-defibrillator; LOE, level of evidence; LV, left ventricular; LVEF, left ventricular ejection fraction.
From Yancy CW, Jessup M, Bozkurt B, et al. 2013 ACCF/AHA guideline for the management of heart failure: a report of the American College of Cardiology Foundation/American Heart Association Task Force on Practice Guidelines. Circulation 2013;128(16):1810–52.

Goals for Treatment

Although there are different drug therapies and interventions for patients with heart failure, the overall goals for treatment remain simple. In general, the primary goal is to improve the symptoms and quality of life for all patients with heart failure. It is also the intent to prolong life by slowing the progression of disease and any other contributing diseases that patients may have. The relief of circulatory congestion and increased tissue perfusion is key as well as reducing vasoconstriction in the innovation of the activation of the RAAS in the SNS. In addition, medical therapy attempts to inhibit the progressive enlargement in remodeling of the ventricles, thus, reducing the overload of the cardiovascular system.

Although medical and interventional therapies are very helpful, key fundamental patient education, adherence, and proper referral to specialists are also components of success. It will be important for the practitioner to recognize when patients' conditions are worsening or problems occur and refer those patients to specialized care when it is needed. This is especially true and referral to heart failure clinics for consideration of devices, such as ventricular assist devices and even heart transplantation. This team effort in the care of patients leads to greater success and outcomes.

Clinical Management

The clinical management for patients with heart failure is multifaceted and complex. Although care is made to make sure that patients improve their quality of life and slow the progression of disease, ongoing clinical evaluations must occur to determine the level of failure patients may be developing. A helpful tool in the assessment of patients with heart failure is the joint American College of Cardiology Foundation (ACCF) and American Heart Association's (AHA) staging for classification of heart failure. This staging evaluates patients relative to their risk for heart failure as well as structural disease that may or may not be present. Stage A starts for those individuals who are at high risk for heart failure but do not exhibit any structural heart disease or symptoms related to heart failure. The stages increase all the way to stage D and change their level of involvement based on the amount of disease patients may have.

In conjunction with the ACCF/AHA's staging, the New York Heart Association (NYHA) established a functional classification for those patients with heart failure. These classifications have to do with the overall physical ability and function of patients' daily activities as well as symptoms, and both association tables take a complementary approach to the management of patients (**Table 5**).[1]

It is important to note that treatment with medications for heart failure is determined algorithmically by the level of classification and staging patients may have. All patients, unless clinically contraindicated, should be initiated on angiotensin-converting enzyme (ACE) inhibitor and beta-blocker therapy. These drugs shall be titrated up as needed for maintenance of blood pressure and heart rate control. As the disease progresses and symptoms continue, additional medications will be added to improve overall function, symptoms, and reduction of morbidity and mortality. The clinician must take care in determining which medications to use, while monitoring for any potential adverse effects, decline in renal function, or worsening of comorbid diseases.[1]

Drug Therapies

A listing of the more commonly used drugs per class is listed as well as therapies (**Tables 6** and **7**).

Table 5
Staging and classification of heart failure

	ACCF/AHA Stage		NYHA Functional Classification
A	At high risk for HF but without structural heart disease or symptoms of HF	None	
B	Structural heart disease but without signs or symptoms of HF	I	No limitation of physical activity HF symptoms not caused by ordinary physical activity
C	Structural heart disease with prior or current symptoms of HF	I	No limitation of physical activity HF symptoms not caused by ordinary physical activity
		II	Slight limitation of physical activity Comfortable at rest, but HF symptoms from ordinary physical activity
		III	Marked limitation of physical activity; comfortable at rest, HF symptoms caused by less than ordinary activity
		IV	Unable to carry on any physical activity without HF symptoms, or symptoms at rest
D	Refractory HF requiring specialized interventions	IV	Unable to carry on any physical activity without HF symptoms, or symptoms at rest

Abbreviation: HF, heart failure.
From Yancy CW, Jessup M, Bozkurt B, et al. 2013 ACCF/AHA guideline for the management of heart failure: a report of the American College of Cardiology Foundation/American Heart Association Task Force on Practice Guidelines. Circulation 2013;128(16):1810–52; with permission.

Table 6 Commonly used drug classes and names	
Drug Class	**Common Drugs Used**
ACE inhibitors	Captopril, lisinopril, ramipril, enalapril
ARBs	Losartan, valsartan, candesartan
Aldosterone antagonists	Spironolactone
β-blockers	Bisoprolol, carvedilol, metoprolol
Digitalis	Digoxin (HFrEF)
Diuretics	Furosemide, torsemide, hydrochlorothiazide, bumetanide
Vasodilators	Isosorbide dinitrate/hydralazine
Statins	Patients with recent/remote history of CAD
ARNI	In place of ACE or ARB, sacubitril-valsartan only approved
Ivabradine	Used in conjunction with maximally tolerated β-blocker

Abbreviations: ARBs, angiotensin receptor blockers; ARNI, angiotensin-receptor neprilysin inhibitor; CAD, coronary artery disease.

Table 7 Therapies for heart failure	
Severity of HF	**Treatment Options**
Stage B, class I	ACE inhibitor or ARB
	β-blocker
Stage C, class I–IV	ACE inhibitor and/or ARB (I–IV)
	β-blocker (I–IV)
	Diuretic (II–IV)
	ARNI (II–III)
	Ivabradine (II–IV)
	Aldosterone antagonist (II–IV)
	Isosorbide dinitrate/hydralazine (I–IV)
	Digoxin (II–IV)
	CRT, ICD (II–III)
Stage D, class IV	All stage C treatments
	Inotropic agents, vasodilators
	Experimental drugs/surgery
	ICD deactivation
	Transplant
	MCS
	Palliative care,
	hospice

Abbreviations: ARB, angiotensin receptor blocker; ARNI, angiotensin-receptor neprilysin inhibitor; CRT, cardiac resynchronization therapy; MCS, mechanical circulatory support.
From Yancy CW, Jessup M, Bozkurt B, et al. 2013 ACCF/AHA guideline for the management of heart failure: a report of the American College of Cardiology Foundation/American Heart Association Task Force on Practice Guidelines. Circulation 2013;128(16):1810–52; and Yancy CW, Jessup M, Bozkurt B. 2016 ACC/AHA/HFSA focused update on new pharmacological therapy for heart failure: an update of the 2013 ACCF/AHA guideline for the management of heart failure. A report of the American College of Cardiology/American Heart Association Task Force on Clinical Practice Guidelines and the Heart Failure Society of America. J Am Coll Cardiol 2016;68(13):1476–88.

Angiotensin-converting enzyme inhibitors

ACE inhibitors are a standard of treatment. Multiple trials related to the use of ACE inhibitors show that this class of drugs in patients with heart failure leads to improvement in patients' symptoms, reduction in hospitalizations, and overall increase in survival rate. Because of this ACE inhibitor should be considered a gold standard of treatment of those patients with heart failure, especially those with HFrEF.

There are multiple agents to choose from; most agents used initially have been linked to randomized clinical trials. ACE inhibitors should be used initially before the initiation of beta-blocker therapy. The drug can be started at low doses to ensure tolerance of the medication and then titrated up for maximum performance. Medications, such as enalapril (Vasotec), captopril (Capoten), lisinopril (Prinivil, Zestril), and several others, can be used for treatment. Practitioners should be aware of the potential side effects that include hypotension, a reduction in renal filtration rate, decreased glomerular filtration rate, hyperkalemia, angioedema, and costs. Periodic monitoring of renal function is key in the use of ACE inhibitors.[1,20]

Angiotensin receptor blockers

Like ACE inhibitors, angiotensin receptor blockers (ARBs) are also a treatment of choice should the practitioner not be able to use ACE inhibitors. Like ACE inhibitors, angiotensin II receptor blockers work by blocking the reading angiotensin aldosterone system. This blockade improves overall morbidity and mortality in patients with heart failure and has been shown to reduce hospitalizations. It is an acceptable alternative for those patients who are not able to take ACE inhibitors. These medications reduce the stimulation of angiotensin II. In patients with HFrEF with current orb symptoms that have been in existence and are intolerant to ACE inhibitors because of cough, ARBs are an acceptable alternative. Concomitant use of ACE inhibitors and ARBs is contraindicated. Although most research trials related to heart failure have shown a reduction in morbidity and mortality with the use of ACE inhibitors, less research has been shown with ARBs. It is likely thought that the mechanism of action a similar; thus, it would be expected that the same or close to similar results would exist with the use of ARBs. Like ACE inhibitors, lower-dose medications are started then titrated up for maximum performance. There is no evidence to show that increasing doses of ARBs reduces overall mortality more than low dose.[1,20]

β-Adrenergic receptor blockers

Beta-blockers are a first-line treatment in heart failure. There are several mechanisms that may have a positive effect and impact on heart failure. There seems to be an overall reduction in the direct impact of catecholamine on the myocardium. Beta-blockers also seem to restore the receptiveness in responsiveness of the beta-receptors. In addition, the drugs help mediate the heart rate by lowering it, which gives beneficial time for greater filling inefficiency of what is already a reduced ejection fraction. They also have an impact and role on levels of vasoconstrictive properties. In patients with ischemic cardiomyopathies, the medications can improve the ability of the heart's myocardial supply and demand mismatches. A role in the antiarrhythmic properties that may occur in patients with arrhythmias is also of benefit. There is also evidence to suggest that beta-blockers reduce the incidence of a likelihood of atrial fibrillation. The most commonly used beta-blockers are bisoprolol (Monocor, Zebeta), carvedilol (Coreg), and metoprolol (Lopressor). Patients are normally started on the lowest dose of the drug and slowly titrated up based on heart rate and blood pressure response.[1]

Contraindications for the use of beta-blockers include those patients who may have second- or third-degree AV block, heart rates less than 50 beats per minute (bpm), hypotension, and those individuals who have a history of asthma. Patients with COPD are not contraindicated for taking beta-blockers. However, care should be given in those individuals to ensure that bronchospasm does not occur.

Hydralazine and nitrates
The use of hydralazine and nitrates is indicated for those patients who have stage C, class I to IV heart failure. There is supporting evidence to show that this combination of drugs provides a reduction in mortality and symptomatic relief in patients with a reduced ejection fraction. The use of hydralazine, which acts as an arterial vasodilator, along with the venous vasodilatation effects of nitrates, gives optimal reduction and preload and afterload effects. This can also reduce filling pressures, which may have a role in cardiac remodeling.

Indications for use of hydralazine and nitrates are for patients with HFrEF. It is specifically indicated for black patients who have NYHA class III to IV heart failure and left ventricular ejection fractions less than 40% who have maximized therapy of their ACE inhibitors and beta-blocker therapy. It is also an alternative for those individuals who are unable to take ACE inhibitors or ARBs because of renal function and/or hypotension.[1]

Diuretics
Diuretics are a class of drugs that are a foundation for the treatment of volume overload and heart failure. The major indication for use of this medication is to relieve the symptoms associated with heart failure, which is volume overload to the lower extremities, congestive symptoms with pulmonary involvement, and elevated jugular venous pressures. Although diuretics are shown to relieve the symptomatic problems related to heart failure, no clinical studies have been done to evaluate any reduction in mortality or morbidity. Although the use of these medications is important for patients' overall quality of life, they should be used in conjunction with modifications in diet and as these are sodium intake equal contributors to the patients' overall volume status.[1,21]

Although the use of diuretics is widespread in the treatment of heart failure, it does have its limitations. Care must be given to patients, especially those who have chronic kidney disease. Regular evaluation of blood urea nitrogen and serum creatinine should be a normal regimen to ensure the use of diuretics is not injuring the kidneys.

The initial treatment of diuretics normally starts with furosemide or torsemide as possible options. These loop diuretics are commonly used and can be adjusted readily. The adjustment is determined based on the response the initial dosing creates and whether or not the patients' renal function has been impaired. It should be noted that, despite increased doses of diuretics with limited production or increases in urine output, the drug should be stopped and an alternative started. In addition to loop diuretics, aldosterone antagonists, such as spironolactone, can be added to therapy. In addition to monitoring of renal function, the practitioner should pay particular attention to any electrolyte imbalances that may occur, especially with hypokalemia and hypomagnesaemia.[21]

Angiotensin II receptor blocker/neprilysin inhibitor
Angiotensin II receptor blockers have widely been known to reduce morbidity and mortality in those patients with heart failure. A newer drug that combines angiotensin II receptor blocker along with the addition of neprilysin, when inhibited, increases the level of brain natriuretic peptides and is now used for those patients with HFrEF. This combination medication acts to selectively bind and prevent the formation of angiotensin II along with increasing levels of BNPs. Sacubitril-valsartan (Entresto) is the only approved medication and is indicated for those patients who have NYHA class

II to IV heart failure. This medication would be used in place of ACE inhibitors or ARBs as part of the component of therapy for heart failure. Patients should not be on this medication and an ACE or ARB together. Those patients wanting to switch from a pure ACE or ARB to the newer therapy should have a 36-hour washout period before initiating treatment.[20,22–24]

There are other considerations that should be made if patients are placed on angiotensin II receptor blocker/neprilysin inhibitors (ARNIs). Contraindications to this drug are hypersensitivity, those with history of angioedema or reaction from ACE or ARB therapy, and those patients with diabetes who are placed on aliskiren. It should also be noted that adjustments in patients' diuretic might be needed given that this drug will have a slow, ongoing diuretic activity.[22,24,25]

Ivabradine
Ivabradine (Corlanor) is a sinus node selective inhibitor, which has been shown to reduce hospital admissions and death from patients with HFrEF. The medication acts by reducing the sinus rate on the "funny pacemaker" at the sinus node. Some patients benefit with slower heart rates to improve filling times and maximizing ejection fraction. Some patients with heart failure will exhibit higher-than-normal resting heart rates, thus, lowering the ability of maximum filling pressures for an already week pumping system. Although beta-blockers also decreased heart rate and improve clinical outcomes, so too does ivabradine by inhibiting the selective sinoatrial pacemaker and prolonging the depolarization phase. Blockade or modulation of the f-current allows for a slowing of the overall heart rate.[20,26]

Indications for this medication are for those patients who have symptomatic, chronic, stable systolic heart failure and left ventricular ejection fraction that is less than 35% and have resting sinus rhythms of 70 bpm or more. It should be noted that patients should already be on ACE inhibitors or an ARB in addition to ivabradine.

Contraindications to this medication are those patients who are exhibiting an acute decompensated heart failure condition, at pressures less than 90 mm Hg systolic, sick sinus syndrome, sinus block, or third-degree AV block unless patients have a functioning demand pacemaker inserted. Those patients with hepatic failure, impairment, or those medications that also use CYP34A need to be carefully considered before being placed on the medication. The most adverse effect would be symptomatic bradycardia; however, this was not seen very often in clinical studies. Visual side effects may also occur, and transient brightness in patients' visual fields or phosphines should be evaluated.[27]

It should be noted that both ARNI therapy and ivabradine are started when both beta-blockers and ACE inhibitors have been done before the initiation of these new medications or if there is a contraindication for patients being on beta-blockers or ACE. Furthermore, maximal therapy should be achieved before starting these newer medications. [20,28]

Lifestyle Modifications

In addition to the medical therapies listed earlier, it is important to also implement lifestyle modifications. Although there has been great advances in success in pharmacologic therapy, the ultimate success of patients being able to stabilize their heart failure lies within their ability to control outside factors that have significant impact on their comorbidities and overall well-being.

Weight and fluid monitoring
It is important to emphasize to every patient the importance of a daily routine of monitoring their weight. A reliable scale along with daily documentation of their weight is

key. Patients should be educated regarding the importance of recording their daily weight at the same time, preferably in the morning, as well as watching for any evidence of increased swelling in the feet, legs, waste, or other signs of fluid retention. A gain of greater than 2 lb over a 24-hour period or greater than 3 lb per week should alert patients to make modifications in their daily diuretic dose and alert their clinician of this change. Fluid intake for these types of patients should be limited to 2 L/d or less.[1]

Sodium restriction and diet
The AHA recommends that sodium restriction be limited to less than 3000 mg per day for patients who have ACCF/AHA stage A or B heart failure. Individuals with stage C or D should be limited to less than 1500 mg per day. These limitations may prevent further volume overload, and individuals with sodium diets that are higher tend to become unresponsive to diuretics.[1]

Blood pressure management
Strict monitoring of blood pressure is critical in the management of heart failure. Hypertension is the most modifiable factor in the prevention of heart failure exacerbations, both HFrEF and HFpEF. Daily monitoring of blood pressure by patients should be part of their regimen, and education regarding adherence to their prescribed medications is paramount.[1]

Activity and exercise
A regular exercise routine of 3 to 5 days a week for up to 30 minutes can significantly improve patients' overall success with heart failure. This routine has proven to improve all-cause mortality and cardiovascular disease mortality and reduce hospitalizations related to heart failure. A decline in patients' overall activity may indicate progression of heart failure. Encouragement of record keeping will help ensure compliance to this therapy.[1]

Additional therapies Additional therapies are also options, as patients' heart failure stages decline. As patients develop stage C HFrEF, some individuals may benefit by certain interventions. These interventions may include cardiac resynchronization therapy, insertion of an in implantable cardiac defibrillator, in some individuals may benefit from revascularization of coronary artery disease or valvular disease. Some individuals may be consideration for heart transplant or left ventricular assist devices. As patients develop within this stage it is important to refer to the individual to an advanced heart failure clinic for consideration of the options.[1] **(Table 8)**

End of Life and Palliative Care
A 77-year-old man who has a ACC/NYHA classification of C/IV presents to the hospital with a refractory heart failure exacerbation, increased shortness of breath, increased tightness to his extremities that are not responsive to high-dose diuretics, in multiple episodes of nonsustained ventricular tachycardia with multiple implantable cardioverter-defibrillator shocks administered. The patient's quality of life has been extremely limited over the last 3 to 6 months, and he is relegated to sitting in a chair and sleeping in a recliner with his head fully elevated. He states that he is at a point where he does not think that he has anymore to give or live for. The resting blood pressure is 90/58 mmHg, pulse is 100 bpm, respiratory rate is 26 bpm, and oxygen saturation is 92% on room air. He exhibits rales halfway up his lung fields, at 3+ pitting edema to his extremities.

Table 8
Goals of heart failure management per New York Heart Association stages

Stage A	Stage B	Stage C: HFpEF	Stage C: HFrEF	Stage D
Goals: • Heart-healthy lifestyle • Prevent vascular, coronary disease • Prevent LV structural abnormalities	Goals: • Prevent HF symptoms • Prevent further cardiac remodeling	Goals: • Control symptoms • Improve HRQOL • Prevent hospitalization • Prevent mortality	Goals: • Control symptoms • Patient education • Prevent hospitalization • Prevent mortality	Goals: • Control symptoms • Improve HRQOL • Reduce hospital admissions • Establish patients' end-of-life goals
Drugs: • ACEI or ARB in appropriate patients for vascular disease or DM • Statins as appropriate	Drugs: • ACEI or ARB as appropriate • Beta-blockers as appropriate	Strategies: • Identification of comorbidities	Drugs for routine use: • Diuretics for fluid retention • ACEI or ARB • Beta-blockers • Aldosterone antagonists	Options: • Advance care measures • Heart transplant • Chronic inotropes • Temporary or permanent MCS • Experimental surgery or drugs • Palliative care and hospice • ICD deactivation
		Treatment: • Diuresis to relieve symptoms of congestion • Follow guideline driven for comorbidities, for example, HTN, AF, CAD, DM	Drugs for use in selected patients: • Hydralazine/isosorbide dinitrate • ACEI or ARB • Digitalis	
			In selected patients: • CRT • ICD • Revascularization or valvular surgery as appropriate	

Abbreviations: ACEI, ACE inhibitor; AF, atrial fibrillation; CAD, coronary artery disease; CRT, cardiac resynchronization therapy; DM, diabetes mellitus; HRQOL, health-related quality of life; HTN, hypertension; ICD, implantable cardioverter-defibrillator; MCS, mechanical circulatory support.

Adapted from Yancy CW, Jessup M, Bozkurt B, et al. 2013 ACCF/AHA guideline for the management of heart failure: a report of the American College of Cardiology Foundation/American Heart Association Task Force on Practice Guidelines. Circulation 2013;128(16):e240–327.

Despite extensive therapy and sometimes intervention for patients with heart failure, the disease progresses and patients develop refractory heart failure. Those patients with ACC/AHA stage D and NYHA class III or IV heart failure may never improve and have poor baseline symptoms even at rest. It is when these extreme limitations in physical activity coupled with symptoms at rest and extensive medical therapy that patients reach an end point. Although difficult, it is incumbent on the practitioner to have serious discussions with patients and their families about end-of-life and palliative care measures. Decisions regarding code status as well as inactivation of implantable defibrillators should be done in advance to respect the wishes of patients. In addition, it may be worthwhile for patients to consider medical power of attorney so that no situation is encountered should patients become incapacitated to make a decision on their own. In addition to conversations with patients and their families, a joint discussion with other members of the team should also commence.

SUMMARY

Heart failure is a complex disease with many contributing factors that make the management complicated and multifaceted. With careful examination, collaboration, and education to both patients and other key stakeholders, the disease can be appropriately managed. Overall goals are directed toward prolonging life, improving adherence, and lengthening survival rates. Frank discussions with patients on expectations and limitations must be done to achieve realistic goals, and eventually preparing for end-of-life discussions is paramount.

REFERENCES

1. WRITING COMMITTEE MEMBERS, Yancy CW, Jessup M, et al. 2013 ACCF/AHA guideline for the management of heart failure: a report of the American College of Cardiology Foundation/American Heart Association Task Force on Practice Guidelines. Circulation 2013;128(16):e240–327.
2. Go AS, Mozaffarian D, Roger VL, et al. Heart disease and stroke statistics- 2014 update: a report from the American Heart Association. Circulation 2014;129(3): e28–292.
3. Prevention, C. f. Centers for Disease Control and Prevention. Division for Heart Disease and Stroke Prevention; 2016. Available at: https://www.cdc.gov/DHDSP/data_statistics/fact_sheets/fs_heart_failure.htm. Available August 28, 2016.
4. Mozzaffarian D, Benjamin EJ, Go AS, et al. Heart disease and stroke statistics- 2015 update: a report from the American Heart Association. Circulation 2015; 131:e29–322.
5. Eichorn EJ, Bristow MR. Medical therapy can improve the biological properties of the chronically failing heart: a new era in the treatment of heart failure. Circulation 1996;94(9):e2285–96.
6. Wong CY, Chaudhry SI, Desai MM, et al. Trends in comorbidity, disability, and polypharmacy in heart failure. Am J Med 2011;124(2):136–43.
7. Braunwald E. Heart failure. J Am Coll Cardiol 2013;1:1–20.
8. Farmakis D, Parissis J, Lekakis J, et al. Acute heart failure: epidemiology, risk factors, and prevention. Rev Esp Cardiol (Engl Ed) 2015;68:245–8.
9. Van Duersen VM, Urso R, Laroche C, et al. Co-morbidities in patients with heart failure: an analysis of the European Heart Failure Pilot Survey. Eur J Heart Fail 2014;16:103–11.

10. Dzau V, Braunwald E. Resolved and unresolved issues in the prevention and treatment of coronary artery disease: a workshop consensus statement. Am Heart J 1991;121:1244–63.
11. Carlson KJ, Lee DC, Goroll AH, et al. An analysis of physicians' reasons for prescribing long-term digitalis therapy in outpatients. J Chronic Dis 1985;38(9):733–9.
12. Di Bari M, Pozzi C, Cavallini MC, et al. The diagnosis of heart failure in the community. Comparative validation of four sets of criteria in unselected older adults: the ICARe Dicomano Study. J Am Coll Cardiol 2004;44(8):1601–8.
13. Shamsham F, Mitchell J. Essentials of the diagnosis of heart failure. Am Fam Physician 2000;61:1319–28.
14. Cowie MR, Collinson PO, Dargie H, et al. Recommendations on the clinical use of B-type natriuretic peptide testing (BNP or NTproBNP) in the UK and Ireland. Br J Cardiol 2010;17:76–80.
15. Cowie MR. Recent developments in the management of heart failure. Practitioner 2012;256:25–9.
16. Rehman SU, Januzzi JL. Natriuretic peptide testing in primary care. Curr Cardiol Rev 2008;4:300–8.
17. Dosh S. Diagnosis of heart failure in adults. Am Fam Physician 2004;70:2145–52.
18. Hobbs FDR, Doust J, Mant J, et al. Diagnosis of heart failure in primary care. Heart 2010;96(21):1773–7.
19. Davie AP, Francis CM, Love MP, et al. Value of the electrocardiogram in identifying heart failure due to left ventricular systolic dysfunction. BMJ 1996;312:222.
20. Yancy CW, Jessup M, Bozkurt B, et al. 2016 ACC/AHA/HFSA focused update on new pharmacological therapy for heart failure: an update of the 2013 ACCF/AHA guideline for the management of heart failure. A report of the American College of Cardiology/American Heart Association Task Force on Clinical Practice Guidelines and the Heart Failure Society of America. J Am Coll Cardiol 2016;68(13):1476–88.
21. Rich MW. Pharmacotherapy of heart failure in the elderly: adverse events. Heart Fail Rev 2012;17(4–5):589–95.
22. Claggett B, Packer M, McMurray JJ, et al. Estimating the long term treatment benefits of sacubitril-valsartan. N Engl J Med 2015;373(23):2289–90.
23. Corporation, N. P. ENTRESTO (sacubitril and valsartan) tablets: prescribing information. East Hanoveer (NJ): Novartis Pharmaceutical Corporation; 2015.
24. Prenner SB, Shah SJ, Yancy CW. Role of angiotensin-neprilysin inhibition in heart failure. Curr Atheroscler Rep 2016;18(8):48.
25. McMurray JJ, Packer M, Desai AS, et al. Angiotensin-neprilysin inhibition versus enalapril in heart failure. N Engl J Med 2014;371(11):993–1004.
26. Savelieva I, Camm AJ. I f inhibition with ivabradine: electrophysiological effects and safety. Drug Saf 2008;31(2):95–107.
27. Amgen I. Corlanor (ivabradine): prescribing information. Thousand Oaks (CA): Amgen, Inc; 2015.
28. Swedberg K, Komajda M, Böhm M, et al. Ivabradine and outcomes in heart failure (SHIFT): a radomised placebo-controlled study. Lancet 2010;376(9744):875–85.

Ischemic Heart Disease

Evaluating for Potential Disease in the Previously Undiagnosed, Those Experiencing Angina, and in Those with Stable Disease

Craig Hricz, MPAS, PA-C[a,b],*

KEYWORDS

- Ischemic heart disease • Stress testing • Coronary artery disease
- Medical management

KEY POINTS

- Determining the appropriate modality for evaluating the patient with potential or existing coronary artery disease is discussed.
- Understanding the advantages and limitations of the various coronary artery disease modalities allows the provider to select the appropriate test and maximize the accuracy of the results.
- The provider should be comfortable with how and when to assess for advancement of coronary artery disease in the patient with an established history.
- Once a diagnosis of coronary artery disease is established, the provider must use the latest recommendations to initiate appropriate medical therapy to slow progression of the disease and improve quality of life.
- The provider should be able to make appropriate adjustments to medical therapy and order the appropriate imaging modality for patients with longstanding coronary artery disease when there is a change in symptoms.

A 55-year-old man presents to the office for evaluation of chest pain. His electrocardiogram (ECG) is unremarkable; however, his described symptoms and his known risk factors make the provider concerned that this could be due to coronary artery disease (CAD). What is the most appropriate testing modality to order? What if the patient has known CAD and is experiencing anginal equivalent pains or has been without symptoms for an extended period? These are common scenarios that the primary care

Disclosure Statement: Nothing to disclose.
[a] School of Physician Assistant Studies, Massachusetts College of Pharmacy and Health Sciences, 1260 Elm Street, Manchester, NH 03101, USA; [b] Emergency Department, Wentworth-Douglass Hospital, 789 Central Avenue, Dover, NH 03820, USA
* School of Physician Assistant Studies, Massachusetts College of Pharmacy and Health Sciences, 1260 Elm Street, Manchester, NH 03101.
E-mail address: craig.hricz@mcphs.edu

Physician Assist Clin 2 (2017) 671–688
http://dx.doi.org/10.1016/j.cpha.2017.06.006
2405-7991/17/© 2017 Elsevier Inc. All rights reserved.

or physician assistant in cardiology encounters on a frequent basis. Having a comfortable knowledge of what diagnostic studies are available, how they are performed, and the basic indications and contraindications of each are essential to providing the patient with the most appropriate and accurate work-up. Once a diagnosis is established, the provider must be familiar with the recommendations for aggressive medical management to minimize further progression of disease.

NONINVASIVE STRESS TESTING MODALITIES: STRESSING METHODS

The following sections summarize the methods used to increase a patient's cardiac demand which, if cardiac in nature, should result in a reproduction in the patient's symptoms and ECG changes consistent with a coronary artery occlusion.

Exercise (Treadmill) Electrocardiogram Stress

Overview

The exercise stress test is the most widely used modality for stress testing. The test can be performed by having the patient walk on a treadmill or by using a stationary bicycle while having ongoing ECG monitoring and blood pressure measurements during each stage of exercise. Both ECG and blood pressure monitoring are continued for at least 5 minutes after completion of exercise.[1] Several protocols have been developed for conducting the exercise stress test, with the Bruce protocol being the most widely used.[2] After completion, the results are analyzed using a prognostic scoring tool, the most popular being the Duke Treadmill Score, which determines the patient's level of risk as low, intermediate, or high.[3]

Indications

Exercise testing is most commonly used to assess for the possibility of CAD as the cause of concerning symptoms in a patient determined to be in the intermediate pre-test probability (PTP) category. Other uses include assessing a patient's response to therapeutic interventions, such as initiation of anti-ischemia therapies or after a revascularization procedure; assessing the possible need for a revascularization procedure in high-risk patients with known CAD; and as a preoperative screening when noncardiac surgery is planned in patients with known CAD or risk factors.[1]

Contraindications

Absolute contraindications include ongoing unstable angina, uncontrolled heart failure or hypertension or arrhythmia, symptomatic aortic stenosis, or severe pulmonary hypertension. The patient should also not have any ongoing pericarditis or myocarditis and, as with other stress modalities, pulmonary embolism and aortic dissection should be excluded from the differential as the cause of the symptoms. Relative contraindications include known left main coronary artery stenosis, outflow tract obstruction, extremes of heart rate, high-degree atrioventricular (AV) block, and abnormal potassium or magnesium levels. The study should be terminated if angina, near-syncope, cyanosis, sustained tachycardia, or significant ST-segment depressions or elevations occur.[1]

Pharmacologic (Chemical) Stress

Overview

This test involves the IV administration of either a vasodilator or a medication with positive inotropic or chronotropic effects in combination with an imaging modality (see later discussion) rather than exercise. Imaging is a necessary component to increase the sensitivity compared with just ECG monitoring. The patient should not eat for at least 2 hours before start of the test and should avoid caffeine and dipyridamole

(Persantine) before testing. Common vasodilators include adenosine, dipyridamole, and regadenoson (Lexiscan). Dobutamine offers both increased rate and contractility effects, whereas atropine provides only increased rate. Dobutamine is the drug of choice if echocardiography is the imaging modality of choice. A vasodilator should be chosen if radionuclide myocardial perfusion imaging (MPI) is planned. The choice of a specific vasodilating agent may be based on a combination of the personal preference of the cardiologist, as well as drug availability on formulary. The patient receives the selected drug via intravenous (IV) infusion. Atropine can be used in conjunction with dobutamine if a patient's target heart rate is not met. Cardiac and blood pressure monitoring occurs in the same manner as during the exercise test.[1,3,4]

Indications

The primary indication for a pharmacologic stress test is the patient's inability to exercise. An exercise stress is preferable to pharmacologic test in patients who are able to adequately exercise because it provides a stronger correlation between symptoms and exertional capacity. In addition to the indications listed for the exercise stress test, it is also used for patients who have a left bundle branch block (LBBB) or a ventricular paced rhythm.[1,3,4]

Contraindications

Vasodilators, specifically adenosine, are contraindicated in patients with systolic blood pressure of less than 90 mm Hg, with a second-degree or third-degree AV block without a pacemaker, or with sick sinus syndrome. These medications should be used with extreme caution in patients with well-controlled asthma or with significant bradycardia. The most common side effects are AV block, bronchospasm, flushing, chest pain, and dyspnea. Indications for ending the study are the same as those listed for the exercise stress. These medications can be quickly reversed with aminophylline; however, this is rarely necessary.[1]

NONINVASIVE STRESS TESTING MODALITIES: IMAGING METHODS

The following is a summary of the methods used to image the effects of increasing cardiac demand by the aforementioned stress modality (exercise or pharmacologic). Changes consistent with a coronary artery occlusion include wall motion abnormalities or areas of decreased perfusion. These changes generally occur within seconds of the development of myocardial ischemia and precede ECG changes.[5] An imaging modality is recommended for patients who

- Belong in the upper half of the intermediate PTP range
- Have an uninterpretable baseline ECG
- Have left ventricular ejection fraction (EF) of less than 50%
- Are undergoing any pharmacologic stress.[2,4]

An imaging modality is also generally recommended for women because ECG stress alone tends to have a high false-positive rate.[6]

Stress Echocardiography

Overview

An echocardiogram is performed before and after either an exercise or a pharmaceutical stress test. If the patient requires a pharmaceutical agent, dobutamine is the drug of choice.[4] Resting images may reveal a pericardial effusion, valvular disorders, or wall motion abnormalities consistent with a prior infarct. Stress images can reveal new wall motion abnormality in the area of reduced blood flow to the myocardium or subendocardium, and increased motion abnormalities in the area of a preexisting infarct. In addition, a stress-related decrease in the global EF can indicate that severe left main coronary artery stenosis or severe multivessel disease is present.[3,4] Echocardiography is generally widely available, avoids radiation exposure, is relatively inexpensive compared with other imaging modalities, and has equal sensitivity and specificity in both men and women.[4,6] Echocardiography can be enhanced with the use of IV contrast agents.

Indications
Echocardiogram is indicated for patients who belong in the middle to upper-end range of the intermediate PTP scale or for patients who require a dobutamine stress test.[2]

Contraindications
There are no absolute contraindications; however, results may be negatively affected by obesity, chronic lung disease, or significantly increased respiratory rate.[4]

Radionuclide Stress Myocardial Perfusion Imaging (Nuclear Stress)

Overview
This imaging modality requires a radioactive tracer injection, which is used to enhance visualization of wall motion abnormalities. If a pharmaceutical stress is required, a vasodilator such as adenosine or dipyridamole is preferred compared with dobutamine. Visualization of wall motion is performed at rest and during stress using either single-photon emission computed tomography (SPECT) or PET. The standard tracer used in an SPECT MPI is usually technetium-based (sestamibi [Cardiolite] or tetrofosmin), but thallium can also be used instead or in conjunction. A PET MPI is performed using a rubidium or ammonia-based radionuclide. The PET version has been less well studied than SPECT and has a more limited availability along with a higher cost; however, it has demonstrated higher diagnostic accuracy, especially in women and obese patients. In addition, PET MPI exposes the patient to lower doses of ionizing radiation. Both studies allow for evaluation of left ventricular function, including calculation of an EF and localized areas of myocardial thickening. PET MPI offers the ability to detect microvascular angina. Left ventricular wall motion abnormalities will generally need to be greater than 3% to 5% to be detected.[3–5]

Indications
SPECT or PET are indicated in patients with LBBB or ventricular pacing. PET is preferred when there is a desire to assess for myocardial viability after a myocardial infarction (MI). Either can be substituted for a stress echocardiogram in patients who have baseline ECG abnormalities.[3]

Contraindications
With the exception of pregnancy, there are no specific contraindications to MPI other than allergy to the pharmaceutical agents or the contraindications specific to exercise or pharmaceutical testing.

Computed Tomographic Coronary Angiography (Cardiac Computed Tomography Angiography)

Overview
Computed tomographic coronary angiography (CTCA) provides a detailed image of coronary artery calcifications (CACs) by combining thin slice computed tomography (CT) in conjunction with IV contrast injection. The more numerous the calcifications, the higher the likelihood that a patients symptoms are related to luminal narrowing. The images are used to calculate a CAC score, which can then be used to risk stratify

the patient. The amount and density of the calcifications is considered when calculating a CAC score, with the Agatston method being a commonly reported score. Agatston scores of lower than 10 equate to minimal calcifications and thus a low risk of an occlusive event. A score higher than 400 indicates extensive disease and is highly correlated to the patient having an occlusive event or requiring a coronary procedure in the near future. These CAC scores are usually calculated for each major vessel and as a total score. The CTCA is not able to adequately detect soft plaques composed of lipid cores, which may have thin caps prone to rupture and does not provide specific functional information regarding the patency of the vessel. The test has a very high negative predictive value but positive results must be followed up with additional testing such as a stress test or cardiac catheterization. For an adequate test, breath must be able to be held for 10 to 30 seconds and the heart rate should be regular and less than 65 beats per minute (bpm), which may require a beta-blocker.[4–8]

Indications
Patients who belong in the lower end of the intermediate PTP spectrum are ideal candidates, assuming there is no associated morbid obesity, arrhythmia, or heart rate higher than 65 despite beta-blocker administration. It is also appropriate for high-risk but asymptomatic women or for patients who have an inconclusive ECG or imaging stress test.[4,5]

Contraindications
This modality should be avoided in patients with compromised renal function, IV contrast allergies, elevated heart rate, nonregular rhythms, or significant obesity. Prior radiation exposures should be considered.[5]

Stress Cardiovascular MRI

Overview
The cardiac MRI is similar to CTCA in that it provides detailed anatomic images; however, it is somewhat inferior to CTCA with regard to visualization of the coronary arteries. This modality can provide information on ventricular function, valvular abnormalities, and infarction size, as well as myocardial perfusion when IV gadolinium and either a vasodilator or dobutamine are added. Limitations to cardiovascular magnetic resonance (CMR) include availability, cost, and that image quality is affected by movement artifact.[3,5,8]

Indications
Due to cost and limited availability or expertise, the CMR is usually not a first-line diagnostic modality for evaluation of CAD. It is a useful alternative to stress echocardiography if body habitus or lung disease limits visualization.[3,4,8]

Contraindications
CMR should not be performed in patients with pacemakers or other metallic devices or foreign bodies. The use of gadolinium should be avoid in patients with compromised renal function. Patients with claustrophobia may require sedation or may not be able to have the procedure at all due to the confining nature of the MRI.[8]

GENERAL CONSIDERATIONS

Exercise stress ECG should be the initial modality considered for patients on the lower end of the intermediate PTP spectrum and without baseline ECG abnormalities due to the following benefits:

- Simplicity

- Lower cost
- Higher availability
- Lack of radiation.

Imaging, either echocardiography or MPI, should be added in any of the following scenarios:

- Pharmacologic stress test is being used
- Patient has resting ECG abnormalities
- Patient is at higher end of the intermediate PTP
- Patient is a woman (in this case, it should be strongly considered).

The addition of an imaging modality improves the sensitivity in these individuals and offers the added benefit of localizing ischemia and providing information regarding other structures and overall function.[3]

With a better understanding of each of these modalities, the following sections discuss the approach to certain patients who may require an evaluation for possible or known CAD.

PATIENTS WITHOUT KNOWN DISEASE

In patients without known CAD, there are 3 questions that the practitioner needs to answer when considering the approach to a work-up:

1. What is the patient's PTP of CAD as the cause of chest pain?
2. What is the patient's exercise capability?
3. Are there any baseline ECG findings, underlying patient factors, or test availability constraints that will dictate which diagnostic modality should be used?[4]

Determining the pretest likelihood of CAD as the cause of chest pain in this previously undiagnosed population is best determined using a table similar to that recommended by the American College of Cardiology and American Heart Association ACC/AHA[2] (**Table 1**).

When using this table, typical angina is defined as having the following 3 traits[2]:

1. Substernal chest discomfort with a characteristic quality and duration
2. Discomfort that is triggered by exertion or emotional stress
3. Symptoms that are alleviated by rest or nitroglycerine.

Table 1
Pretest likelihood of coronary artery disease

Age (y)	Nonanginal Pain		Atypical Angina		Typical Angina	
	Men (%)	Women (%)	Men (%)	Women (%)	Men (%)	Women (%)
30–39	4	2	34	12	76	26
40–49	13	3	51	22	87	55
50–59	20	7	65	31	93	73
60–69	27	14	72	51	94	86

Adapted from Fihn SD, Gardin JM, Abrams J, et al. 2012 ACCF/AHA/ACP/AATS/PCNA/SCAI/STS guideline for the diagnosis and management of patients with stable ischemic heart disease: a report of the American College of Cardiology Foundation/American Heart Association Task Force on Practice Guidelines, and the American College of Physicians, American Association for Thoracic Surgery, Preventive Cardiovascular Nurses Association, Society for Cardiovascular Angiography and Interventions, and Society of Thoracic Surgeons. J Am Coll Cardiol 2012;60(24):e44–164.

Atypical angina is defined as having 2 of the 3 traits, whereas nonanginal pain has 1 or none of these traits. The predictive accuracy increases if any of the following are present: history of diabetes with fasting glucose greater than 140 mg/dL, cholesterol greater than 250 mg/dL, recent or active smoking, and Q-wave or ST-T-wave changes on ECG. Interestingly enough, hypertension and a family history of early ischemic heart disease did not demonstrate any additional accuracy in predicting CAD as the underlying cause of symptoms.[2] The calculated probability places the patient into 1 of 3 categories: low (<10%), intermediate (10%–90%), or high probability (>90%).[9] For those in the low probability category with an unremarkable ECG, no further testing is warranted. Patients who belong in the intermediate category require noninvasive diagnostic testing to assess for ischemia. It should be noted that another reported probability calculator gives men ages 30 to 39 years with nonanginal pain an 18% PTP; therefore, any man older than 30 years will always belong in the intermediate category at the very least.[4] High PTP patients are probably best served by having a cardiac catheterization.[10]

When the patient's PTP has been determined to be in the intermediate category requiring noninvasive testing, the next step is to determine the individual's exercise capacity. Ability to exercise will help to determine which testing modality is most appropriate. Exercise capacity is considered among the highest prognostic indicators of long-term risk.[2] Standardized exercise or activity questionnaires are available for this purpose; however, a less formal conversation with the patient is usually sufficient. If the patient reports the ability to "walk for more than 5 minutes on flat ground or up 1 to 2 flights of stairs without needing to stop," they should be able to perform an exercise stress test to a reasonable enough degree to provide reliable results.[3]

Finally, consider other factors that would dictate using one modality over another or require the addition of imaging to a standard exercise stress test. The following list is a summary of factors (see previous discussion of each modality) that can affect the interpretability of some modalities and require consideration when deciding on which modality to order[2–4]:

- Morbid obesity: consider stress radionuclide myocardial perfusion with PET, avoid coronary CT angiography (CTA)
- Bronchospasm or advanced lung disease history: avoid vasodilator stress with bronchospasm history, avoid coronary CTA with chronic lung disease if breath holding is limited
- Hypotension: avoid vasodilator stress
- Hypertension greater than 180 mm Hg: avoid dobutamine stress
- Renal insufficiency or failure: avoid CTCA or CMR with gadolinium
- Theophylline or significant caffeine use: hold for 48 hours and 12 hours, respectively, before vasodilator stress
- Digoxin use: stress with imaging modality needed
- Beta-blocker use: dobutamine stress may not adequately increase heart rate, hold for 48 hours
- Symptomatic aortic stenosis: avoid dobutamine
- ECG abnormalities
  - Sick sinus syndrome, high-degree AV block: avoid vasodilator stress
  - Frequent ventricular arrhythmias or rapid atrial fibrillation: avoid dobutamine
  - Left ventricular hypertrophy with associated ST-T abnormalities, LBBB, Wolff-Parkinson-White syndrome, resting ST depression greater than 1 mm: add

nuclear or echocardiography imaging to stress test without dobutamine or consider coronary CTA
- ○ LBBB or ventricular paced rhythms: use vasodilator radionuclide with SPECT or PET
- ○ Nonsinus rhythm or heart rate greater than 65 bpm after beta-blocker: avoid coronary CTA.

Local test availability, as well as radiology and cardiology expertise, may dictate which modality will be most appropriate.

When considering how urgently the selected test should be performed, the patient's symptoms should dictate the timeframe. Chest pain accompanied by 1 or more of the following symptoms is more highly associated with CAD:

- Exertional component
- Radiation to the arms or neck
- Diaphoresis
- Vomiting.

If these symptoms have been progressing in frequency or intensity, the possibility of noncompliance, inadequate treatment, or advancing disease should be considered. Indications for immediate emergency department referral include[11]

- Symptoms at rest
- Unstable vital signs
- ECG changes.

In patients whose symptoms are stable and other differential diagnoses have been excluded, outpatient stress testing is reasonable and should usually take place within 1 week. Validated clinical decision-making tools for chest pain complaints are very useful in the office or emergency department setting. The Marburg Heart Score developed by Bösner and colleagues can help determine the likelihood that the reported symptoms are indeed cardiac in nature by answering 5 simple questions related to the patient's known risk factors and description of symptoms. It has been validated to have a sensitivity near 90% if the patient has 3 or more points out of the 5 total and a negative predictive value in excess of 97% if the score is 2 or lower.[12] Another clinical decision tool, the HEART score developed by Barbra Backus, MD, PhD, predicts the likelihood of having a major adverse cardiac event within the next 6 weeks. A score of 4 or more out of 15 points has a 58% sensitivity and an 85% specificity for a cardiac event occurring within the next 6 weeks. A score of 3 or lower was associated with a less than 1% event rate.[13]

It should be noted that the National Institute for Health and Care Excellence, based in England, has recommended coronary angiography as the first-line modality for patients without known disease but who have a pretext probability of 61% to 90% and an abnormal resting ECG (pathologic Q-waves, LBBB, ST-segment abnormalities, or T-wave abnormalities). If the probability is 30% to 60%, an imaging stress is recommended, and if the probability is only 10% to 29%, CTCA is advised.[14]

PATIENTS WITH NEWLY DIAGNOSED DISEASE: MEDICAL MANAGEMENT

Once the diagnosis of atherosclerotic coronary disease has been made, immediate medical intervention should occur with the goals being to improve the patient's quality of life and minimize or prevent further progression of the disease. The following is a list of recommendations from the AHA/ACC that can be remembered using the mnemonic "ABCDE"[15]:

A. Aspirin, antianginals, and angiotensin-converting enzyme (ACE) inhibitors
B. Beta-blockers and blood pressure
C. Cholesterol and cigarettes
D. Diet, diabetes, and depression
E. Education and exercise.

Aspirin

Inhibiting platelet aggregation at plaque sites is very important for successful management of CAD. Aspirin is the most commonly used medication for this purpose and should be started in all patients diagnosed with CAD unless contraindicated. A dose of 81 mg daily provides adequate inhibition. The main side effect is the potential to develop gastric bleeding. Clopidogrel 75 mg daily should be substituted if an aspirin allergy exists; however, it has not shown any benefit in outcomes for patients with stable CAD and should not be combined with aspirin except in patients with an acute coronary syndrome.[2]

Antianginals

Short-acting nitrates should be added when a patient has persistent angina despite adequate beta-blocker dosing. Sublingual tablets or oral sprays are the most commonly used preparations and both are available at 0.4 mg per dose. Headache, hypotension, and lightheadedness are common side effects.[2]

Angiotensin-Converting Enzyme Inhibitors

ACE inhibitors are recommended for patients diagnosed with CAD who have diabetes or left ventricular dysfunction. They are also recommended in any patient who has had a MI and should be the second-line option for blood pressure management after beta-blockers. Cough and angioedema are the potential side effects. If an ACE inhibitor is not well tolerated, an angiotensin receptor blocker, such as losartan or valsartan, should be substituted.[2]

Blood Pressure and Beta-blockers

Attempts should be made to achieve a blood pressure of 130/80 mm Hg or lower in patients with CAD with 55 mm Hg being the minimal diastolic pressure. Blood pressure reduction improves mortality rates and anginal symptoms by decreasing oxygen demand, and can prevent or slow the development of left ventricular hypertrophy. A beta-blocker is the drug of choice for patients with CAD and is even recommended in patients without hypertension, if tolerated. Carvedilol, metoprolol succinate, and bisoprolol are examples of beta-blockers commonly used in the treatment of CAD and have demonstrated an improvement in the morbidity rates in these patients. Patients with severe asthma or chronic obstructive pulmonary disease (COPD) should not be prescribed beta-blockers. However, mild asthmatics may tolerate labetalol or carvedilol and individuals with mild COPD may tolerate atenolol or metoprolol. Fatigue and exacerbation of peripheral artery disease are the more common side effects and beta-blocker use should not be stopped abruptly if at all possible to avoid rebound hypertension. If beta-blockers are contraindicated or not well-tolerated, a calcium channel blocker such as amlodipine should be substituted.[2,16]

Cholesterol

Low-density lipoprotein (LDL) cholesterol should be lowered to less than 100 mg/dL in patients with CAD, and an attempt should be made to achieve less than 70 mg/dL for patients at very high risk. Simvastatin, pravastatin, and atorvastatin have all been studied extensively and can be effective. Side effects include elevated liver function tests, myalgias, and rhabdomyolysis. Once LDL has been addressed, an effort should be made to decrease triglyceride levels to less than 200 mg/dL and increase high-density lipoprotein (HDL) levels to higher than 40 mg/dL. Nicotinic acid is recommended for this purpose.[2]

Cigarettes

Smoking cessation should be strongly emphasized and patients should also be counseled on the importance of avoiding second-hand smoke. There are numerous options available to assist in smoking cessation but the process starts, and is most effective, when the provider educates the patient and family members on the negative impacts, assists in the development of a plan for cessation, and frequently follows-up with and encourages progress. Formal self-help programs or behavioral therapy sessions are good options. Pharmacologic options include the numerous nicotine replacement therapies available, as well as medications such as bupropion sustained-release and varenicline. Most patients will benefit from a combination of these interventions. Along similar lines, patients should be encouraged to avoid prolonged or excessive exposure to air pollution due to its oxidative and inflammatory effects.[2]

Diet

A body mass index of 18.5 to 24.9 kg/m^2 and a waist circumference less than 40 inches for men or 35 inches for women is recommended. Patient's should be encouraged to have a diet that emphasizes fruits, grains, vegetables, and lean meats while avoiding foods that are high in saturated fats, transfats, cholesterol, or sodium. Alcohol should be limited to 1 drink per day for women and no more than 2 per day for men. Small quantities of alcohol can increase HDL levels, lower insulin levels, increase insulin sensitivity, and provide some anti-inflammatory effects but large quantities on a regular basis have been shown to increase mortality.[2]

Diabetes

The goal of diabetes management for patients with CAD should be a hemoglobin A1c of 7% to 9%, ideally at the lowest end of this range, especially for younger individuals. The specific management of diabetes is beyond the scope of this article.[2]

Depression (Added to Mnemonic by this Author)

It is recommended that patients with CAD also be screened for depression due to a possible link between depression and poor outcomes. It also stands to reason that a depressed patient will have a lower compliance with the recommended therapies listed in this section. The Patient Health Questionnaire is the recommended screening tool. Medications, referral for counseling, or referral to a psychiatrist are all reasonable options if the screening is positive.[2]

Education

Explain the importance of strict medication, dietary, and lifestyle modification adherence in a manner that is understandable based on the patient's level of intelligence. Providing statistics from studies may also help to emphasize these points. The patient should also be instructed to report any new or worsening symptoms, as well as any medication issues such as side effects or cost that might delay appropriate care.[2]

Exercise

Regular exercise can reduce mortality and improve lifestyle in patients with CAD and should be strongly encouraged. Recommendations are for 30 to 60 minutes of moderate-intensity aerobic activity at least 5 days per week. In addition, some degree of muscle strengthening exercise should be encouraged for at least 2 days per week. An exercise stress test may be beneficial in determining the patient's physical work capacity. Medically supervised exercise programs (cardiac rehabilitation) or scheduled sessions with certified trainers are good ways to ensure compliance and achieve goals.[2]

Other

The World Health Organization and AHA recommend an annual influenza vaccine for patients with CAD.

PATIENTS WITH KNOWN DISEASE: STABLE VERSUS UNSTABLE ANGINA

In patients with known CAD, stable angina is generally defined as

- Deep, vague chest and/or arm pain occurring secondary to exertion or emotional stress
- Symptoms relieved in less than 5 minutes after cessation of activity or use of nitroglycerine.

An anginal equivalent is considered to be dyspnea on exertion without chest pain but with discomfort in 1 or more of the following areas

- Upper extremity
- Back
- Neck or jaw
- Epigastrium.

Other potential anginal equivalents are

- Unexplained nausea or vomiting
- Diaphoresis
- General fatigue
- Syncope.

Unstable angina refers to an exacerbation, either in severity or duration, of these symptoms with less exertion, no exertion, or requiring more nitroglycerine than what the patient has been previously accustomed to. Unstable angina may be associated with ECG changes such as ST depression or T-wave inversions but there should not be an elevation in cardiac biomarkers, which distinguishes unstable angina from a non-ST elevation MI.[17]

Patients who have been diagnosed with CAD require aggressive medical management (see previous discussion) and, depending on the severity of disease, may require percutaneous coronary intervention (PCI), such as angioplasty and stenting, or coronary artery bypass grafting (CABG). After diagnosis and appropriate treatment has been initiated, the patient should be followed by the primary care provider or cardiologist every 4 to 6 months for the first year and then annually thereafter.[2,17] If the patient's symptoms are stable, it is reasonable to consider a stress test to assess for possible subclinical advancement of occlusive disease. If testing is considered, it should be performed at least 5 years after CABG or at least 2 years after PCI.[3] In these

Table 2
Canadian Cardiovascular Society grading scale for angina pectoris

Class I	Usual physical activity (walking, climbing stairs) does not evoke angina, only strenuous or rapid work or recreation
Class II	Slight limitation of ordinary activities (walking 2 blocks, climbing 1 flight of steps) under normal circumstances, postprandial, in a cold or windy environment, in the morning, or during emotional stress
Class III	Marked limitation of ordinary activities under normal circumstances
Class IV	Unable to carry out any physical activity without angina or angina at rest

Adapted from Kaul P, Naylor CD, Armstrong PW, et al. Assessment of activity status and survival according to the Canadian Cardiovascular Society angina classification. Can J Cardiol 2009;25(7):e225–31.

circumstances any stress modality is appropriate, including stress ECG, assuming the criteria for the specific study are met.[9]

New or evolving angina or anginal equivalent symptoms require repeat testing and consideration of advancing medical therapies, as well as possible intervention therapy. The Canadian Cardiovascular Society (CCS) Grading Scale is commonly used to classify the severity of angina (**Table 2**).[18] **Table 3** summarizes the American College of Cardiology Foundation's recommendations for testing in these individuals.[9]

Patients with progressive angina or who have developed unstable angina should be evaluated for the possibility of having an interventional procedure, either PCI or CABG. Medical therapy in these patients should also be reassessed. Ensuring that the patient is prescribed all of the recommended therapies previously mentioned and is compliant should be the first step. Next, medications should be maximized to target goals. For

Table 3
Testing recommendations in patients with known coronary artery disease

Prior Test Results (Without Prior Revascularization)	Exercise ECG	Stress MPI	Stress Echocardiogram	Stress CMR	CTCA	Cardiac Catheterization
Normal exercise ECG	M	A	A	A	A	M
Normal stress imaging or nonobstructive disease on catheterization	M	A	A	A	R	M
Abnormal exercise ECG	R	A	A	A	A	A
Abnormal stress imaging	R	M	M	M	A	A
Obstructive disease on CTCA	M	A	A	A	R	A
Obstructive disease on catheterization	A	A	A	M	R	A
Abnormal CAC score (>100)	A	A	A	A	M	A
Prior revascularization	M	A	A	A	M	A

Abbreviations: A, appropriate; M, may be appropriate; R, rarely appropriate.
Adapted from Wolk MJ, Bailey SR, Doherty JU, et al. ACCF/AHA/ASE/ASNC/HFSA/HRS/SCAI/SCCT/SCMR/STS 2013 multimodality appropriate use criteria for the detection and risk assessment of stable ischemic heart disease. J Am Coll Cardiol 2014;63(4):380–406.

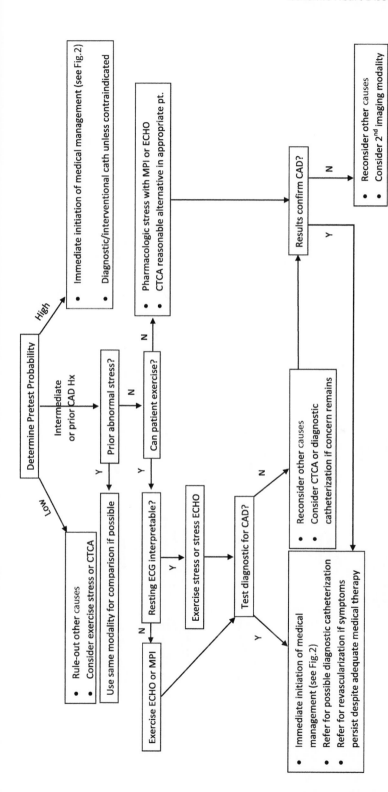

Fig. 1. Stable chest pain modality decision tree. cath, catheterization; ECHO, echocardiogram; Hx, history; pt, patient. (*Data from* Montalescot G, Udo S, Stephan A, et al. 2013 ESC guidelines on the management of stable coronary artery disease. Eur Heart J 2013;34(38):2949–3003; and Qaseem A, Fihn S, Williams S, et al. Diagnosis of stable ischemic heart disease: summary of a clinical practice guideline from the American College of Physicians/American College of Cardiology Foundation/American Heart Association/American Association for Thoracic Surgery/Preventive Cardiovascular Nurses Association/Society of Thoracic Surgeons. Ann Inter Med 2012;157(10):729–34.)

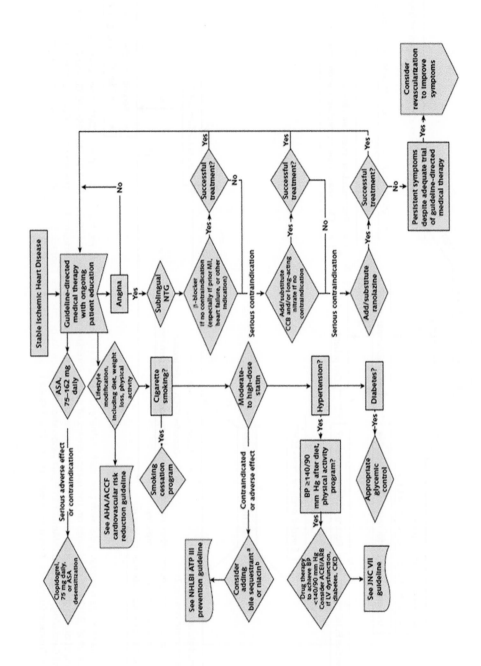

example, beta-blockers should be titrated not only to the blood pressure goals previously mentioned but also to a target heart rate of 50 to 60 bpm.[19] Consider having the patient use nitroglycerine in a preventative manner 5 to 10 minutes before activity. Finally, consider the addition of other medications.

Long-Acting Nitrates

Long-acting nitrates, such as isosorbide mononitrate tablets or nitroglycerine paste, are effective options and should be started at low doses and titrated as needed for symptom control. Patients should be advised to have a nitrate-free period of 10 to 14 hours per day to avoid developing a tolerance. As with short-acting nitrates, phosphodiesterase inhibitors should be strictly avoided within 24 hours of taking a long-acting nitrate (48 hours in the case of tadalafil) to avoid severe hypotension.[2]

Ranolazine

Ranolazine prevents the late influx of sodium into the myocardium and ultimately results in improved oxygen utilization within the tissue. Studies have shown improved exercise tolerance and decreased frequency of angina episodes while on the drug, as well as an improvement in glycemic control. The drug causes minimal changes to both heart rate and blood pressure and does not require dosage adjustments for sex, heart failure, or diabetes. Elderly patients or those with kidney disease or taking diltiazem, verapamil, aprepitant, erythromycin, fluconazole, simvastatin, or digoxin should be prescribed a low dose, not to exceed 500 mg twice daily. It should be avoided in patients with a prolonged QT interval, hepatic failure, or with the drugs itraconazole, ketoconazole, phenobarbital, carbamazepine, phenytoin, clarithromycin, rifampin, St. John's wort, or certain protease inhibitors. The main side effects are constipation, nausea, headache, and dizziness.[2]

Ivabradine

Ivabradine acts on the sinoatrial node to reduce heart rate, which allows for a longer diastolic period, ultimately resulting in increased oxygenation to the myocardium. It has been shown to improve exercise capacity and decrease anginal events compared with beta-blockers; however, it has shown no reduction in mortality rates or hospital admission rates; therefore, it is mostly used to improve patients' quality of life. With regard to chronic angina, ivabradine is generally only recommended for use in patients who also have a history of heart failure. It is contraindicated with the

◄─────────────────────────────────

Fig. 2. Guideline-directed medical therapy for patients with stable ischemic heart disease. ACCF, American College of Cardiology Foundation; ACEI, ACE inhibitor; ATP III, adult treatment panel III; ASA, aspirin; BP, blood pressure; CCB, calcium-channel blocker; CKD, chronic kidney disease; JNC VII, Seventh Report of the Joint National Committee on Prevention, Detection, Evaluation, and Treatment of High Blood Pressure; LV, left ventricular; NHLBI, National Heart, Lung, and Blood Institute. [a] The use of bile acid sequestrant is relatively contraindicated when triglyceride levels are 200 mg/dL or greater and is contraindicated when triglyceride levels are 500 mg/dL or greater. [b] Dietary supplement niacin must not be used as a substitute for prescription niacin. (*From* Qaseem A, Fihn S, Dallas P, et al. Management of stable ischemic heart disease: summary of a clinical practice guideline from the American College of Physicians/American College of Cardiology Foundation/American Heart Association/American Association for Thoracic Surgery/Preventive Cardiovascular Nurses Association/Society of Thoracic Surgeons. Ann Intern Med 2012;157(10):735–43.)

drugs listed for ranolazine and the primary side effect is transient visual disturbances.[2]

Alternative Treatment Modalities

Chronic angina that is refractory to maximized medical therapy and interventional therapy may benefit from several nontraditional treatment modalities. Enhanced external counterpulsation is a method that uses sequentially inflatable cuffs around the calves and thighs to increase venous return, resulting in an increased preload and ultimately an increase in the coronary artery perfusion pressure. Transmyocardial revascularization uses a laser to increase microvascular circulation and denervate ischemic myocardium. Spinal cord stimulation at the level of T1 has been shown to improve anginal pain, reduce the number of reported anginal events, and improve exercise duration and decrease ST depression events. These 3 modalities are class IIb recommendations. Acupuncture has been given a class III recommendation and is not currently recommended for the treatment of chronic angina. This is primarily due to a lack of studies. Other therapies in the class III (no benefit) category include estrogen, vitamin, or mineral supplementation; chelation therapy; and other agents, such as garlic and coenzyme Q10.[2]

PATIENTS WITH KNOWN DISEASE: STABLE ISCHEMIC HEART DISEASE

The primary emphasis for managing a patient with stable disease should be frequent attempts to reeducate and encourage strict adherence to the established plan to slow any advancement of the disease and lead to a longer period of a high quality of life. Communication at office visits or by telephone, email, or mailings can be used as continued reminders of the importance of medication compliance and smoking cessation, as well as adherence to the prescribed dietary and exercise recommendations.

The practitioner should regularly monitor blood pressure, lipids, and a hemoglobin A1c, if applicable, and maintain tight control by making dietary and medication adjustments. It is imperative for the practitioner to maintain his or her own education on the latest guidelines from the major organizations on these topics whenever they are released (**Figs. 1** and **2**). (See Craig Hricz's article, "Acute Coronary Syndrome: Care After a Patient Event and Strategies to Improve Adherence," in this issue.)

Regarding repeat stress testing, consideration should be given to when a noninvasive study is warranted and which modality is most appropriate. An alternative angina scoring system to the CCS angina scale mentioned earlier is the Seattle angina questionnaire (SAQ).[20] This tool may provide a more reproducible and sensitive way of quantifying patients' angina symptoms and quality of life, and can be a useful tool in determining when a patient with known disease requires repeat testing. In general, new symptoms or a worsening of chronic symptoms requires immediate evaluation. Patients who are at high risk (EF<50%, significant multivessel disease, history of diabetes) or who have had a prior silent ischemic event should have an exercise ECG performed at roughly 1-year intervals or a stress imaging modality at 2-year intervals. These timeframes may be lengthened depending on degree of concern and adequacy of medical and lifestyle interventions. Other indications for repeat testing are incomplete revascularization attempt, change in risk profile, or if a major surgery is being scheduled. Any of the previously discussed modalities can be used for reassessment, including a standardized exercise ECG test. If possible, it is advised to use the same modality that was initially used to diagnose the patient's disease. This allows for a more reliable comparison of findings. In patients who have undergone stenting or have vascular clips, CTCA results may be limited due to the amount of artifact that these devices may generate.[2]

REFERENCES

1. Practice points: pharmacologic and exercise stress tests. Available at: https://www. asnc.org/files/Practice%20Resources/Practice%20Points/PPStressTests081511 [1].pdf. Accessed August 18, 2016.

2. Fihn SD, Gardin JM, Abrams J, et al. 2012 ACCF/AHA/ACP/AATS/PCNA/SCAI/ STS guideline for the diagnosis and management of patients with stable ischemic heart disease: a report of the American College of Cardiology Foundation/American Heart Association Task Force on Practice Guidelines, and the American College of Physicians, American Association for Thoracic Surgery, Preventive Cardiovascular Nurses Association, Society for Cardiovascular Angiography and Interventions, and Society of Thoracic Surgeons. J Am Coll Cardiol 2012;60(24):e44–164.

3. Askew JW, Chareonthaitawee P, Arruda-Olson AM. Selecting the optimal cardiac stress test. In: Post TW, editor. UpToDate. Waltham (MA): UpToDate. Accessed July 28, 2016.

4. Koskinas KC. Appropriate use of non-invasive testing for diagnosis of stable coronary artery disease. 2014. Available at: https://www.escardio.org/guidelines. Accessed August 16, 2016.

5. Kontos M, Diercks DB, Kirk JD. Emergency department and office-based evaluation of patients with chest pain. Mayo Clin Proc 2010;85(3):284–99.

6. Wyant A, Collett D. Identifying and managing CP in women. J Am Acad Physician Assist 2015;28(1):48–52.

7. Hoffmann U, Brady TJ, Muller J. Cardiology patient page. Use of new imaging techniques to screen for coronary artery disease. Circulation 2003;108(8):e50–3.

8. Chizner MA. Clinical cardiology made ridiculously simple. Miami (FL): MedMaster; 2012.

9. Wolk MJ, Bailey SR, Doherty JU, et al. ACCF/AHA/ASE/ASNC/HFSA/HRS/SCAI/ SCCT/SCMR/STS 2013 Multimodality appropriate use criteria for the detection and risk assessment of stable ischemic heart disease. J Am Coll Cardiol 2014; 63(4):380–406.

10. New criteria provide guidance about when (and when not) to use cardiac catheterization to look for heart problems. 2012. Available at: http://www.scai.org/ press/detail.aspx?cid=2a6e4faa-36f7-4487-ac5f-24db55fa2856#.v7rxo6ld37w. Accessed August 17, 2016.

11. Yelland YJ. Outpatient evaluation of the adult with chest pain. In: Post TW, editor. UpToDate. Waltham (MA): UpToDate. Available at: https://www.uptodate.com/ contents/outpatient-evaluation-of-the-adult-with-chest-pain?source=search_ result&search=outpatient%20evaluation%20of%20the%20adult%20with%20chest %20pain&selectedTitle=1~150. Accessed July 28, 2016.

12. Cayley WE Jr. Chest pain–tools to improve your in-office evaluation. J Fam Pract 2014;63(5):246–51. Expanded Academic ASAP.

13. Mahler SA, Hiestand BC, Goff DC, et al. Can the HEART score safely reduce stress testing and cardiac imaging in patients at low risk for acute coronary syndrome? Crit Pathw Cardiol 2011;10(3):128–33.

14. Chest pain of recent onset: assessment and diagnosis. NICE. Available at: https:// www.nice.org.uk/guidance/cg95/chapter/1-guidance. Accessed September 1, 2016.

15. Amsterdam EA, Wenger NK, Brindis RG, et al. 2014 AHA/ACC guideline for the management of patients with non-st-elevation acute coronary syndromes: executive summary: a report of the American College of Cardiology/American Heart Association Task Force on Practice Guidelines. Circulation 2014;130(25): 2354–94.

16. Podrid P. Major side effects of beta blockers. In: Post TW, editor. UpToDate. Waltham (MA): UpToDate. Available at: https://www.uptodate.com/contents/major-side-effects-of-beta-blockers?source=search_result&search=major%20side%20effects%20of%20beta%20blockers&selectedTitle=1~150. Accessed September 2, 2016.

17. National Guideline Clearinghouse (NGC). Guideline summary: stable coronary artery disease. In: National Guideline Clearinghouse (NGC). Rockville (MD): Agency for Healthcare Research and Quality (AHRQ); 2013. Available at: https://www.guideline.gov/summaries/summary/46241/stable-coronary-artery-disease. Accessed September 01, 2016.

18. Kaul P, Naylor CD, Armstrong PW, et al. Assessment of activity status and survival according to the Canadian Cardiovascular Society angina classification. Can J Cardiol 2009;25(7):e225–31.

19. Fraker TD Jr, Fihn SD, Gibbons RJ, et al. 2007 chronic angina focused update of the ACC/AHA 2002 guidelines for the management of patients with chronic stable angina: a report of the American College of Cardiology/American Heart Association Task Force on Practice Guidelines Writing Group to develop the focused update of the 2002 Guidelines for the management of patients with chronic stable angina. Circulation 2007;116(23):2762–72 [Erratum appears in Circulation 2007;116(23):e558].

20. Chan PS, Jones PG, Arnold SA, et al. Development and validation of a short version of the Seattle angina questionnaire. Circulation 2014;7(5):640–7.

Approaches to Valvular Heart Disease in the Primary Care Setting

Classic Presentations and Current Management Guidelines

Dan Tzizik, MPAS, PA-C

KEYWORDS

- Valvular heart disease • Aortic stenosis • Aortic regurgitation • Mitral stenosis
- Mitral valve prolapse • Mitral regurgitation • Tricuspid stenosis
- Tricuspid regurgitation

KEY POINTS

- Valvular heart disease is a common subset of cardiac disease whose prevalence significantly increases with age.
- Valvular heart disease often presents with classic history and physical examination findings that are essential to its ultimate diagnosis.
- Careful consideration of risk/benefit analysis with the patient is key to determining the ultimate course of patients diagnosed with valvular heart disease.
- Symptoms of valvular heart disease often precedes significant irreversible hemodynamic dysfunction.

INTRODUCTION

In general, valvular heart disease (VHD) can manifest as stenosis, regurgitation, or both of the aortic, mitral, tricuspid, or pulmonic valves. In addition to those conditions, mitral valve prolapse (MVP) can also occur. VHD is a common condition in developed and developing countries, although the cause and epidemiology differ greatly between the two socioeconomic states. Rheumatic heart disease (RHD) was the typical cause of VHD worldwide. However, over the last 6 decades, a drastic change in the cause has occurred. In developed industrialized nations, RHD has become exceedingly

Conflicts of Interest: The author has no financial disclosures or conflicts of interest.
Department of Physician Assistant Studies, Massachusetts College of Pharmacy and Health Sciences, 1260 Elm Street, Manchester, NH 03101, USA
E-mail address: dan.tzizik@mcphs.edu

Physician Assist Clin 2 (2017) 689–713
http://dx.doi.org/10.1016/j.cpha.2017.06.009
2405-7991/17/© 2017 Elsevier Inc. All rights reserved.

rare and, as such, has been replaced by calcific degenerative causes with postinterventional, infective endocarditis and connective tissue disorders contributing as well.[1] RHD is still the chief cause in developing countries where rheumatic fever is still prevalent.[1] In the United States, the prevalence of VHD in the population as a whole is approximately 2.5%.[2] Further, in developed countries, because of the predominance of degenerative causes, the prevalence of moderate to severe VHD increases precipitously with age (**Fig. 1**). According to one meta-analysis of sampled database populations, a prevalence of 0.3% was found in the 18 to 44 years old age bracket but increases dramatically to 11.7% in people aged 75 years and older (see **Fig. 1**).[2] In addition, in the group aged 75 years or older, the most common valvular disorder by far was mitral regurgitation (9.3%), followed by aortic stenosis (AS) (2.8%), aortic regurgitation (2.0%), and mitral stenosis (0.2%).[2] The age adjusted prevalence of the population as a whole followed this same hierarchy although the prevalence of each was lower because of the lower prevalence in younger age groups. The effect of these conditions on mortality is not negligible, with a population-adjusted risk ratio of 1.36.[2] The Euro Heart Survey studied a pool of 5001 patients, 18 years of age and older, who were encountered in clinics or hospitalized and who underwent screening echocardiography. Those who had evidence of primary and significant valve disease were included. Of those patients who had no previous valve surgery, AS was most common (33.9%) with mitral regurgitation (24.9%), multiple (20.2%), aortic regurgitation (10.4%), and mitral stenosis (9.5%).[3] Isolated right-sided valve disorders were seen in only 0.8% of the population, with approximately 85% and 9.7% of these having isolated tricuspid valve regurgitation and isolated pulmonic involvement respectively.[3] What can be concluded is that, generally, VHD in the developed world is

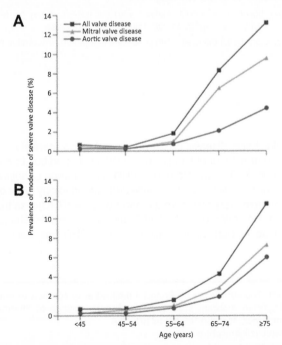

Fig. 1. Age-stratified prevalence of VHD. (*A*) Frequency in Population Based Studies (*B*) Frequency in Olmstead County (MN) community. (*Data from* Nkomo VT, Gardin JM, Skelton TN, et al. Burden of valvular heart disease: a population-based study. Lancet 2006:368(9540):1005–11.)

common, its prevalence increases significantly with age, and it is mainly degenerative in cause. Further, although moderate to severe mitral regurgitation tends to be most common in the general population, significant AS is most common in the population that is seen in clinics or hospitalized. Mitral regurgitation still represents a significant portion of this population and isolated right-sided valve disease is rare. The presence of VHD can adversely influence the clinical outcomes of patients and places them in a higher risk category.

Aortic Stenosis

Case scenario: a 73-year-old man presents to his primary care office complaining of progressively worse dyspnea on exertion for the last 6 months. This patient, who rarely seeks medical care, had a witnessed syncopal event while on his usual 3.2-km (2-mile) walk. This event, which scared him considerably, motivated him to make this appointment. His past medical history is significant for hypertension and hypercholesterolemia. Social history is significant for 22 pack-years of cigarette smoking, which he quit 10 years ago. On physical examination, vital signs are stable other than a blood pressure of 155/124 mm Hg. A 4/6 late peaking ejection systolic murmur is detected and best heard at the cardiac base. The murmur has never been documented. Pitting edema rated 2+ is noted in bilateral lower extremities.

AS is the most common valvular abnormality in patients who present for medical care. Having the knowledge of presenting symptoms, risk factors, diagnostic evaluation, appropriate management based on diagnostic findings, and possible sequelae is crucial in the primary care setting. There are 3 main causes of AS: calcification of a morphologically normal valve, calcification of a congenital bicuspid valve, and RHD. These causes are shown in **Fig. 2**.

Risk factors for aortic stenosis

Understanding who is at risk is of critical importance in order to screen patient populations appropriately and assess the importance of presenting symptoms. The risk factors for aortic valve sclerosis and, ultimately, AS closely mirror those of coronary artery atherosclerosis.[4] Age, gender (male), body mass index, hyperlipidemia, smoking status, hypertension, increased lipoprotein A level, and increased low-density lipoprotein (LDL) cholesterol level have been found to be independent risk factors for degenerative aortic valve disease.[4] The magnitude of risk was less for LDL cholesterol than for the other risk factors and the magnitudes of the associations of all the risk factors were similar to those of coronary artery atherosclerosis in the elderly.[4] Further, once the provider has identified those patients who are at risk, knowing those factors that contribute to the progression of disease process is also of import. The risk factors for a faster progression of AS can be subdivided into patient-related, hemodynamics-related, and valve-related factors. Significant patient-related factors include older age, cigarette smoking, hypertension, obesity, diabetes, lipid abnormalities, chronic renal failure, symptom appearance or worsening, and concomitant coronary artery disease.[5] Significant hemodynamically related factors include left ventricular systolic dysfunction and/or low cardiac output, hemodynamic changes during exercise, and dialysis.[5] In addition, inherent valve-related factors include bicuspid aortic valve, degenerative AS, valve calcification and regurgitation, and mild-moderate stenosis at initial presentation.[5] Recent studies have indicated that other associations may exist. Lower socioeconomic status has been implicated as having a higher prevalence of AS.[6] Racial predisposition continues to be difficult to assess. Depending on whether echocardiography is used as a screening tool, black patients may have the same or lower prevalence of AS than white patients but may have a higher degree of valve

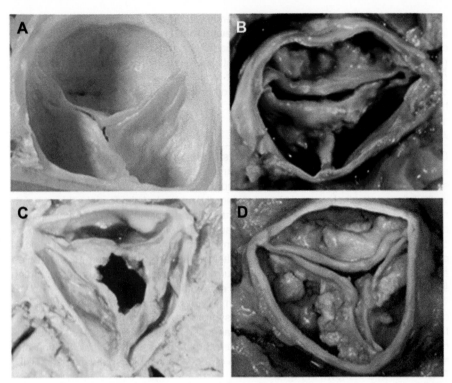

Fig. 2. Major pathologic variants of AS. (*A*) Normal trileaflet aortic valve. (*B*) Calcific bicuspid aortic valve stenosis. (*C*) Rheumatic aortic valve stenosis. (*D*) Calcific degenerative aortic valve stenosis.

degradation before valve replacement.[6] Practitioners must also be aware of the growing body of evidence that supports drug-induced iatrogenic causes of AS. Fenfluramine derivatives, ergot alkaloids, and pergolide are known to be valvulopathic with resultant regurgitation. However, Ennezat and colleagues[7] recently reported evidence to support the possibility of AS being caused by such exposure. More investigation is needed in this area.

Presentation and natural history of aortic stenosis

The presentation of AS is a spectrum with some patients being diagnosed serendipitously and others presenting with symptoms directly related to their AS. Knowing the classic physical examination findings and the natural history is essential for practitioners.

Key features of the physical examination:[8]

- Carotid upstroke: slow increasing, low amplitude, late peaking.
- Low pulse pressure.
- Cardiac impulse and palpation: impulse is displaced inferiorly and laterally. A thrill may be palpated in the right second intercostal space; leaning forward with expiration may accentuate the thrill.
- Murmur: ejection, systolic, and late peaking best heard at the cardiac base. Accentuated with squatting, reduced with standing or Valsalva maneuvers. Concomitant diastolic crescendo-decrescendo murmur of aortic regurgitation may be present.

- Heart failure signs and symptoms: always examine for signs and symptoms of heart failure that include orthopnea, dyspnea, edema, S_3 heart sound, increased jugular venous pressure, pulmonary rales, and positive hepatojugular reflex.

Key features of the history:[8]
- Exertional dyspnea: may reflect symptoms related to pulmonary congestion resulting from increased end-diastolic pressures caused by a worsening obstructive AS and a maladaptive, stiff, hypertrophied left ventricle. As well, may be related to decreased cardiac output with exertion.
- Angina: outflow obstruction by a stenotic aortic valve leads to adaptive concentric hypertrophy, which in turn leads to increased oxygen demand with decreased cardiac output.
- Syncope: inadequate cerebral perfusion caused by decreased cardiac output, particularly with exertion.
- Heart failure: a combination of worsening outflow obstruction and maladaptive hypertrophy leads to increased end-diastolic pressures that, in turn, lead to pulmonary edema and heart failure.

Natural history Symptom onset was identified long ago as a serious prognostic finding and predicted an average survival of 2 to 3 years following this onset.[9] Thus, a careful history and physical examination can detect patients with asymptomatic AS and afford the opportunity for prompt radiographic staging, closer follow-up appointments, monitoring of telltale symptoms, and definitive intervention (discussed later). Asymptomatic patients are not usually given the option of definitive care (ie, valve replacement). However, recent studies indicate that the asymptomatic group may be heterogeneous and there may be subsets of asymptomatic patients with severe stenosis and normal left ventricular function who could benefit from early intervention.[10] Although the risk of death is lower in asymptomatic patients, there is still demonstrable risk, particularly with hemodynamically significant AS. In this population, the probability of remaining free of cardiac symptoms steadily declines to approximately 33% in 5 years.[11] In addition, the risk of sudden death in asymptomatic hemodynamically significant patients is approximately 1% per year.[11]

Evaluation and grading of aortic stenosis
The evaluation of AS is performed by echocardiography, which has largely replaced cardiac catheterization over the last 30 years for this purpose.[12] Transthoracic echocardiography (TTE) is the standard initial test of choice.[13] TTE can generally measure aortic jet velocity, aortic valve area, severity of calcification and underlying anatomy, ejection fraction, possibility of concomitant mitral valve disease, and mean transaortic pressure gradient.[8] Doppler data are used to measure the transaortic jet velocity, aortic orifice area, and transaortic pressure gradient. Echocardiographic measurement of aortic jet velocity, aortic valve area, and rate of change of velocity over time are reliable predictors of clinical outcome.[14] The grading scale endorsed jointly by the American College of Cardiology (ACC) and the American Heart Association (AHA) is shown in **Table 1**. This grading scale was devised to guide therapeutic options with individual patients. Severe AS is defined as an aortic velocity of 4.0 m/s or mean pressure gradient 40 mm Hg by the 2014 guidelines.[13]

Treatment: surgical versus nonsurgical
The stage of the patient ultimately determines the therapeutic options that are available. The 2014 ACC/AHA guidelines also address timing and choice of intervention (**Tables 2** and **3** respectively). However, many other factors come into play when

Table 1
Grading scale

Stage	Definition	Valve Anatomy	Valve Hemodynamics	Hemodynamic Consequences	Symptoms
A	At risk of AS	• Bicuspid aortic valve (or other congenital valve anomaly) • Aortic valve sclerosis	• Aortic V_{max} <2 m/s	• None	• None
B	Progressive AS	• Mild to moderate leaflet calcification of a bicuspid or trileaflet valve with some reduction in systolic motion or • Rheumatic valve changes with commissural fusion	• Mild AS: aortic V_{max} 2.0–2.9 m/s or mean ΔP <20 mm Hg • Moderate AS: aortic V_{max} 3.0–3.9 m/s or mean ΔP 20–39 mm Hg	• Early LV diastolic dysfunction may be present • Normal LVEF	• None
C: Asymptomatic Severe AS					
C1	Asymptomatic severe AS	• Severe leaflet calcification or congenital stenosis with severely reduced leaflet opening	• Aortic V_{max} $\geq$4 m/s or mean ΔP $\geq$40 mm Hg • AVA typically is $\leq$1.0 cm^2 (or AVAi $\leq$0.6 cm^2/m^2) • Very severe AS is an aortic V_{max} $\geq$5 m/s or mean ΔP $\geq$60 mm Hg	• LV diastolic dysfunction • Mild LV hypertrophy • Normal LVEF	• None: exercise testing is reasonable to confirm symptom status
C2	Asymptomatic severe AS with LV dysfunction	• Severe leaflet calcification or congenital stenosis with severely reduced leaflet opening	• Aortic V_{max} $\geq$4 m/s or mean ΔP $\geq$40 mm Hg • AVA typically $\leq$1.0 cm^2 (or AVAi $\leq$0.6 cm^2/m^2)	• LVEF <50%	• None

D: Symptomatic Severe AS

Stage	Definition	Valve anatomy	Valve hemodynamics	Hemodynamic consequences	Symptoms
D1	Symptomatic severe high-gradient AS	• Severe leaflet calcification or congenital stenosis with severely reduced leaflet opening	• Aortic V_{max} ≥4 m/s or mean ΔP ≥40 mm Hg • AVA typically ≤1.0 cm² (or AVAi ≤0.6 cm²/m²) but may be larger with mixed AS/AR	• LV diastolic dysfunction • LV hypertrophy • Pulmonary hypertension may be present	• Exertional dyspnea or decreased exercise tolerance • Exertional angina • Exertional syncope or presyncope
D2	Symptomatic severe low-flow/low-gradient AS with reduced LVEF	• Severe leaflet calcification with severely reduced leaflet motion	• AVA ≤1.0 cm² with resting aortic V_{max} <4 m/s or mean ΔP <40 mm Hg • Dobutamine stress echocardiography shows AVA ≤1.0 cm² with V_{max} ≥4 m/s at any flow rate	• LV diastolic dysfunction • LV hypertrophy • LVEF <50%	• HF • Angina • Syncope or presyncope
D3	Symptomatic severe low-gradient AS with normal LVEF or paradoxic low-flow severe AS	• Severe leaflet calcification with severely reduced leaflet motion	• AVA ≤1.0 cm² with aortic V_{max} <4 m/s or mean ΔP <40 mm Hg • Indexed AVA ≤0.6 cm²/m² and • Stroke volume index <35 mL/m² • Measured when patient is normotensive (systolic BP <140 mm Hg)	• Increased LV relative wall thickness • Small LV chamber with low stroke volume • Restrictive diastolic filling • LVEF ≥50%	• HF • Angina • Syncope or presyncope

Abbreviations: AR, aortic regurgitation; AS, aortic stenosis; AVA, aortic valve area; AVAi, aortic valve area indexed to body surface area; BP, blood pressure; HF, heart failure; LV, left ventricular; LVEF, left ventricular ejection fraction; ΔP, pressure gradient; V_{max}, maximum aortic velocity.

Data from Nishimura RA, Otto CM, Bonow RO, et al. 2014 AHA/ACC guideline for the management of patients with valvular heart disease: a report of the American College of Cardiology/American Heart Association Task Force on practice guidelines. J Am Coll Cardiol 2014;63:e57–185.

Table 2
Summary of recommendations for aortic stenosis: timing of intervention

Recommendations	COR	LOE	References
AVR is recommended for symptomatic patients with severe high-gradient AS who have symptoms by history or on exercise testing (stage D1)	I	B	10
AVR is recommended for asymptomatic patients with severe AS (stage C2) and LVEF <50%	I	B	
AVR is indicated for patients with severe AS (stage C or D) when undergoing other cardiac surgery	I	B	
AVR is reasonable for asymptomatic patients with very severe AS (stage C1, aortic velocity ≥5.0 m/s) and low surgical risk	IIa	B	
AVR is reasonable in asymptomatic patients (stage C1) with severe AS and decreased exercise tolerance or an exercise decrease in BP	IIa	B	27,38
AVR is reasonable in symptomatic patients with low-flow/low-gradient severe AS with reduced LVEF (stage D2) with a low-dose dobutamine stress study that shows an aortic velocity ≥4.0 m/s (or mean pressure gradient ≥40 mm Hg) with a valve area ≤1.0 cm² at any dobutamine dose	IIa	B	
AVR is reasonable in symptomatic patients who have low-flow/low-gradient severe AS (stage D3) who are normotensive and have an LVEF ≥50% if clinical, hemodynamic, and anatomic data support valve obstruction as the most likely cause of symptoms	IIa	C	NA
AVR is reasonable for patients with moderate AS (stage B) (aortic velocity 3.0–3.9 m/s) who are undergoing other cardiac surgery	IIa	C	NA
AVR may be considered for asymptomatic patients with severe AS (stage C1) and rapid disease progression and low surgical risk	IIb	C	NA

Abbreviations: AVR, aortic valve replacement by either surgical or transcatheter approach; COR, class of recommendation; LOE, level of evidence; NA, not applicable.

Data from Nishimura RA, Otto CM, Bonow RO, et al. 2014 AHA/ACC guideline for the management of patients with valvular heart disease: a report of the American College of Cardiology/American Heart Association Task Force on practice guidelines. J Am Coll Cardiol 2014;63:e57–185.

determining which treatment will be best for the patient: nonsurgical versus surgical and, if surgical, whether it is to be surgical aortic valve replacement (SAVR) or the less invasive transcatheter aortic valve replacement (TAVR). AS is a progressive disease process whose pathogenesis is caused by outflow obstruction and, thus, the most definitive intervention is removing the obstruction. Determining the correct strategy for each individual patient, while weighing risks versus benefits, is important. The most recent estimates indicate that approximately 75.6% of elderly patients with severe AS are symptomatic and 40.5% of those are not treated surgically.[15] Of those not treated surgically, 40.3% were potential TAVR candidates.[15] A recent study found a 14% to 16% lower 1-year survival rate of those treated conservatively (nonsurgical) compared with TAVR/SAVR.[16] Further, the Placement of Aortic Transcatheter Valve 1 study showed an approximately 22% higher 5-year risk of death for nonsurgical therapy compared with TAVR and a statistically similar 5-year risk of death of patients who received TAVR versus SAVR.[17,18] Therefore, when counseling patients on risks and benefits of surgical intervention versus the nonsurgical approach, there is substantial evidence that a higher risk is incurred with the nonsurgical strategy and, with the advent of TAVR, increasing experience of valve teams with the use of TAVR, and improving technologies, the threshold for surgical treatment has lowered. Comorbidities and absence of relevant symptoms have been shown to be common reasons for

Table 3
Summary of recommendations for aortic stenosis: choice of surgical or transcatheter intervention

Recommendations	COR I	LOE	References
Surgical AVR is recommended in patients who meet an indication for AVR (Section 3.4) with low or intermediate surgical risk (Section 2.5 in the full-text guideline)	I	A	
For patients in whom TAVR or high-risk surgical AVR is being considered, members of a heart valve team should collaborate to provide optimal patient care	I	C	NA
TAVR is recommended in patients who meet an indication for AVR for AS who have a prohibitive surgical risk and a predicted post-TAVR survival >12 mo	I	B	
TAVR is a reasonable alternative to surgical AVR in patients who meet an indication for AVR (Section 3.4) and who have high surgical risk (Section 2.5 in the full-text guideline)	IIa	B	
Percutaneous aortic balloon dilatation may be considered as a bridge to surgical or transcatheter AVR in severely symptomatic patients with severe AS	IIb	C	NA
TAVR is not recommended in patients in whom existing comorbidities preclude the expected benefit from correction of AS	III: no benefit	B	

Abbreviation: TAVR, transcatheter aortic valve replacement.
Data from Nishimura RA, Otto CM, Bonow RO, et al. 2014 AHA/ACC guideline for the management of patients with valvular heart disease: a report of the American College of Cardiology/American Heart Association Task Force on practice guidelines. J Am Coll Cardiol 2014;63:e57–185.

choosing the nonsurgical approach.[16] A shared, informed approach by patients and the medical team on patient-defined goals may aid in the decision-making process. Goals, such as enjoying favorite activities and spending time with loved ones, rather than goals related to heart failure, seem to be more common when patients consider therapeutic options.[19]

Aortic Regurgitation

Case scenario: A 52-year-old man presents with a complaint of dyspnea on exertion and lower extremity edema for the last month. He complains of occasional exertional midsubsternal chest tightness that is relieved with rest. No significant past medical history. Vital signs include a pulse of 110 beats/min and a blood pressure of 180/62 mm Hg. Physical examination reveals a crescendo-decrescendo diastolic murmur with a late diastolic rumbling that radiates to the neck. A precordial heave and strong, sudden radial pulse with sharp drop-off is noted also.

Pure aortic valve regurgitation (AR) is much less prevalent than AS in those patients presenting for medical care. AR arises from incomplete approximation of the aortic leaflets resulting in diastolic regurgitant backflow of stroke volume. Patients typically develop AR younger than AS, although the two conditions can coexist.[8] AR comes in 2 general forms: chronic and acute. The two entities differ in presentation because of hemodynamics, causes, and treatment. Chronic AR is a state of increasing end-diastolic volumes and cardiac output with resultant adaptive eccentric cardiomyopathy to manage the higher volume. This adaptation develops over time. Acute AR is a condition in which the myocardium does not have the opportunity to adapt. Therefore, both the regurgitant stroke volume and diastolic atrial filling volume contribute to fluid overload of the left ventricle. In chronic AR, the left ventricle adapts to the regurgitant volume by increasing the cavity size and the cardiac output in an attempt to maintain homeostasis. This adaptation is seen in asymptomatic younger patients with AR. Men and women aged 21 to 35 years with AR had echocardiographic evidence of increased left ventricular dimensions and mass.[20] Acute AR leads to a sudden increase in diastolic volume, leading to reduced cardiac output.

Risk factors for aortic regurgitation
Chronic
- Congenital bicuspid aortic valve[21]
- Aortic root dilatation/disease
- Degenerative calcific primary valve disease

Acute
- Infective endocarditis[8]
- Trauma
- Aortic dissection
- After balloon dilatation or TAVR[13]

Presentation and natural history of aortic regurgitation
The presentation of AR depends largely on the type (chronic or acute). Chronic regurgitation tends to be more insidious because cardiac remodeling compensates for the regurgitant volume for many years. However, acute regurgitation can suddenly lead to hypotension and cardiogenic shock.

Key features of the physical examination
Chronic
- Crescendo-decrescendo diastolic murmur directly proceeding A_2, which is best heard on the left sternal border (primary valve disease) and right sternal border (ascending aorta dilatation cause) at the level of the third and fourth intercostal spaces.[8] A harsh systolic murmur radiating to the carotid may be heard and is attributable to the increased cardiac output. The duration and intensity of the murmur are directly related to the severity of disease.
- Austin-Flint murmur: a mid to late diastolic apical rumbling.
- Widened pulse pressure.
- Chest heave.
- Signs of congestive heart failure may be present in advanced cases.
- Water hammer (sudden increase and abrupt collapse) and bisferiens pulse (double peaked).
- Quincke sign: pulsations in the capillaries of the nail beds.

Acute
- Ill appearance
- Cyanosis
- Tachycardia
- Murmurs: same as chronic but usually shorter in duration
- Pulse pressure: slightly widened or normal
- Hypotension
- Peripheral signs: vasoconstriction, edema may be present

Key features of the history
Chronic
- Angina/myocardial ischemia: usually only in later stages[8]
- Orthopnea

- Exertional dyspnea
- Paroxysmal nocturnal dyspnea

Acute
- Acutely ill
- Sudden onset

Natural history The natural history of pure AR presents some treatment, monitoring, and diagnostic challenges. This history refers to AR that was evident early in life but the underlying theme is applicable to the process whose onset occurs later in life. More than 40 years ago, the insidious nature of AR was evident. In one mixed prospective/retrospective study in 1973, younger patients were generally symptom free.[22] Disability developed in the fourth and fifth decades of life.[22] Hemodynamic dysfunction usually precedes the onset of symptoms.[22] Patients who develop asymptomatic regurgitation experience reduced survival percentage, which is particularly accentuated after the age of 50 years (**Fig. 3**).[23] Hemodynamic ventricular dysfunction combined with the extensive cardiac remodeling and adaptation that occur before symptom onset puts these patients at risk for postoperative heart failure and death.[24]

Evaluation and staging of aortic regurgitation
Diagnostics
- Electrocardiogram (ECG): a left ventricular strain pattern indicates dilatation and hypertrophy. There is often T-wave inversion and ST depression.[8]
- Chest radiograph: cardiomegaly, pulmonary edema, and left atrial enlargement may be seen. Aortic valve calcification may be seen in mixed stenosis and regurgitation.
- Cardiac MRI: the most accurate means of assessing severity and flow/mass parameters. Indicated when echocardiography in inadequate or with moderate to severe regurgitation.[13]
- Echocardiography: TTE is usually the initial test of choice. Transesophageal echocardiography (TEE) is sometimes used to optimize the imaging. Can detect most of the aortic and valve/leaflet anatomy. Doppler and color flow echocardiography are very sensitive and accurate for the quantification of valve orifice size

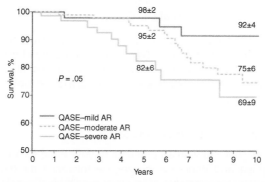

Fig. 3. Survival in asymptomatic patients with aortic regurgitation. QASE, Quantitative American Society of Echocardiography. (*Data from* Detaint D, Messika-Zeitoun D, Maalouf J, et al. Quantitative echocardiographic determinants of clinical outcome in asymptomatic patients with aortic regurgitation: a prospective study. JACC Cardiovasc Imaging 2008;1:1–11.)

and regurgitant volume and are the basis for the current grading scheme (mild, moderate, severe).

Staging Grading of regurgitation is based on anatomic and hemodynamic parameters and is used in the ultimate staging of the patient's condition and timing and degree of intervention. The staging of chronic AR is complicated and depends on specific valve anatomy and hemodynamics, degree of ventricular dilatation, degree of ventricular systolic competence, and symptoms (**Table 4**).[13] Accurate staging of established disease determines the level of intervention. Therefore, careful and meticulous history and physical examination are necessary. The grading scheme is based on the Quantitative American Society of Echocardiography (QASE) scale, with severe defined as regurgitant volume greater than or equal to 60 mL/beat or effective regurgitant orifice (ERO) greater than or equal to 30 mm^2, mild AR as regurgitant volume less than 30 mL/beat and ERO less than 10 mm^2, and moderate as everything in between these two boundaries.

Treatment: surgical and pharmacologic

The timing and type of intervention are outlined in the 2014 AHA/ACC guidelines. Intervention for AR does not just depend the onset of symptoms. As stated previously, a large degree of irreversible adaptive anatomic remodeling with ultimate systolic dysfunction can occur before the onset of symptoms. The importance of this fact cannot be overstated. The current guidelines consider this fact; they advocate safe, preemptive intervention to lessen the ultimate maladaptation that occurs. Functional status and symptomatic status are key to evaluating the possible morbidity and mortality. Comparing New York Heart Association (NYHA) class I/II and III/IV, the 10-year survival rates after aortic valve replacement (AVR) are 78% and 45% respectively.[13] This finding further shows that symptoms are a late finding in the disease process and have potentially dire consequences. If NYHA class III or IV patients are not corrected surgically, they incur a mortality of 24.6% per year.[13] Valve replacement is the ultimate treatment of these patients.

Acute aortic regurgitation Emergent surgery is indicated.[13] These patients are often very ill and unstable.

Chronic aortic regurgitation

Pharmacologic Dihydropyridine calcium channel blockers or angiotensin-converting enzyme inhibitors (ACEI)/angiotensin receptor blockers (ARBs) are recommended for stages B and C (see **Table 4**).[13]

Surgical Aortic valve repair has been attempted with a lack of reproducibility.[13] Most patients need replacement via SAVR. TAVR is an option for regurgitant aortic valves but there are several challenges. The anatomic changes, to include aortic dilatation, make this approach more challenging. Needing a larger replacement valve size restricts the use of TAVR as well.[21]

Mitral Regurgitation and Mitral Valve Prolapse

Case scenario: a 34-year-old woman presents to your clinic for the first time with a complaint of dyspnea and decrease in exercise tolerance for the last 3 months. Past medical history is unremarkable. Vital signs are stable. Grossly, the patient has somewhat marfanoid features to your estimation. Auscultation yields 2 midsystolic clicks with a late systolic crescendo rumble that gets later and more intense with isometrics.

Table 4
Stages of chronic aortic regurgitation

Stage	Definition	Valve Anatomy	Valve Hemodynamics	Hemodynamic Consequences	Symptoms
A	At risk of AR	• Bicuspid aortic valve (or other congenital valve anomaly) • Aortic valve sclerosis • Diseases of the aortic sinuses or ascending aorta • History of rheumatic fever or known RHD • IE	• AR severity: none or trace	• None	• None
B	Progressive AR	• Mild to moderate calcification of a trileaflet valve bicuspid aortic valve or other congenital valve anomaly • Dilated aortic sinuses • Rheumatic valve change • Previous IE	• Mild AR: ○ Jet width <25% of LVOT ○ Vena contracta <0.3 cm ○ RVol <30 mL/beat ○ RF <30% ○ ERO <0.10 cm^2 ○ Angiography grade 1+ • Moderate AR: ○ Jet width 25%–64% of LVOT ○ Vena contracta 0.3–0.6 cm ○ RVol 30–59 mL/beat ○ RF 30%–49% ○ ERO 0.10–0.29 cm^2 ○ Angiography grade 2+	• Normal LV systolic function • Normal LV volume or mild LV dilatation	• None

(continued on next page)

Table 4
(continued)

Stage	Definition	Valve Anatomy	Valve Hemodynamics	Hemodynamic Consequences	Symptoms

C	Asymptomatic severe AR	• Calcific aortic valve disease
		• Bicuspid valve (or other congenital abnormality)
		• Dilated aortic sinuses or ascending aorta
		• Rheumatic valve changes
		• IE with abnormal leaflet closure or perforation
			• Severe AR:
			  ○ Jet width ≥65% of LVOT
			  ○ Vena contracta >0.6 cm
			  ○ Holodiastolic flow reversal in the proximal abdominal aorta
			  ○ RVol ≥60 mL/beat
			  ○ RF ≥50%
			  ○ ERO ≥0.3 cm^2
			  ○ Angiography grade 3+ to 4+
			  ○ In addition, diagnosis of chronic severe AR requires evidence of LV dilatation
				C1: normal LVEF (≥50%) and mild to moderate LV dilatation (LVESD ≤50 mm)
				C2: abnormal LV systolic function with depressed LVEF (<50%) or severe LV dilatation (LVESD >50 mm or indexed LVESD >25 mm/m^2)
					• None; exercise testing is reasonable to confirm symptom status

D	Symptomatic severe AR	• Calcific valve disease
		• Bicuspid valve (or other congenital abnormality)
		• Dilated aortic sinuses or ascending aorta
		• Rheumatic valve changes
		• Previous IE with abnormal leaflet closure or perforation
			• Severe AR:
			  ○ Doppler jet width ≥65% of LVOT
			  ○ Vena contracta >0.6 cm
			  ○ Holodiastolic flow reversal in the proximal abdominal aorta
			  ○ RVol ≥60 mL/beat
			  ○ RF ≥50%
			  ○ ERO ≥0.3 cm^2
			  ○ Angiography grade 3+ to 4+
			  ○ In addition, diagnosis of chronic severe AR requires evidence of LV dilatation
				• Symptomatic severe AR may occur with normal systolic function (LVEF ≥50%), mild to moderate LV dysfunction (LVEF 40%–50%), or severe LV dysfunction (LVEF <40%)
				• Moderate to severe LV dilatation is present
					• Exertional dyspnea or angina or more severe HF symptoms

Abbreviations: ERO, effective regurgitant orifice; IE, infective endocarditis; LVESD, left ventricular end-systolic dimension; LVOT, left ventricular outflow tract; RF, regurgitant fraction; RVol, regurgitant volume.

Data from Nishimura RA, Otto CM, Bonow RO, et al. 2014 AHA/ACC guideline for the management of patients with valvular heart disease: a report of the American College of Cardiology/American Heart Association Task Force on Practice Guidelines. J Am Coll Cardiol 2014;63:e57–185.

Owing to mitral regurgitation (MR) being the most common valvular abnormality, its pathogenesis and treatment are active areas of research, which continues to evolve. In general, MR involves the retrograde flow of blood from the left ventricle to the left atrium through an incompetent mitral valve during systolic contraction of the left ventricle. Two subcategories comprise MR: primary and secondary. Primary MR results from an inherent defect in the valve structure or associated apparatus that interferes with its function. Secondary MR results from abnormal left ventricular architecture or a process that interferes with the function of an anatomically normal valve. The most common cause of primary MR is myxomatous degenerative valvular disease with postinflammatory steady decline.[25] Secondary MR is a pathologic process involving a normal mitral valve whose function is impaired by a dysfunctional left ventricle.[26] MVP is addressed here along with MR because of their propensity to coexist.

Causes of mitral regurgitation
Primary
- Degenerative myxomatous valve disease[26]
- RHD
- Healed infective endocarditis
- Related to systemic disease
- MVP

Secondary
- Left ventricular dilatory processes, ischemic or otherwise

Presentation and natural history of mitral regurgitation
Key features of the physical examination
- Partial to holosystolic murmur best heard at the base and apex. Differentiation of this murmur with the murmur of AS can be accomplished by palpation of the carotid pulse, which is sharp, brisk, and hyperdynamic in MR but slow and delayed in AS.[8] The murmur is diminished with sudden standing and augmented with squatting. It has been suggested that mid to late systolic murmurs of MR related to MVP, compared with holosystolic murmurs, have more benign consequences and outcomes.[27] However, the same question was addressed by Ahmed and colleagues,[28] who found that there was no difference in critical markers of left ventricular dysfunction, related to isolated degenerative MR, between holosystolic and mid to late systolic murmurs. Further, late systolic murmurs of MR should not be considered evidence of unimportant regurgitation.[28]
- Right-sided heart failure[8]: hepatomegaly, edema, and ascites can be seen in acute MR are is not as marked in chronic severe MR because of compensatory enlargement of the left atrium, which reduces the pulmonary resistance and, thus, the signs of right-sided heart failure.

Key features of the history
- Chronic weakness[8]
- Fatigue
- Dyspnea on exertion, related to both decreased cardiac output and increased pulmonary hypertension and congestion

Natural history Most patients who develop chronic primary MR remain asymptomatic for many years.[26] Those with severe MR undergo left ventricular remodeling and dilatation with left atrial enlargement, which compensates for increased diastolic volume.[26] Eventually these changes become maladaptive and the patient becomes symptomatic. Severe primary MR has a high morbidity and mortality, with an excess mortality risk of 6.3% per year.[26] As in AR, in its chronic state, MR is compensated for such that significant dysfunction can occur before the onset of symptoms. However, similar to AR, in its acute state (resulting from myocardial infarction, infective endocarditis, or chordal rupture), the condition is not well tolerated because of the suddenly heightened diastolic filling volumes and pressures with concomitant decreased cardiac output and increased pulmonary pressures.[29] Secondary MR owes its natural history to both the underlying ventricular process and the resultant MR. However, the left ventricular dysfunction of secondary MR usually precedes the regurgitation, with the two processes eventually having additive effects.[29] Secondary MR tends to have a poorer prognosis.[13]

Evaluation and staging of mitral regurgitation
Diagnostic evaluation

- Echocardiography: TTE, particularly with Doppler and color flow, is usually the initial test of choice. Occasionally TEE is used to further show valve detail.[8]
- ECG: left atrial enlargement and atrial fibrillation are the most frequent findings, although evidence of ventricular hypertrophy is common.[8]
- Chest radiography: cardiomegaly and left atrial enlargement are commonly found, shown by Kerley B lines and evidence of pulmonary edema both in acute MR (sudden increase in pulmonary back pressure) and chronic decompensating MR (progressive decrease in efficiency of eccentric left ventricular hypertrophy causing increased pressure upstream of the left atrium).[8]
- Cardiac magnetic resonance: can estimate regurgitant volume accurately.[8]
- Angiography.

Staging of mitral regurgitation Per the AHA/ACC guidelines, the staging of MR is based on several hemodynamic and anatomic criteria. The staging includes differentiation by the designation of primary and secondary. One of the defining criteria is that of severe regurgitation, which is greater than 50% of the regurgitant fraction.[26] Staging the degree of MR is critical from a surgical perspective but also to gauge the amount of dysfunction that is implied by hemodynamic and anatomic data. **Tables 5** and **6** show the current staging criteria of both primary and secondary MR.

Treatment: surgical and pharmacologic
Acute mitral regurgitation Easily titratable vasodilator therapy with nitroprusside or nicardipine.[13] Intra-aortic balloon counterpulsation can be useful as well. Surgical intervention with repair or replacement is most often required.

Chronic primary mitral regurgitation
Pharmacologic According to the 2014 AHA/ACC guidelines, pharmacologic therapy in this subset of patients with MR is indicated in those patients who are symptomatic but do not undergo surgery.[13] However, in severe cases, other investigators have indicated that no medical therapy has altered outcome but afterload reduction and diuretic therapy may help symptomatically.[26] There is evidence to support that beta$_1$-adrenergic receptor blockade positively affects the course of MR through increased left ventricular function.[30] ACEIs may be effective as well.[13]

Surgical Choices include either mitral valve repair or replacement. The choice depends on the anatomy of the valve dysfunction. Ultimately, either repair or replacement is needed to alter the course of the process significantly.[13]

Table 5
Stages of primary mitral regurgitation

Grade	Definition	Valve Anatomy	Valve Hemodynamics[a]	Hemodynamic Consequences	Symptoms
A	At risk of MR	• Mild MVP with normal coaptation • Mild valve thickening and leaflet restriction	• No MR jet or small central jet area <20% LA on Doppler • Small vena contracta <0.3 cm	• None	• None
B	Progressive MR	• Severe MVP with normal coaptation • Rheumatic valve changes with leaflet restriction and loss of central coaptation • Prior IE	• Central jet MR 20%–40% LA or late systolic eccentric jet MR • Vena contracta <0.7 cm • Regurgitant volume <60 mL • Regurgitant fraction <50% • ERO <0.40 cm² • Angiographic grade 1–2+	• Mild LA enlargement • No LV enlargement • Normal pulmonary pressure	• None
C	Asymptomatic severe MR	• Severe MVP with loss of coaptation or flail leaflet • Rheumatic valve changes with leaflet restriction and loss of central coaptation • Prior IE • Thickening of leaflets with radiation heart disease	• Central jet MR >40% LA or holosystolic eccentric jet MR • Vena contracta ≥0.7 cm • Regurgitant volume ≥60 mL • Regurgitant fraction ≥50% • ERO ≥0.40 cm² • Angiographic grade 3–4+	• Moderate or severe LA enlargement • LV enlargement • Pulmonary hypertension may be present at rest or with exercise • C1: LVEF >60% and LVESD <40 mm • C2: LVEF ≤60% and LVESD ≥40 mm	• None
D	Symptomatic severe MR	• Severe MVP with loss of coaptation or flail leaflet • Rheumatic valve changes with leaflet restriction and loss of central coaptation • Prior IE • Thickening of leaflets with radiation heart disease	• Central jet MR >40% LA or holosystolic eccentric jet MR • Vena contracta ≥0.7 cm • Regurgitant volume ≥60 mL • Regurgitant fraction ≥50% • ERO ≥0.40 cm² • Angiographic grade 3–4+	• Moderate or severe LA enlargement • LV enlargement • Pulmonary hypertension present	• Decreased exercise tolerance • Exertional dyspnea

Abbreviations: LA, left atrium/atrial; LVESD, left ventricular end-systolic dimension.

[a] Several valve hemodynamic criteria are provided for assessment of MR severity, but not all criteria for each category are present in each patient. Categorization of MR severity as mild, moderate, or severe depends on data quality and integration of these parameters in conjunction with other clinical evidence.

Data from Nishimura RA, Otto CM, Bonow RO, et al. 2014 AHA/ACC guideline for the management of patients with valvular heart disease: a report of the American College of Cardiology/American Heart Association Task Force on practice guidelines. J Am Coll Cardiol 2014;63:e57–185.

Table 6
Stages of secondary mitral regurgitation

Grade	Definition	Valve Anatomy	Valve Hemodynamics[a]	Associated Cardiac Findings	Symptoms
A	At risk of MR	• Normal valve leaflets, chords, and annulus in a patient with coronary disease or cardiomyopathy	• No MR jet or small central jet area <20% LA on Doppler • Small vena contracta <0.30 cm	• Normal or mildly dilated LV size with fixed (infarction) or inducible (ischemia) regional wall motion abnormalities • Primary myocardial disease with LV dilatation and systolic dysfunction	• Symptoms caused by coronary ischemia or HF may be present that respond to revascularization and appropriate medical therapy
B	Progressive MR	• Regional wall motion abnormalities with mild tethering of mitral leaflet • Annular dilatation with mild loss of central coaptation of the mitral leaflets	• ERO <0.20 cm[2b] • Regurgitant volume <30 mL • Regurgitant fraction <50%	• Regional wall motion abnormalities with reduced LV systolic function • LV dilatation and systolic dysfunction caused by primary myocardial disease	• Symptoms caused by coronary ischemia or HF may be present that respond to revascularization and appropriate medical therapy
C	Asymptomatic severe MR	• Regional wall motion abnormalities and/or LV dilatation with severe tethering of mitral leaflet • Annular dilatation with severe loss of central coaptation of the mitral leaflets	• ERO ≥0.20 cm[2b] • Regurgitant volume ≥30 mL • Regurgitant fraction ≥50%	• Regional wall motion abnormalities with reduced LV systolic function • LV dilatation and systolic dysfunction caused by/because of primary myocardial disease	• Symptoms caused by/because of coronary ischemia or HF may be present that respond to revascularization and appropriate medical therapy
D	Symptomatic severe MR	• Regional wall motion abnormalities and/or LV dilatation with severe tethering of mitral leaflet • Annular dilatation with severe loss of central coaptation of the mitral leaflets	• ERO ≥0.20 cm[2b] • Regurgitant volume ≥30 mL • Regurgitant fraction ≥50%	• Regional wall motion abnormalities with reduced LV systolic function • LV dilatation and systolic dysfunction caused by primary myocardial disease	• HF Symptoms caused by MR persist even after revascularization and optimization of medical therapy • Decreased exercise tolerance • Exertional dyspnea

[a] Several valve hemodynamic criteria are provided for assessment of MR severity, but not all criteria for each category are present in each patient. Categorization of MR severity as mild, moderate, or severe depends on data quality and integration of these parameters in conjunction with other clinical evidence.
[b] The measurement of the proximal isovelocity surface area by two-dimensional TTE in patients with secondary MR underestimates the ERO because of the crescentic shape of the proximal convergence.

Data from Nishimura RA, Otto CM, Bonow RO, et al. 2014 AHA/ACC guideline for the management of patients with valvular heart disease: a report of the American College of Cardiology/American Heart Association Task Force on Practice Guidelines. J Am Coll Cardiol 2014;63:e57–185.

Chronic secondary mitral regurgitation

Pharmacologic Diuretics, β-blockers, ACEIs/ARBs, and aldosterone antagonists are advocated for the treatment of failure symptoms.[13]

Surgical Either repair or replacement is recommended depending on the staging of the patient. However, because of the underlying left ventricular process, which causes a morphologically normal left atrium to become dysfunctional, surgical intervention has not been shown conclusively to prolong life or improve symptoms in this group of patients.[13] The presence of regurgitation may contribute to the degradation of an already dysfunctional ventricle or may simply be a sign of a more dysfunctional ventricle. Thus, it is debatable whether intervention alters the course.[31]

Surgical mitral valve repair/replacement versus transcatheter mitral valve repair

Repair, rather than replacement, of the mitral valve in regurgitation is usually preferred. Owing to the complexity of the anatomy, the transcatheter approach to mitral valve repair in regurgitation is difficult and is limited to the Mitraclip.[26] Surgical mitral valve repair/replacement (SMVR) is still the gold standard. However, if the patient's risk profile makes SMVR prohibitive, transcatheter mitral valve repair has been shown to improve functional status and quality of life.[32]

Mitral valve prolapse

MVP affects approximately 2.4% of the general population and is twice as frequent in women as in men.[8] MVP is the most important cause of MR in the United States.[8] MVP is typically a primary syndrome not related to other cardiac processes. There are familial and nonfamilial associations of MVP.[33] Connective tissue disorders such as Ehlers-Danlos syndrome, Marfan syndrome, pseudoxanthoma elasticum, and osteogenesis imperfecta have all been linked to MVP.[33] Although the syndrome is more common in women, it is more common for severe myxomatous changes, commonly requiring surgery, to occur in older men.[8] Most patients remain asymptomatic.

Key features of the history and physical examination

- Syncope/presyncope, palpitations, fatigue, dyspnea, exercise intolerance, apical chest pain.[8]
- Patients are often of lighter weight, and have a higher incidence of scoliosis and pectus excavatum.
- Auscultation: typical nonejection systolic clicks, often followed by a mid to late crescendo systolic murmur. Straining of Valsalva or sudden standing moves the click and murmur earlier in systole. Sudden supine position, maximal isometrics, or post-Valsalva can delay the click and murmur. Isometrics increase the intensity and post-Valsalva reduces the intensity.

Complications Because of the lack of approximation of the valve leaflets and the billowing of either 1 or both into the atrium, it is intuitive that regurgitation would be common in MVP. However, studies have found further associations between MVP and MR. Primary MVP with MR, through distortion of the structures of the valve by compensatory left ventricular dilatation, further exacerbates regurgitation, creating a positive feedback loop.[34] Early surgical intervention may break this feedback loop.[34] MVP is defined as retrograde displacement of the mitral valve leaflets into the left atrium past the annular plane during systole.[35] The frequency of coexistent MVP and clinically significant regurgitation depends on the specific leaflet that is prolapsing.[36] The proportion of moderate to severe regurgitation is significantly higher with posterior leaflet prolapse than with anterior.[36] Further, the occurrence of atrial fibrillation, congestive heart failure, and chordal rupture are also significantly higher with posterior leaflet prolapse.[36] The severity of the regurgitation was a strong prognostic indicator for complications.[36]

Sudden cardiac death has an association with myxomatous MVP. In a recent study by Narayanan and colleagues,[37] patients with MVP with sudden cardiac arrest were studied to determine their frequency of MR. Approximately 82% of patients with MVP who had sudden cardiac arrest had coexistent MR, 58.8% of the regurgitation being moderate to severe. Patients tended to be younger and with fewer cardiovascular risk factors.[37] The incidence of sudden cardiac death in patients with MVP is twice that of the population as a whole.[38] Severe MR with a flail segment has approximately a 2% per year risk of sudden cardiac death.[39] Thus, the increased risk in this subset of patients demands increased vigilance and possibly early repair.

An increased risk of infectious endocarditis (IE) is associated with MVP. Recent studies show a strong correlation with MVP and viridans group streptococci endocarditis.[40] The risk of IE in patients with MVP with moderate or greater regurgitation is approximately 0.3%.[41] However, this risk doubles in the setting of a flail segment, showing that the risk of IE directly correlates with the degree of regurgitation.[41] This finding contrasts with an incidence of 1.5 to 6 per 100,000 patient years in the general population.[42]

Mitral Stenosis

RHD is by far the most common cause of mitral stenosis (MS), with approximately 99% of stenotic mitral valves having evidence of RHD on excision.[8,43] Thus, with the observed decline of RHD in developed nations, the prevalence of MS has declined steadily.[44] The decline in developed nations is in stark contrast with the prevalence in developing nations. The prevalence of RHD in Cambodia and Mozambique are 21.5 and 30.4 per 1000 respectively, whereas they are 0.5 per 1000 in developed nations.[44] Rothenbuhler and colleagues[45] describe RHD as "a physical manifestation of poverty and social inequality." However, as discussed previously, the Euro Heart Survey noted an MS prevalence of 9.5% of those individuals encountered in a medical visit.[3] Therefore, although the prevalence of MS has declined, it is still encountered with regularity. The cause of MS in developed nations is primarily degenerative calcification of the mitral annulus with resultant stenosis.[26] In addition, the prevalence of MS still mirrors that of RHD and thus it is still encountered in developing nations and immigrants from these nations.

Presentation and natural history of mitral stenosis

MS is an obstructive process leading to several hemodynamic sequelae that explain the history and physical examination. The presentation of patients with MS can vary greatly depending on the compensatory mechanisms that predominate. Patients can present with symptoms of pulmonary congestion/hypertension with normal cardiac output because of increased left atrial pressure. This increase in pressure pushes more blood across the stenotic valve, thus preserving cardiac output at the expense of increased upstream pulmonary pressures.[8] However, in some, the left atrial pressure does not increase appreciably, which spares the upstream pulmonary pressures but results in reduced cardiac output.[8] The reduction in cardiac output is exacerbated as the heart rate increases because of reduced diastolic filling times.[8] Patients often improve when the ventricular rate is controlled.[8]

Key features of the physical examination

- Murmur: presence of an opening snap followed by a low diastolic rumble best heard at the apex[8]
- Mitral facies: pinkish to purplish patches on the cheeks caused by systemic vasoconstriction and low cardiac output

- Irregular pulse: atrial fibrillation, which may predispose to thrombus formation[29]
- Signs of left and right heart failure

Key features of the history
- Dyspnea: often caused by pulmonary edema[8]
- Hemoptysis: sudden increase in pulmonary vascular pressure
- Chest pain: may be a result of concomitant coronary artery atherosclerosis but is often unexplained

Natural history The natural history of MS is usually one of a prolonged asymptomatic period followed by steady deterioration. The normal mitral valve orifice area is usually 4 to 5 cm^2 and symptoms usually do not begin until a reduction in area to 2 cm^2.[29] Further, a yearly reduction of 0.1 to 0.3 cm^2 occurs, which explains the prodromal asymptomatic period and steady decline.[29] However, the left ventricle is usually morphologically and functionally normal. Without intervention by either valve repair or replacement, the 5-year survival rate is 44% for symptomatic patients overall and worsens with NYHA class III and IV.[8]

Evaluation and staging of mitral stenosis

- Echocardiography: the most accurate mode of evaluation; can measure valve orifice area, atrial size, and pulmonary artery pressure[8]
- Chest radiograph: usually shows left atrial enlargement
- ECG: not sensitive for detection but can show left atrial enlargement and right ventricular hypertrophy

Staging of mitral stenosis Staging is essential for determination of the timing of intervention and is based on hemodynamic, anatomic, and symptomatic factors.

Treatment: surgical and pharmacologic
Surgical Intervention is usually delayed until the onset of symptoms. This delay is justified considering the sparing of any pathogenicity to the left ventricle and the slow advance of the disease process.[13] Commissurotomy is indicated if the commissure is fused causing decreased motion of the leaflets.[26]

- Percutaneous mitral balloon commissurotomy[13]: usually initial intervention of choice for symptomatic patients with severe MS and no anatomy that would preclude the procedure. Not indicated if there is no evidence of commissure fusion. Not indicated for degenerative stenosis or annular calcification.[26]
- Mitral valve surgery: repair, commissurotomy, or replacement is indicated if the patient's anatomy is not favorable for balloon commissurotomy, the patient has had a failed balloon, or the patient is having cardiac surgery for another indication.[13]
- Transcatheter valve implantation: some of the limitations alluded to earlier in relation to MR apply to stenosis as well. Attempts have yielded success rates of 90% but a 30-day mortality of 35%.[26] Trials are ongoing to further explore this possibility. In the future, this approach holds much promise for those patients in whom balloon commissurotomy is not indicated and who are at high risk for complications with surgery.

Pharmacologic
- Anticoagulation: patients with uncorrected MS are at a higher risk of embolic events. Hemostasis caused by the propensity for atrial fibrillation in addition to the downstream obstructive process is causal. Those patients with a history

of atrial fibrillation, prior embolic events, or left atrial embolus should be anticoagulated.[13]

- Heart rate control: atrial fibrillation and other arrhythmias may increase the ventricular response rate, with a resultant decreased diastolic filling time and increased upstream pulmonary pressures, and can lead to pulmonary edema. Heart rate control may be beneficial in these patients.[13] Cardioversion may be required. In addition, treatment of patients with symptoms brought on by exercise should be considered.[13]

Tricuspid Regurgitation and Stenosis

Tricuspid regurgitation

Malfunctioning of the tricuspid valve leading to regurgitation may be either primary or functional (secondary; the result of pathologic process involving right ventricular pressure or volume overload).[26] Most tricuspid regurgitation (TR) is functional.[13] Symptoms are usually well tolerated and clinically silent. However, when mixed with pulmonary hypertension, TR can lead to symptoms related to right-sided heart failure.[8] Physical examination may include a systolic thrill and murmur in the neck in addition to hepatomegaly, ascites, and peripheral edema. Intervention depends on whether the process resulting in TR is primary or functional. For example, the TR resulting from the pulmonary hypertension of MS usually resolves with mitral repair or replacement.[8] When the tricuspid apparatus is distorted and/or the regurgitation is severe, choices of intervention include annuloplasty, mechanical valve, or bioprosthesis. Loop diuretics may improve symptoms.[13]

Tricuspid stenosis

Almost all tricuspid stenosis (TS) is rheumatic in origin and coexists with MS.[8] TS is rare, even in areas where RHD is prevalent, representing 0.3% of valve lesions in those areas.[46] There is often some degree of TR associated with TS. TS is often missed during evaluation because of usual left-sided valve involvement. Particularly during physical examination, the murmur of MS usually overshadows that of TS. The murmur of TS can be heard as a soft crescendo-decrescendo systolic murmur best heard at the left lower sternal border, sometimes preceded by a scratchy noise or opening snap.[8] The symptoms are similar to the those of TR (discussed earlier). Loop diuretics may improve symptoms.[13] Intervention is recommended when performing interventions for left-sided valvular disease or symptomatic severe isolated TS and is usually repaired, although replacement may be necessary.[13]

Pulmonic Regurgitation and Stenosis

Pulmonic regurgitation

The most common causes include being a sequela of long-standing pulmonary hypertension, IE, carcinoid syndrome, and postsurgical repair of tetralogy of Fallot.[8] The murmur of pulmonary regurgitation is a high-pitched, blowing diastolic decrescendo best heard at the second to fourth intercostal spaces near the left parasternal border.[8] Signs and symptoms include those of right ventricular overload but often it is well tolerated for years. Surgical intervention is considered if there is evidence of significant right ventricular dysfunction, although addressing the cause of pulmonary hypertension, if present, is advised.[13]

Pulmonic stenosis

Pulmonic stenosis is a rare condition that is overwhelmingly a primary congenital disorder.[8,13] However, malignant carcinoid can cause stenosis of the valve with accumulation. Interventions include percutaneous balloon pulmonic valve commissurotomy and valve replacement.[13]

REFERENCES

1. Boudoulas KD, Borer JS, Boudoulas H. Etiology of valvular heart disease in the 21st century. Cardiology 2013;126:139–52.
2. Nkomo VT, Gardin JM, Skelton TN, et al. Burden of valvular heart disease: a population-based study. Lancet 2006;368(9540):1005–11.
3. Iung B, Baron G, Tornos P, et al. Valvular heart disease in the community: a European experience. Curr Probl Cardiol 2007;32(11):609–61.
4. Stewart BF, Sicovick D, Lind B, et al. Clinical factors associated with calcific aortic valve disease. J Am Coll Cardiol 1997;29(3):630–44.
5. Faggiano P, Antonini-Canterin F, Baldessin F, et al. Epidemiology and cardiovascular risk factors of aortic stenosis. Cardiovasc Ultrasound 2006;4(27):1–5.
6. Beydoun HA, Beydoun MA, Liang H, et al. Sex, race, and socioeconomic disparities in patients with aortic stenosis (from a nationwide inpatient sample). Am J Cardiol 2016;118(6):860–5.
7. Ennezat PV, Bruneval P, Czitrom D, et al. Drug-induced aortic valve stenosis: an under recognized entity. Int J Cardiol 2016;220:429–34.
8. Mann D, Zipes D, Libby P, et al. Braunwald's heart disease: a textbook of cardiovascular medicine. Philadelphia: Elsevier Health Sciences; 2015.
9. Ross J Jr, Braunwald E. Aortic stenosis. Circulation 1968;38:61–7.
10. Sathyamurthy I, Jayanthi K. Asymptomatic severe aortic stenosis with normal left ventricular function-a review. Indian Heart J 2016;68:576–80.
11. Pellikka PA, Sarano ME, Nishimura RA, et al. Outcome of 622 adults with asymptomatic, hemodynamically significant aortic stenosis during prolonged followup. Circulation 2005;111(24):3290–5.
12. Popovic AD, Thomas JD, Cosgrove DM, et al. Time-related trends in the prospective evaluation of patients with valvular stenosis. Am J Cardiol 1997;80(11):1464–8.
13. Nishimura RA, Otto CM, Bonow RO, et al. 2014 AHA/ACC guideline for the management of patients with valvular heart disease: a report of the American College of Cardiology/American Heart Association Task Force on Practice Guidelines. J Am Coll Cardiol 2014;63:e57–185.
14. Otto CM, Burwash IG, Legget ME, et al. Prospective study of asymptomatic valvular aortic stenosis. Clinical, echocardiographic and exercise predictors of outcome. Circulation 1997;95:2262–70.
15. Osnabrugge RL, Mylotte D, Head SJ, et al. Aortic stenosis in the elderly: disease prevalence and number of candidates for transcatheter aortic valve replacement: a meta-analysis and modeling study. J Am Coll Cardiol 2013;62:1002–12.
16. Gonzalez-Saldivar H, Rodriguez-Pascual C, de la Morena G, et al. Comparison of 1-year outcome in patients with severe aorta stenosis treated conservatively or by aortic valve replacement or by percutaneous transcatheter aortic valve implantation (data from a multicenter Spanish registry). Am J Cardiol 2016;118:244–50.
17. Kapadia SR, Leon MB, Makkar RR, et al. 5-year outcomes of transcatheter aortic valve replacement compared with standard treatment for patients with inoperable aortic stenosis (PARTNER 1): a randomised controlled trial. Lancet 2015;385(9986):2485–91.
18. Mack MJ, Leon MB, Smith CR, et al. 5-year outcomes of transcatheter aortic valve replacement or surgical aortic valve replacement for high surgical risk patients

with aortic stenosis (PARTNER 1): a randomised controlled trial. Lancet 2015;385: 2477–85.

19. Coylewright M, Palmer R, O'Neill E, et al. Patient-defined goals for the treatment of severe aortic stenosis: a qualitative analysis. Health Expect 2015;19:1036–43.
20. Reid CL, Anton-Culver A, Yunis C, et al. Prevalence and clinical correlates of isolated mitral, isolated aortic regurgitation, and both in adults aged 21 to 35 Years (from the CARDIA Study). Am J Cardiol 2007;99(6):830–4.
21. Bonow RO, Leon MB, Doshi D, et al. Management strategies and future challenges for aortic valve disease. Lancet 2016;387:1312–23.
22. Goldschlager N, Pfeiffer J, Cohn K, et al. The natural history of aortic regurgitation: a clinical and hemodynamic study. Am J Med 1973;54(5):577–88.
23. Detaint D, Messika-Zeitoun D, Maalouf J, et al. Quantitative echocardiographic determinants of clinical outcome in asymptomatic patients with aortic regurgitation: a prospective study. JACC Cardiovasc Interv 2008;1:1–11.
24. Bonow RO. Aortic regurgitation: time to reassess timing of valve replacement? JACC Cardiovasc Interv 2011;4(3):231–3.
25. Olson LJ, Subramanian R, Ackermann DM, et al. Surgical pathology of the mitral valve: a study of 712 cases spanning 21 years. Mayo Clin Proc 1987;62:22–34.
26. Nishimura R, Vahanian A, Eleid MF, et al. Mitral valve disease-current management and future challenges. Lancet 2016;387:1324–34.
27. Topilsky Y, Michelena H, Bichara V, et al. Mitral valve prolapse with mid-late systolic mitral regurgitation pitfalls of evaluation and clinical outcome compared with holosystolic regurgitation. Circulation 2012;125:1643–51.
28. Ahmed MI, Sanagala T, Denney T, et al. Mitral valve prolapse with a late-systolic regurgitant murmur may be associated with significant hemodynamic consequences. Am J Med Sci 2009;338(2):113–5.
29. Ray R, Chambers J. Mitral valve disease. Int J Clin Pract 2014;68(10):1216–20.
30. Ahmed MI, Aban I, Lloyd SG, et al. A randomized controlled phase IIb trial of beta1-receptor blockade for chronic degenerative mitral regurgitation. J Am Coll Cardiol 2012;60(9):833–8.
31. Bonow RO. The saga continues: does mitral valve repair improve survival in secondary mitral regurgitation? JACC Cardiovasc Interv 2014;7(8):882–4.
32. Lim DS, Reynolds MR, Feldman T, et al. Improved functional status and quality of life in prohibitive surgical risk patients with degenerative mitral regurgitation after transcatheter mitral valve repair. J Am Coll Cardiol 2014;64(2):182–92.
33. Rajamannan NM. Myxomatous mitral valve disease bench to bedside: LDL-density-pressure regulates Lrp5. Expert Rev Cardiovasc Ther 2014;12(3): 383–92.
34. Otani K, Takeuchi M, Kaku K, et al. Evidence of a vicious cycle in mitral regurgitation with prolapse secondary tethering attributed to primary prolapse demonstrated by three-dimensional echocardiography exacerbates regurgitation. Circulation 2012;126(suppl 1):S214–21.
35. Shah PM. Current concepts in mitral valve prolapse-diagnosis and management. J Cardiol 2010;56:125–33.
36. Kuroda K, Nishinaga M, Yamasawa M, et al. Relationship between severity of mitral regurgitation and prognosis of mitral valve prolapse: Echocardiographic follow-up study. Am Heart J 1996;132(2 pt 1):348–55.
37. Narayanan K, Uy-Evanado A, Teodorescu C, et al. Mitral valve prolapse and sudden cardiac arrest in the community. Heart Rhythm 2016;13(2):498–503.
38. Hayek E, Gring CN, Griffin BP. Mitral valve prolapse. Lancet 2005;365:507–18.

39. Grigioni F, Enriquez-Sarano M, Ling LH, et al. Sudden death in mitral regurgitation due to flail leaflet. J Am Coll Cardiol 1999;34:2078–85.
40. DeSimone DC, DeSimone CV, Tleyjah IM, et al. Association of mitral valve prolapse with infective endocarditis due to viridans group streptococci. Clin Infect Dis 2016;61(4):623–5.
41. Katan O, Michelena HI, Avierinos JF, et al. Incidence and predictors of infective endocarditis in mitral valve prolapse: a population-based study. Mayo Clin Proc 2016;91(3):336–42.
42. Mylonakis E, Calderwood SB. Infective endocarditis in adults. N Engl J Med 2001; 345:1318–30.
43. Chambers JB, Bridgewater B. Epidemiology of valvular heart disease. In: Otto CM, Bonow RO, editors. Valvular heart disease: a companion to Braunwald's heart disease. 4th edition. Philadelphia: Saunders; 2013. p. 1–13.
44. Iung B. Mitral stenosis still a concern in heart valve diseases. Arch Cardiovasc Dis 2008;101(10):597–9.
45. Rothenbuhler M, O'Sullivan CJ, Stortecky S, et al. Active surveillance for rheumatic heart disease in endemic regions: a systematic review and meta-analysis of prevalence among children and adolescents. Lancet Glob Health 2014; 2(12):717–26.
46. Manjunath CN, Srinivas P, Ravindrinath K, et al. Incidence and patterns of valvular heart disease in a tertiary care high-volume cardiac center: a single center experience. Indian Heart J 2014;66(3):320–6.

Syncope: Primary Care Office Evaluation and Workup

Craig Hricz, MPAS, PA-C*, Dan Tzizik, MPAS, PA-C

KEYWORDS

- Syncope • Neurally mediated syncope • Orthostatic syncope • Vasovagal syncope
- Cardiovascular syncope • Long QT syndrome • Brugada syndrome
- Postural orthostatic tachycardia syndrome

KEY POINTS

- The cause of syncope is usually neural, orthostatic, or cardiovascular.
- Cardiovascular syncope can be a result of arrhythmias, structural abnormalities, or indirect causes.
- Overall, neurally mediated syncope is most common; however, cardiovascular syncope is very common in patients younger than 65 years and orthostatic syncope in those older than 65 years.
- The cause of syncope can often be distinguished by history alone without further testing, but testing should be performed if the cause is in doubt.

INTRODUCTION

Syncope, as defined by *Harrison's Principles of Internal Medicine*, is "A transient, self-limited loss of consciousness due to acute global impairment of cerebral blood flow. The onset is rapid, duration brief, and recovery spontaneous and complete."[1] Although the causes of syncope are many, a detailed history and specific findings on the physical examination can lead to a specific diagnosis in many cases and guide additional workups in others. The causes of syncope belong in 3 broad categories: neurally mediated, orthostatic, and cardiovascular. Neurally mediated causes are the most common among all age ranges, including up to 80% of causes in children. Cardiovascular causes are the second most common in adults younger than 65 years; however, orthostatic causes surpass cardiovascular in those older than 65 years. Over

The authors have no financial or conflict of interest to disclose.
School of Physician Assistant Studies, Massachusetts College of Pharmacy and Health Sciences, 1260 Elm Street, Manchester, NH 03101, USA
* Corresponding author.
E-mail address: craig.hricz@mcphs.edu

all age ranges there is still a relatively high percentage of cases classified as of unknown cause despite an adequate evaluation. Understanding the pathophysiology of each of these is crucial in being able to determine the cause of the event because specific aspects of the history and physical examination are highly associated with specific causes. In many cases a cause can be reliably determined based on the history and the physical without additional workup. In cases in which the cause is less certain, the provider needs to be able to account for specific causes of concern and be able to determine the appropriate workup.[2]

CAUSES

Table 1 provides a general list of causes subdivided by category type.[2–4] Each broad cause subtype is further expanded on within the appropriate discussion in the sections that follow.

NEURAL CAUSES

Case scenario: A 40-year-old woman presents for evaluation of rectal pain and bleeding. She is 10 days status post fistula-in-ano repair with seton. She states that the area abruptly became more painful with significant bleeding just before arrival. Initial vital signs are stable; however, the patient appears anxious. On examination of the rectal area, the patient experiences significant pain with palpation at the surgical site where moderate bleeding is also present. As the patient continues to complain of pain, she begins to hyperventilate and has a syncopal event resulting in a very brief seizure with a quick return to baseline mental status. She later reports that a similar event related to pain had happened once before.

Neurally mediated syncope, sometimes referred to as reflex syncope, is caused by an inappropriate autonomic reflex response that results in generalized vasodilation (hypotension) and bradycardia ultimately leading to cerebral hypoperfusion. This reflex is self-limiting, which allows for both the blood pressure (BP) and pulse (P) to return to normal in a relatively quick timeframe.

Key symptoms include

- Lightheadedness
- Blurred or tunnel vision
- Nausea
- Diaphoresis
- Vague prodromal abdominal pain
- Postsyncopal reflex anoxic seizure.

Table 1			
Syncope categories and causes			
Neural	**Orthostatic**	**Cardiovascular**	**Other**
Vasovagal event	Volume deficit	Arrhythmia	Transient ischemic attack or cerebrovascular accident
Carotid sinus sensitivity	Medication-related	Structural abnormalities	Psychogenic
Situational	Autonomic failure	Indirect (vascular)	Bilateral carotid stenosis
Postexertional	Septic shock		Epidural hemorrhage

Data from Refs.[2–4]

Key features of the history include asking what the patient was doing or what type of environment they were in at the time of the event:

- Fearful, painful, or emotionally stressful event
- Crowded or excessively hot spaces
- Excessive coughing or laughing
- Urinating or defecating
- Recent exercise or eating
- Prolonged standing
- Events related to manipulation of the neck, for example, movement, fastening a tight collar, or shaving.

Neurally mediated syncope is an unlikely diagnosis if the patient was in a supine position at the time of symptom onset.[3,4] The following sections give specific examples for each neurally mediated subcategory.

Vasovagal

Vasovagal syncope is usually directly related to an emotional stressor, such as fear of crowded spaces or an emotionally stressful, anxiety-provoking event. Excessive heat exposure or exposure to a noxious odor are also possibilities.[3,4]

Carotid Sinus Sensitivity

Although relatively rare (approximately 1% of syncope cases), carotid sinus hypersensitivity and diseased sinus nodes may be responsible for a fair amount of unexplained syncope cases, especially in patients older than 50 years. Events such as rotating or hyperextending the head, shaving, or wearing a tightly collared shirt can trigger a syncopal event related to the carotid sinus. Carotid sinus sensitivity is among the few neurally mediated causes that is directly tested for. A carotid massage is recommended when considering carotid sinus sensitivity as the possible cause or in unexplained cases to rule it out. The procedure requires applying 10 seconds of pressure over the carotid bifurcation just below the angle of the mandible, immediately followed by the same procedure on the opposite side. It can be performed while the patient is supine but is most accurate with the patient in the erect position with the use of a tilt-table. The test is positive if any of the following occur: systolic BP drop of at least 50 mm Hg, pause in the heart rate of at least 3 seconds, or a combination of these. Pacemaker placement will reduce events by approximately 70%.[3]

Situational

Syncope preceded by coughing or sneezing, as well as a bowel movement or micturition, belongs in the situational category. Weightlifting, eating a large meal, or the sight of a needle or blood are other examples that could trigger a situational syncope episode.[3,4]

Postexertional

Postexertional syncope occurs when vigorous cardiovascular exercise stops and the lack of muscle contraction in the legs minimizes the amount of venous blood returning to the heart in relation to the rate and contractility of the heart. The end result is a transient decrease in oxygenated blood to the brain. The same pathophysiology can be seen in individuals with hypertrophic cardiomyopathy and aortic stenosis, but these cases would belong with the cardiovascular type.[3]

With the exception of carotid sinus sensitivity, these types of syncope can be difficult to test for and even more difficult to treat. Avoidance of the triggering event can be challenging, if not impossible, in most of these cases and can be very disconcerting for these patients. Physical isometric counterpressure maneuvers, such as crossing the legs or making a fist, at the onset of presyncope symptoms can be useful.[2]

ORTHOSTATIC CAUSES

Case scenario: A 86-year-old man presents to emergency department (ED) complaining of multiple episodes of passing out over the past 2 weeks. Events are almost daily and generally associated with standing. His wife reports that he stops responding to her, then passes out and has to be caught to prevent him from falling. She notices he also becomes stiff. He has struck his head at least once but not today. He denies palpitations, vomiting, diarrhea, or dark stools. His medical history is positive for coronary artery bypass grafting, atrial fibrillation, heart failure, cerebrovascular accident, and prior gastrointestinal bleed. Medications include amiodarone, metoprolol, and warfarin. Examination is unremarkable, including a negative stool guaiac test. Orthostatic vital signs are as follows: supine, BP 132/59, P 52; standing, BP 84/43, P 57.

A low volume of venous blood returning to the heart causes orthostatic syncope. Under normal physiologic conditions, approximately 25% to 30% of venous blood pools in the pelvic and lower extremity veins within a few minutes of standing, followed by the autonomic system increasing vasoconstriction and heart rate in an effort to maintain adequate blood flow to the brain and organs. If the autonomic system is incapable of initiating these changes or if there is an inadequate intravascular volume to allow these changes to be effective, hypotension and, ultimately, syncope will result. Most of these patients will be older than 40 years and may have 1 or more medical conditions (see later discussion). Patients who have had a syncopal event secondary to orthostatic causes will generally report that the episode occurred shortly after standing or having recently started a new medication (see later discussion). They may also report symptoms consistent with gastrointestinal bleeding or poor oral intake that has led to dehydration. The patient or a bystander may report that pallor and diaphoresis were present at the time of the event.[3,4] The following sections discuss specific examples for each orthostatic subcategory.

Volume Deficit

The 2 main causes of volume deficit are hemorrhage (primarily a gastrointestinal bleed) and dehydration. Patients may report noticing black, tarry stools or vomiting coffee-ground material. Normal-appearing stools do not rule out a bleed as the cause and should be confirmed with a stool guaiac test. Several reasons can contribute to a patient being dehydrated, including excess exercise or heat exposure, vomiting or diarrhea, use of diuretics, and poor oral intake secondary to a lack of access to fluids or a lack of desire to drink, which is usually found in the elderly who may be depressed or have some degree of dementia. Treatment options include a blood transfusion for hemorrhagic causes or administering intravenous fluids in cases of dehydration. Fludrocortisone 0.1 to 0.3 mg daily to expand fluid volume is also an option for the latter.[2,4]

Medications

Several medication classes can be responsible for orthostatic syncope, many of which are used in the treatment of various cardiovascular diseases. These classes include beta-blockers, diuretics, vasodilators, and nitroglycerine. Others possible classes include antidepressants and phenothiazines. Inquiring about new medications or recently increased dosages of these medications is an important component of the medical history. Reducing the dosage or replacing the medication with a different class will usually address the problem.[4,5]

Autonomic Failure

Chronic medical conditions that can led to an autonomic disruption include renal failure, hepatic failure, diabetes, amyloidosis, spinal cord injuries, alcoholism, and Parkinson disease. Postural orthostatic tachycardia syndrome (POTS) also involves autonomic dysfunction (see later discussion). Improved control of these underlying disorders, in addition to the isometric counterpressure maneuvers mentioned earlier and compression stockings for those with venous pooling, can help to minimize the frequency of syncopal events. Midodrine at doses of 5 to 20 mg every 8 hours has proven effective in the treatment of syncope related to autonomic failure.[2,4,5]

Shock

Shock is defined as an inadequate tissue perfusion and can be secondary to several causes within each underlying shock category (hypovolemic, cardiogenic, obstructive, neurogenic, and distributive).[1] Almost all of these causes result in hypotension, which leads to syncope with positional changes. Distributive shock secondary to sepsis is an important cause to consider in cases of syncope, especially in the elderly or immunocompromised. These patients can have multiple comorbid medical problems, polypharmacy, and/or unreliable histories, which can make this cause challenging to diagnose if it is not considered as part of the initial differential diagnosis. Septic shock is managed with intravenous antibiotics, aggressive fluid administration, and vasopressors.[6]

Syncope that is secondary to an orthostatic cause can usually be determined by performing orthostatic vital signs. The Centers for Disease Control and Prevention recommends the following procedure for assessing orthostatic vital signs. First, the patient should be lying supine for at least 5 minutes. Next, record the supine BP and P. Third, stand the patient upright and repeat BP and P assessments at 1 and 3 minutes. In the normal individual, standing should produce a minimal change in the systolic BP and an approximate 5 mm Hg increase in diastolic BP. An abnormal test, which generally signifies a hypovolemic state, is when the systolic BP drops by at least 20 mm Hg or the diastolic BP drops by at least 10 mm Hg by the 3-minute mark. This is usually accompanied by lightheadedness, blurred vision, or possibly a syncopal event. The heart rate response to standing can also be a clue as to the underlying cause. A normal response to standing is a 10 to 20 beats per minute (bpm) increase in heart rate. Elevations above these levels usually indicate hypovolemia and more extreme elevations are associated with POTS, whereas elevations of less than 10 bpm are frequently seen in patients with autonomic failure secondary to central or peripheral nervous system disease. Beta blocker use should not significantly affect the reliability of heart rate changes with orthostatics.[7–10]

CARDIOVASCULAR CAUSES

Case scenario: A 76-year-old man presents to the ED for evaluation of syncope. He had apparently finished eating dinner, stood up, became diaphoretic, and passed out. There was no reported seizure activity and no injuries. He states he has been having episodes of shortness of breath over the past several weeks, with associated dizziness and lightheadedness. Last week he presented to another hospital and a cardiac catheterization was performed that showed no significant disease. He was discharged with an event monitor, which he is still wearing. Since then, he has had 2 episodes of dizziness and weakness. Physical examination reveals cyanosis of the fingers and toes, otherwise he is normal. Vital signs were as follows: BP 64/43, P 46, respiration 16, temperature 97.5, and Po_2 94% on 3L/min on nasal cannula.

Cardiovascular syncope occurs when there is a direct cardiac or vascular cause that prohibits oxygenated blood from reaching the brain. Although cardiovascular syncope is not nearly as common as neurally mediated causes or, in some cases, orthostatically mediated, it has the highest potential for mortality. Common symptoms that a patient with cardiovascular syncope might report are palpitations, chest pain, and/or shortness of breath. In some cases, an exertional component may also be present. These patients will frequently have a cyanotic appearance at the time of the event as opposed to the pale and diaphoretic appearance seen with most cases of neurally or orthostatically mediated syncope.[3,4] The following sections give specific examples for each cardiovascular subcategory.

Arrhythmias

Although the syncope or near-syncope event may have been related to an arrhythmia, more often than not the arrhythmic event will have resolved by the time the patient is seen by a provider. Careful assessment of the electrocardiogram (ECG) can reveal clues to an underlying pathologic condition responsible for these paroxysmal brady or tachy-arrhythmias. It is recommended that the provider familiarize him or herself with the ECG findings specific to these causes.[2,3,5]

Sinus bradycardia and heart blocks

The cause of syncope in the context of a conduction block is usually bradycardia.[11] Sick sinus syndrome is an cause known to contribute to presyncope or frank syncope, and is an umbrella term that ultimately refers to sinus node dysfunction. Sick sinus syndrome can manifest as sinus bradycardia, sinus arrest, sinoatrial block, and alternating bradycardia or tachycardia.[12] Beta blocker use is also responsible for sinus bradycardia. A dosage adjustment or alternative medication should be considered if near syncope or frank syncope is occurring in a patient on a beta blocker with bradycardia.

Congenital long QT syndrome and secondary QT prolongation

QT segment prolongation can both be inherited or secondary to exogenous stimuli. QT prolongation leads to runs of torsades de pointe that reduce cardiac output, resulting in syncope. The ventricular tachycardia can degrade to ventricular fibrillation, resulting in sudden death.[13] The diagnosis of long QT syndrome, a congenital syndrome, can be established with a reproducible QTc of 480 to 499 ms with repeated unexplained episodes of syncope without a secondary cause.[13] A major cause of secondary or acquired QTc prolongation are medications. A long list of medications has been shown to facilitate QTc prolongation.[14]

Brugada syndrome

Brugada syndrome is a group of heritable dysrhythmias that can lead to syncope via ventricular fibrillation and sudden cardiac death. Brugada syndrome was first described in 1992 by Brugada and Brugada.[15] Since then, much work has been performed to elucidate the pathogenesis, epidemiology, and genetics. Thirteen mutations of sodium, calcium, or potassium channels have been identified that can lead to Brugada syndrome.[16] The heart is structurally normal but the channel mutations lead to the dysrhythmogenesis. Classic findings on ECG include right bundle branch block with ST segment elevations in the anterior precordial leads. There are 3 distinct patterns termed types 1, 2, and 3 (**Fig. 1**).

Type 1   Type 2   Type 3

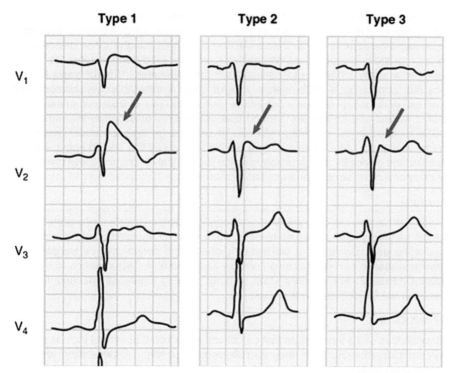

Fig. 1. Brugada patterns. *From* Mann D, Zipes D, Libby P, et al. Braunwald's heart disease: a text-book of cardiovascular medicine. Philadelphia: Elsevier Health Sciences; 2015. Figure E37-5.

Other potential arrhythmia causes to consider

Other potential causes of arrhythmia to consider are supraventricular tachycardia, ventricular tachycardia, Wolf-Parkinson-White, and arrhythmogenic right ventricular dysplasia.

Postural orthostatic tachycardia syndrome

POTS is defined as the increase in heart rate greater than 30 bpm or persistent standing heart rate of greater than 120 bpm in a symptomatic patient when changing from a supine to standing position.[17] Normally, with this change of position a sub-stantial amount of venous pooling occurs due to gravitational influences. In response to this, the heart rate, as well as the systolic and diastolic BPs rise, which augments venous return and cardiac output. Vasoconstriction provides shunting of blood to necessary organs and vital signs normalize. POTS patients have a noncompensatory increase in venous return, resulting in the heart rate continuing to rise. BP often does not rise with heart rate, which is among several factors affecting venous return.[17] Most these patients are female and white. Patients often present with lightheaded-ness, palpitations, exercise intolerance, and syncope (approximately 30%). Roughly 50% of these patients will also experience dependent acrocyanosis, a dark reddish to blue discoloration, of the lower legs.[18] Unfortunately, according to a 2013 study, the average delay to diagnosis is nearly 6 years.[19] Obtaining a detailed history and considering POTS in the syncope differential diagnosis are critical to making this diagnosis in a timely fashion and will result in a positive impact on the patient's qual-ity of life.

Pacemaker or automatic implantable cardioverter defibrillator

Many patients at risk for malignant arrhythmias have internal pacemakers or automatic implantable cardioverter defibrillators (AICDs). The functioning of these devices may be appropriate or inappropriate, and each circumstance may lead to episodes of syncope. In a study by Kou and colleagues,[20] approximately 12% of patients who received spontaneous high-energy shocks from implantable defibrillators had syncopal episodes. In a large study of the malfunction rate of both pacemakers and AICDs, Maisel and colleagues[21] found that only 0.39% of pacemakers and 2% of AICDs malfunctioned, requiring removal. Thus, although syncope could occur due to malfunctioning of these devices, the likelihood is low. If this should occur, interrogation of the device by the cardiology service is essential to determine whether a malfunction or a more serious process has occurred.

Structural

A variety of causes can belong in this category, including myocardial infarction; hypertrophic cardiomyopathy; cardiac masses, such as atrial myxomas and tumors; pericardial disease, consisting of cardiac tamponade and constrictive pericarditis; and valvular disease.[2,5] (See discussion of Dan Tzizik's article, "Approaches to Valvular Heart Disease in the Primary Care Setting: Classic Presentations and Current Management Guidelines," in this issue.)

Indirect Cardiac

Abnormalities of the vasculature that can directly affect cardiac output include pulmonary embolus, thoracic aortic aneurysm dissection, pulmonary hypertension, and subclavian steal syndrome.[2,5]

WORKUP

As evident by the descriptions of the typical histories that occur with either neural or orthostatic causes, many cases of syncope can readily be diagnosed on the history alone. Confirmation of the suspected cause can often be easily made with simple techniques such as orthostatic vital signs or carotid sinus massage. Cases of suspected cardiovascular or unknown origin and syncope in patients with other comorbidities usually require a more extensive workup using 1 or more tests.

Laboratory Testing

A complete blood count to evaluate the patient's hemoglobin and hematocrit for evidence of anemia is the most useful laboratory test. A B-type natriuretic peptide test is useful if the patient has a history or risk factors for heart failure, and it is also used in the Risk Stratification of Syncope in the Emergency Department (ROSE) rule clinical decision-making tool. Other specific studies, such as a D-dimer for pulmonary embolus, Lyme titer for cases of heart block in which Lyme disease is a concern, pregnancy test if ruptured ectopic is suspected, or cardiac enzymes to evaluate for a myocardial infarction are examples of some tests that are appropriate in select cases. A basic metabolic panel is usually obtained to assess for electrolyte and blood sugar abnormalities but generally provides little value in determining the underlying cause of syncope.[4]

Electrocardiogram and Telemetry

An ECG should be ordered for every patient with syncope. Not only will this detect an arrhythmia occurring at the time of the ECG but it will also reveal abnormal interval lengths that may represent an increased risk of arrhythmia. The ECG may also reveal other causes responsible for the syncopal event, including myocardial infarction, pulmonary embolus, and hypertrophic cardiomyopathy. Specific ECG findings were previously discussed and illustrated. To capture any potential paroxysmal arrhythmias, continuous telemetry should be used on all syncope patients while in the ED or if admitted to the hospital.[4]

Holter Monitor

The Holter monitor is used to continuously monitor the heart for a period of 24 to 72 hours. It is most useful for patients who report frequent, daily symptoms of palpitations or near syncope. If the patient suffers an event while on the monitor and no arrhythmia is recorded, it is likely that the patient's symptoms are related to a psychogenic cause.[2]

Event Monitor

An event monitor is similar to the Holter monitor but used over a 4-week timeframe. This additional time will ensure that most arrhythmias are captured. It also allows for the patient to manually record a time period when they are actively experiencing symptoms and allow the cardiologist to assess if a cardiac cause was responsible. In cases in which the event monitor did not successfully capture an arrhythmia and the patient continues to experience symptoms without another cause identified, an implanted loop recorder can be considered for a 1-year to 2-year period.[2]

Electrophysiologic Study

An electrophysiologic study (EP) study attempts to elicit an underlying arrhythmia and potentially locate its source. The 2 primary indications for performing an EP study are (1) palpitations, presyncope, or syncope in a patient with a prior myocardial infarction and (2) syncope of uncertain origin in a patient with compromised left ventricular function or structural heart disease. An EP study can also be considered in patients with a bundle branch block whose symptoms have not been diagnosed with traditional noninvasive testing. In appropriate cases, an EP can establish a diagnosis in 50% of cases of palpitations that had not been captured by ECG or extended monitoring. The highest yield is seen in patients older than 50 years with a history of structural heart disease who report lengthy events with sudden terminations and palpitations felt in the neck. In some cases, the results of an EP study can be used to perform a cardiac ablation in the hopes of treating the cause of the arrhythmia. Contraindications include unstable angina, coagulopathy, and uncontrolled heart failure.[22–25]

Tilt-Table Testing

The tilt-table test can be a valuable tool in the assessment of syncope, particularly to confirm a vasovagal cause or in cases of unexplained syncope. The test has a specificity of 90% for vasovagal syncope. It is the test of choice for suspected cases of POTS and is useful for detecting reflex syncope related to bradycardia and hypotension.[2,3]

Echocardiogram

An echocardiogram study can determine if structural causes are responsible for a syncopal event, including severe aortic stenosis or dissection, hypertrophic cardiomyopathy, tamponade, and congenital coronary artery anomaly.[2,25]

Stress Test

An exercise stress test has some merit for cases of exertional syncope but has an overall yield of less than 5%.[3]

Head Computed Tomography

In general, head computed tomography is of little value in the workup of syncope except under the following circumstances: associated head trauma (before or as a result of the syncope), syncope associated with a seizure, change in mental status, or a new neurologic defecit.[26]

Fig. 2 gives a summary of the workup recommendations.

DISPOSITION

The basic treatment options have been discussed and a suggested workup flowsheet is included in **Fig. 2**. Much of the decision-making centers around deciding which patients require hospitalization to obtain a more urgent workup. Several risk stratification tools have been created over the years in an effort to assist the provider in this process; however, none of these tools have been classified as level 1 evidence for use and only the San Francisco Syncope Rule and the Osservatorio Epidemiologicosulla Sincope nel Lazio (OESIL) risk score have been validated in multiple settings and are considered level 2 for use as general guidance; however, these are not substitutes for solid clinical judgment. A newer tool that shows promise is the Canadian Syncope Risk Score, which requires further validation. In general, syncope associated with the following risk factors should be considered high risk for adverse events: confirmed or suspicion of acute coronary syndrome, heart failure or structural heart disease history, new ECG changes, anemia, and/or unstable vital signs.[27–30]

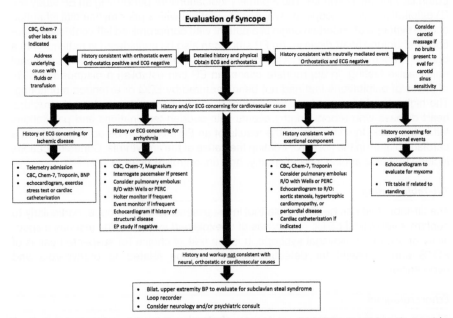

Fig. 2. Syncope workup. bilat, bilateral; BP, blood pressure; BNP, B-type natriuretic peptide test; CBC, complete blood count; Chem-7, basic metabolic panel; eval, evaluate EP, electro-physiology study; PERC, pulmonary embolism rule-out criteria; R/O, rule-out.

REFERENCES

1. Freeman R. Syncope. In: Harrison TR, Kasper DL, Fauci AS, et al, editors. Harrison's principles of internal medicine. 18th edition. New York: McGraw Hill Education; 2012. p. 171–7.

2. Moya A, Sutton R, Ammirati F, et al. Guidelines for the diagnosis and management of syncope (version 2009): The Task Force for the Diagnosis and Management of Syncope of the European Society of Cardiology (ESC). Eur Heart J 2009; 30(21):2631–71.

3. Hanna EB. Syncope: etiology and diagnostic approach. Cleve Clin J Med 2014; 81(12):755–66.

4. Gauer RL. Evaluation of Syncope. Am Fam Physician 2011;84(6):640–50.

5. Syncope Evaluation. In DynaMed [database online]. EBSCO Information Services. 2016. Available at: http://www.dynamed.com/login.aspx?direct=true& site=DynaMed&id=113862. Accessed October 17, 2016.

6. Peeters SY, Hoek AE, Mollink SM, et al. Syncope: risk stratification and clinical decision making. Emerg Med Pract 2014;16(4):1–22.

7. STEADI materials for health care providers. 2016. Centers for Disease Control and Prevention. Available at: http://www.cdc.gov/steadi/materials.html. Accessed October 14, 2016.

8. Shibao C, Lipsitz LA, Biaggioni I. ASH position paper: evaluation and treatment of orthostatic hypotension. J Clin Hypertens 2013;15(3):147–53.

9. Raj SR. Postural Tachycardia Syndrome (POTS). Circulation 2013;127(23): 2336–42.

10. Maeder MT, Zurek M, Rickli H, et al. Prognostic value of the change in heart rate from the supine to the upright position in patients with chronic heart failure. J Am Heart Assoc 2016;5(8):e003524.

11. Kearney K, Ellingson S, Stout K, et al. From bradycardia to tachycardia: complete heart block. Am J Med 2015;128(7):702–6.

12. Adan V, Grown L. Diagnosis and treatment of sick sinus syndrome. Am Fam Physician 2003;67(8):1725–32.

13. Priori S, Wilde A, Horie M, et al. HRS/EHRA/APHRS Expert consensus statement on the diagnosis and management of patients with inherited primary arrhythmia syndromes. J Arrhythmia 2014;30:1–28.

14. Woosley RL, Romero KA. Available at: www.Crediblemeds.org. Accessed November 12, 2016. QTdrugs List, AZCERT, Inc. 1822 Innovation Park Dr., Oro Valley, AZ 85755.

15. Brugada P, Brugada J. Right bundle branch block, persistent ST segment elevation and sudden cardiac death: A distinct clinical and electrocardiographic syndrome. A multicenter report. J Am Coll Cardiol 1992;20(6):1391–6.

16. Mann D, Zipes D, Libby P, et al. Braunwald's Heart Disease: a textbook of cardiovascular medicine. Philadelphia: Elsevier Health Sciences; 2015.

17. Johnson J, Mack K, Kuntz N, et al. Postural orthostatic tachycardia syndrome: a clinical review. Pediatr Neurol 2011;42(2):77–85.

18. Raj SR. The Postural Tachycardia Syndrome (POTS): pathophysiology, diagnosis & management. Indian Pacing Electrophysiol J 2006;6(2):84–99.

19. Physician Patient Interaction in Postural Orthostatic Tachycardia Syndrome. In: Dysautonomia International. Available at: http://www.dysautonomiainternational. org/pdf/PhysicianPatientInteractionInPOTS.pdf. Accessed November 17, 2016.

20. Kou WH, Calkins H, Lewis RR, et al. Incidence of loss of consciousness during automatic implantable cardioverter-defibrillator shocks. Ann Intern Med 1991; 115(12):942–5.
21. Maisel WH, Moynahan M, Zuckerman BD, et al. Pacemaker and ICD generator malfunctions: analysis of Food and Drug Administration annual reports. JAMA 2006;295(16):1901–6.
22. Hilfiker G, Schoenenberger AW, Erne P, et al. Utility of electrophysiological studies to predict arrhythmic events. World J Cardiol 2015;7(6):344.
23. Linzer M, Yang EH, Estes NA 3rd, et al. Diagnosing syncope. Part 2: unexplained syncope. Clinical Efficacy Assessment Project of the American College of Physicians. Ann Intern Med 1997;127:76.
24. Brembilla-Perrot B, Sellal JM, Olivier A, et al. Electrophysiological study generally is negative in patients <40years suspected of supraventricular tachycardia but also complaining of chest pain and/or syncope. Int J Cardiol 2016;203:1109–13.
25. Tracy CM, Akhtar M, DiMarco JP, et al. American College of Cardiology/American Heart Association 2006 update of the clinical competence statement on invasive electrophysiology studies, catheter ablation, and cardioversion: a report of the American College of Cardiology/American Heart Association/American College of Physicians Task Force on Clinical Competence and Training developed in collaboration with the Heart Rhythm Society. J Am Coll Cardiol 2006;48:1503.
26. Goyal N, Donnino MW, Vachhani R, et al. The utility of head computed tomography in the emergency department evaluation of syncope. Intern Emerg Med 2006;1(2):148–50.
27. Serrano LA, Hess EP, Bellolio MF, et al. Accuracy and quality of clinical decision rules for syncope in the Emergency Department: a systematic review and meta-analysis. Ann Emerg Med 2010;56(4):362–73.e1.
28. Thiruganasambandamoorthy V, Kwong K, Wells GA, et al. Development of the Canadian Syncope Risk Score to predict serious adverse events after emergency department assessment of syncope. Can Med Assoc J 2016;188(12):E289–98.
29. Costantino G, Casazza G, Reed M, et al. Syncope risk stratification tools vs clinical judgment: an individual patient data meta-analysis. Am J Med 2014;127(11). 1126.e13-25.
30. Puppala VK, Dickinson O, Benditt DG. Syncope: classification and risk stratification. J Cardiol 2014;63(3):171–7.

Pulmonary Hypertension and Thrombembolism— Long-Term Management and Chronic Oral Anticoagulation

Eric W. Cucchi, MS, PA-C[a,b,]*, Jillian Levy, MS, PA-C[c]

KEYWORDS

- Pulmonary hypertension • Pulmonary artery hypertension • Anticoagulation
- Warfarin

KEY POINTS

- Pulmonary hypertension (PH) is a complex disease that is characterized by an elevated mean pulmonary arterial pressure of greater than or equal to 25 mm Hg.
- PH has a wide variety of etiologies, all with specific therapies.
- Presenting symptoms are generally nonspecific and can include fatigue, lethargy, angina, weakness, signs of right heart failure, and increasing shortness of breath.
- Pulmonary artery hypertension is associated with increased thrombosis and disrupted coagulation and fibrinolysis, making anticoagulation an attractive and frequently used therapeutic modality.
- Pulmonary vasodilator therapy and oral anticoagulation are the main tools of long-term medical therapy.

INTRODUCTION

Pulmonary hypertension (PH) is a complex disease that is characterized by an elevated mean pulmonary arterial pressure (mPAP) of greater than or equal to 25 mm Hg (**Table 1**). In the United States, there are approximately 200,000 hospitalized patients annually who have PH as a primary or secondary diagnosis.[1] Before introducing new treatments, the average life expectancy of the patients with PH was 2.5 years.[2] Due to the complexity of the disease and the multiple etiologies of

Disclosure Statement: Neither author has any financial or conflict of interest to disclose.
[a] Affiliate Practitioner Critical Care Residency Program, Critical Care, UMass Memorial Medical Center, The Graduate School of Nursing, University of Massachusetts Medical School, 55 Lake Avenue North, HA318, Worcester, MA 01655, USA; [b] Physician Assistant Studies, Bay Path University, Longmeadow, MA, USA; [c] UMass Memorial Medical Center, eICU, 281 Lincoln Street, Worcester, MA 01605, USA
* Corresponding author. UMass Memorial Medical Center, 55 Lake Avenue North, HA318, Worcester, MA 01655.
E-mail address: Eric.Cucchi2@umassmemorial.org

Physician Assist Clin 2 (2017) 727–741
http://dx.doi.org/10.1016/j.cpha.2017.06.008
2405-7991/17/© 2017 Elsevier Inc. All rights reserved.

physicianassistant.theclinics.com

Table 1
Right heart catheterization evaluation

Hemodynamic Parameter	Hemodynamic Cutoff	Diagnosis
mPAP	<20 mm Hg	Normal
PAWP	≤15 mm Hg	Normal, when mPAP <25 mm Hg
mPAP	≥25 mm Hg	PH
PAWP	≤15 mm Hg	Precapillary PH[a]
PAWP	>15 mm Hg	Postcapillary PH [a]
Transpulmonary pressure gradient (mPAP-PAWP)	≤12 mm Hg	Passive postcapillary PH
Transpulmonary pressure gradient (mPAP-PAWP)	>12 mm Hg	Reactive postcapillary PH
PVR	>3 Wood units	PAH[b]

[a] When mPAP is ≥25 mm Hg.
[b] When mPAP is ≥25 mm Hg and PAWP <15 mm Hg.

the disease, the World Health Organization (WHO) has classified PH into 5 classes with the purpose of helping guide diagnosis and treatment (**Table 2**). There has been a total of 5 World Symposia on PH since 1973.[3–8] The most recent, the Nice Classification in 2013, has further refined previous works to develop the new clinical classification of PH. In this classification there are 5 major groupings and several subgroups that further define etiology with the aim to guide diagnosis and treatment.

GROUP 1—PULMONARY ARTERY HYPERTENSION

Pulmonary artery hypertension (PAH) is defined by a pulmonary vascular resistance (PVR) greater than 3 Wood units with mPAP greater than or equal to 25 mm Hg and pulmonary artery wedge pressure (PAWP) less than 15 mm Hg[9] determined by a right heart catheterization (RHC) at rest.

PAH affects the small pulmonary arteries with vascular obstruction by intimal and media proliferation and increased vascular resistance though complex multifactorial pathways. This results in increased right ventricular afterload and eventual failure.[10]

The cardiopulmonary effects of PAH can be debilitating and worsen health-related quality of living,[11] resulting in inactive lifestyles.[2]

In the REVEAL[12] study of 2176 patients enrolled with PAH, the 1-year survival rate with PAH at 1 year after enrollment was 91%. Increased mortality is seen with PVR of greater than 32 Wood units, portal hypertension, modified New York Heart Association (NYHA)/WHO functional class IV, men greater than 60 years old, and family history of PAH. Connective tissue disease, renal insufficiency, modified NHYA/WHO functional class III (**Table 3**), resting systolic blood pressure of less than 110 mm Hg, resting heart rate greater than 92 beats per minute, 6-minute walk distance less than 165 m, B-type natriuretic peptide (BNP) greater than 180 pg/mL, presence of pericardial effusion, percent predicted diffusing capacity of the lungs for carbon monoxide (D_{LCO}) less than or equal to 32%, and mean right arterial pressure greater than 20 mm Hg within the year preceding enrollment.

Conversely, a modified NHYA/WHO functional class I, 6-minute walk distance greater than or equal to 440 m, BNP less than 50 pg/mL, and D_{LCO} greater than or equal to 80% have an increased 1-year survival rate.[12]

PAH is a broad term is further characterized by several subgroups based on etiology that have recently been updated by the Nice Classification.[7]

Table 2	
Fifth World Congress classification for pulmonary hypertension	
1	Pulmonary artery hypertension
1.1	Idiopathic PAH
1.2	Heritable PAH
1.2.1	BMPR2
1.2.2	ALK1, endoglin, Smad9, CAV1, KCNK3
1.2.3	Unknown
1.3	Drug and toxin induced
1.4	Associated with...
1.4.1	Connective tissue disease
1.4.2	HIV infection
1.4.3	POPH
1.4.4	CHD
1.4.5	Schistosomiasis
1'	Pulmonary veno-occlusive disease and/or pulmonary capillary hemagniomatosis
1"	Persistent PH of the newborn
2	PH owing to left heart disease
2.1	Left ventricular systolic dysfunction
2.2	Left ventricular diastolic dysfunction
2.3	Valvular disease
2.4	Congenital/acquired left heart inflow/outflow tract obstruction and congenital cardiomyopathies
3	PH owing to lung diseases and/or hypoxia
3.1	COPD
3.2	ILD
3.3	Other pulmonary diseases with mixed restrictive and obstructive pattern
3.4	Sleep-disordered breathing
3.5	Alveolar hypoventilation disorders
3.6	Chronic exposure to high altitude
3.7	Developmental abnormalities
4	CTEPH
5	PH with unclear multifactorial mechanisms
5.1	Hematologic disorders, chronic hemolytic anemia, myeloproliferative disorders, splenectomy
5.2	Systemic disorders: sarcoidosis, pulmonary Langerhans cell histocytosis, lymphangioleiomyomatosis, neurofibromatosis, vasculitis
5.3	Metabolic disorders: glycogen storage disease, Gaucher disease, thyroid disorders
5.4	Others: tumoral obstruction, fibrosing mediastinitis, chronic renal failure, segmental PH

From Simonneau G, Gatzoulis MA, Adatia I, et al. Updated clinical classification of pulmonary hypertension. J Am Coll Cardiol 2013;62(25 Suppl):D34–41.

Group 1.1—Idiopathic Pulmonary Arterial Hypertension

When there is an isolated or unclear etiology of PAH and no hereditary influence known, then a patient is considered to have an idiopathic PAH. The estimated

Table 3
Modified New York Heart Association/World Health Organization classification for pulmonary hypertension

Class I	Patients with PH but without resulting limitation of physical activity. Ordinary physical activity does not cause undue dyspnea or fatigue, chest pain, or near syncope.
Class II	Patients with PH resulting in slight limitation of physical activity. They are comfortable at rest. Ordinary physical activity causes undue dyspnea or fatigue, chest pain, or near syncope
Class III	Patients with PH resulting in marked limitation of physical activity. They are comfortable at rest. Less than ordinary activity causes undue dyspnea or fatigue, chest pain, or near syncope
Class IV	Patient with PH with inability to carry out physical activity without symptoms. These patients manifest signs of right heart failure. Dyspnea and/or fatigue may even present at rest. Discomfort is increased by any physical activity.

From Montani D, Gunther S, Dorfmuller P, et al. Pulmonary arterial hypertension. Orphanet J Rare Dis 2013;8:97; with permission.

incidence of IPAH is 5.8 per million.[13] The mean survival rate with patients with idiopathic PAH is 2.8 years.[14]

Group 1.2—Heritable Pulmonary Arterial Hypertension

Hereditary PAH is a term that includes both familial PAH and de novo mutation resulting in PAH. Bone morphogenetic protein receptor type 2 (BMPR2) (Group 1.2.1) gene mutations account for 80% of heritable PAH.[15] Patients with BMPR2 mutation may have a more severe disease. Much less common heritable sources of PAH include activin receptor-like kinase type 1 (ALK-1), endoglin, mothers against decapentagplegic 9 (Smad 9), caveolin-1 (CAV1), and KCNK3 or transforming growth factor β signaling family (Group 1.2.2). These types of heritable pulmonary arterial hypertension may coexist with hereditary hemorrhagic telangiectasia.[16–25] There is also a subset of patients with an unknown (Group 1.2.3) heritable mutations resulting in PAH.

Group 1.3—Drugs and Toxin Induced

There are several drugs and toxins that can result in PAH. Aminorex; benfluorex[26,27]; fenfluramine; dexfenfluramine[7]; selective serotonin reuptake inhibitors late in pregnancy, which can result in persistent PH of the newborn[28]; and toxic rapeseed oil are considered definite risks of PAH. Amphetamines, L-tryptophan, dasatinib,[29] and methamphetamines are considered likely causes of PAH. Cocaine, phenylpropanolamine, St. John's wort, chemotherapeutic agents, amphetamine-like drugs, and interferon α and interferon β[27,30,31] are considered to have a possibility of causing PAH. Oral contraceptives, estrogen, and cigarette smoking are unlikely causes of PAH.[3,4,7,32–34]

Group 1.4—Associated with

Group 1.4.1—Connective tissue disease

There is a prevalence of 13% of patients with connective tissue disease (CTD) who may have PAH.[35] Systemic sclerosis is often the most associated PAH; however, there is a subset of patients with systemic sclerosis who have PH from other causes. Patients with systemic sclerosis and a mPAP between 21 mm Hg and 24 mm Hg are at high risk for PAH within 3 years.[36] PAH has also been described in several other connective tissue disorders, such as systemic lupus erythematosus and mixed connective tissue disorder.[37–40] The 1-year mortality rate for patients with idiopathic PAH is 15%[41] compared with PAH from scleroderma, which is 30%.[42]

Group 1.4.2—HIV infection
The pathophysiology of HIV causing PAH is unclear but the prevalence of PAH in patients with HIV infection is 0.46%.[43] Additionally, patients on highly active antiretroviral therapy have a 70% survival rate at 5 years[44]; therefore, treating the underlying HIV infection is imperative.

Group 1.4.3—Portal hypertension
Porto-PH (POPH) rather than cirrhosis is risk factor for developing PAH. Patients with POPH have a worse prognosis than those with idiopathic PAH.[44,45]

Group 1.4.4—Congenital heart disease
Congenital heart disease (CHD), especially in patients with residual systemic to pulmonary shunting, can eventually lead to increased PVR and reversal of flow. When this reversal of flow results in cyanosis it is called Eisenmenger syndrome, which is the most severe form of PAH in CHD.[46,47] The 2013 Nice Classification has added 4 further classifications of PAH associated with CHD. These new classifications are Eisenmenger syndrome, left-to-right shunts, PAH with coincidental CHD, and postoperative PAH.[7]

Group 1.4.5—Schistosomiasis
Schistosoma eggs can cause occlusions in the pulmonary vascular but the etiology of the PAH is more likely a multifactorial inflammatory process.[48]

Group 1'
Pulmonary veno-occlusive disease and/or pulmonary capillary hemangiomatosis are uncommon causes of PAH.[6]

GROUP 1"
Persistent PH of the newborn has its own category because it has more differences than similarities compared with the other PAH subgroups.[7]

GROUP 2—PULMONARY HYPERTENSION DUE TO LEFT HEART DISEASE
PH secondary to left heart disease is the most common cause of PH.[49] Elevated left atrial pressure is transmitted retrograde into the pulmonary venous system and the pulmonary arteries resulting in an increased pressure. PVR remains normal or near normal.

PH due to left heart disease is further subdivided into PH due to left ventricular systolic dysfunction (Group 2.1), left ventricular diastolic dysfunction (Group 2.2), valvular disease (Group 2.3), and congenital/acquired left heart inflow/outflow tract obstruction and congenital cardiomyopathies (Group 2.4).[7]

GROUP 3—PULMONARY HYPERTENSION DUE TO LUNG DISEASES AND/OR HYPOXIA
PH due to lung disease and/or hypoxia is further divided by the Nice Classification into chronic obstructive pulmonary disease (COPD) (Group 3.1), interstitial lung disease (ILD) (Group 3.2), other pulmonary diseases with mixed restrictive and obstructive pattern (Group 3.3), sleep-disordered breathing (Group 3.4), alveolar hypoventilation disorders (Group 3.5), chronic exposure to high altitude (Group 3.6), and

developmental lung diseases (Group 3.7). Alveolar hypoxia secondary to lung disease, ventilatory defects or high altitude is the most common cause of PH in this category. In patients with parenchymal disease, the PH is moderate (25–35 mm Hg).[50] The survival rate at 5 years is 36% in patients with COPD and an mPAP greater than or equal to 25 mm Hg[51,52] and in 40% of patients with left lateral decubitus PH.

Sleep-disordered breathing is common in patients with PH. Central sleep apnea and Cheyne-Stokes respirations are more common in the younger population with PH and right-sided heart failure, whereas obstructive sleep apnea (OSA) is frequently found in older, obese male patients with PH.[53] There is a high incidence of increased mPAP in OSA, and treatment of OSA can improve the mPAP.[54,55] Evidence suggests that in patients with OSA, the presence of obesity, daytime hypoxia and hypercapnia, abnormal pulmonary function testing, and nocturnal oxygen desaturation strongly correlates with PH.[53]

GROUP 4—CHRONIC THROMBOEMBOLIC PULMONARY HYPERTENSION

Chronic thromboembolic PH (CTEPH) may be a frequent cause of PH and is caused by obstruction of the pulmonary arteries by thromboemboli, tumors, or foreign bodies.[6] Groups of concern are those patients who recently had an acute pulmonary embolism (PE). CTEPH can occur in 4% of patients after an acute PE.[56,57] The curative treatment of CTEPH is pulmonary thromboendarterectomy and, therefore, should be referred appropriately.[6]

GROUP 5—PULMONARY HYPERTENSION WITH UNCLEAR MULTIFACTORIAL MECHANISMS

Groups 5 is the most diverse of the WHO groups. The first subgroup includes hematologic disorders that may result in PH (Group 5.1). Included in this group are myeloproliferative disorders, splenectomy, and chronic hemolytic anemias, such as sickle cell disease, thalassemia, hereditary spherocytosis, stomatocytosis, and microangiopathic hemolytic anemia.[58–63] The cause of PH in this group is unclear and likely multifactorial due to chronic thromboembolism, high cardiac output, left heart disease, and hyperviscosity.[64,65] The second subgroups in WHO Group 5 are the systemic disorders (Group 5.2), such as sarcoidosis, pulmonary histocytosis, and lymphangioleiomyomatosis. Metabolic disorders (Group 5.3), such as glycogen storage disease, Gaucher disease, and thyroid disorders, make up the third subgroup. Thyroid disorders may account of 21.6% of all PAH.[66] The fourth and final subgroup is others (Group 5.4), which includes fibrosing mediastinitis, chronic renal failure, and segmental PH.[7]

Symptoms

Presenting symptoms are generally nonspecific and can include fatigue, lethargy, angina, weakness, signs of right heart failure, and increasing shortness of breath[67,68]; 75% of patients may present late with modified NHYA/WHO functional class III or IV[13] (see **Table 3**). Hoarseness of the voice may be noted and this is due to compression of the left laryngeal nerve by the dilated pulmonary artery (Ortner syndrome).[10]

NHYA/WHO functional testing, a 6-minute walk, and exercise testing can evaluate the severity of symptoms.

Evaluation and Screening

Evaluating patients for PH requires both confirmation of the presence of an elevated mPAP and a determination of the underlying cause.[68] The underlying cause then guides the treatment and management of the patient. When considering etiology of PH in patients with an elevated mPAP, cardiac (Group 2) or pulmonary (Group 3) disease should be considered first, given these are the more common etiologies of PH.

The initial screening tools include blood tests. Basic metabolic chemistries, complete blood cell counts, hepatic function, BNP, and thyroid testing should be obtained to begin the diagnostic evaluation.

Echocardiography is considered the screening tool of choice. The maximum velocity of the tricuspid regurgitant jet can estimate pulmonary arterial systolic pressure. Left ventricular systolic and diastolic function, the cardiac valves, and inflow/outflow tract can also be evaluated by echocardiography. It is also helpful in assessing right ventricular systolic dysfunction that may have resulted secondary to PH.[68]

Early screening with echocardiography is recommended for high-risk groups, which include CTD patients, CHD patients, portal hypertension patients, recent PE patients, chronic hemolysis patients, HIV-infected patients,[68] and patients with systemic sclerosis for at least 3 years.[69]

The most common supraventricular tachycardia in PH is atrial flutter followed by atrial fibrillation, with an annual risk of 2.8%.[70] Therefore, an electrocardiogram should be obtained to screen for arrhythmias as well as underlying structural abnormalities.

A chest radiograph should be obtained to help determine underlying pulmonary and/or cardiac disease; 90% of cases of idiopathic PAH are abnormal at the time of the diagnosis,[67] characterized by central pulmonary arterial dilation with loss of peripheral blood vessels. Right atrial and right ventricular enlargement can be seen in advanced PH.

Pulmonary function testing, including D_{LCO}, can be helpful in evaluating for underlying lung disease. Forced expiratory volume in the first second of expiration, functional vital capacity, and total lung capacity can be helpful in determining underlying COPD or ILD. D_{LCO} has been shown helpful in evaluating PAH in patients with underlying systemic sclerosis.[69]

Another diagnostic test that should be consider is a sleep study, given the association of OSA and PH as well as a high-resolution chest CT, which can reveal detailed information regarding the pulmonary and cardiac anatomy. It may how pulmonary artery disease in CTEPH.

If no heart or lung disorders are found, then CTEPH is next to consider, especially in a patient with a recent PE. A ventilation/perfusion scan can be performed to help establish a diagnosis.

Lastly, if no diagnosis has been established, then PAH should be considered. Evaluation for PAH can include the above but, additionally, if a patient's presenting symptoms warrant further investigation, then testing for connective tissue disorders, hemolysis, thrombophilia, HIV, parasitic infection, and genetic testing may be required. An abdominal ultrasound with Doppler should be performed in patients suspect of portal hypertension.

An RHC is not always needed but confirms diagnosis and can evaluate prognosis based on severity of hemodynamic parameters.[68] A left heart catheterization is not needed unless clinically warranted. An RHC may also be required to determine the severity of PH.

A normal mPAP is less than or equal to 20 mm Hg[71,72] and PH is defined by an increase in mPAP to greater than or equal to 25 mm Hg and a PAWP less than or equal to 15 mm Hg at rest as assessed by RHC.[8] Patients with an mPAP of 21 mm Hg to 24 mm Hg need to be monitored more frequently and there is at this no consensus on management until further studies are performed.[68]

The RHC can help further differentiate the etiology of the PH based on the parameters found. An mPAP greater than or equal to 25 mm Hg and PAWP less than or equal to 15 mm Hg can suggest precapillary PH, which can be found in WHO Groups 1, 3, 4, and 5, and an mPAP of greater than or equal to 25 mm Hg and a PAWP of greater than 15 mm Hg suggest postcapillary source of hypertension, which can be found in Groups 2 and 5.[9] Postcapillary PH can be further defined as passive and reactive based on the transpulmonary pressure gradient (mPAP–pulmonary capillary wedge pressure) of less than or equal to or greater than 12 mm Hg, respectively.[10] Using the RHC to determine PVR is useful in determining PAH. A PVR greater than 3 Wood units with mPAP greater than or equal to 25 mm Hg and PAWP less than or equal to 15 is diagnostic for PAH (WHO Group 1)[9] (see **Table 1**).

In addition to hemodynamic measurements, the RHC allows for vasoreactivity testing to determine which patients may respond to calcium channel blockers. The gold standard agent is inhaled nitrous oxide but other agents have been used, such as intravenous (IV) epoprostenol, IV adenosine, and inhaled iloprost.[9]

Treatment and Management of Pulmonary Artery Hypertension

PH has a wide variety of etiologies, all with specific therapies. Managing the underlying cause of PH often secondarily improve the PH. Therapies specific to PAH are discussed.

Patients who enter strenuous activities (eg, exercise) have peripheral vasodilatation and increased demand on the heart, which can increase the risk of acute heart failure and syncope. Patients should refrain from aggressive physical activity.[10] Vasoconstriction can occur as a result of hypoxia and, therefore, patients traveling by air (above 1500–2000 m) should travel with supplemental oxygen.[73]

Pregnancy is associated with a 30% to 50% mortality rate[73] and is contraindicated in women with PAH. Contraception is recommended in these patients[74,75] and due to the prothrombotic risk associated with hormonal therapy, mechanical contraception (eg, intrauterine device or surgical sterilization) should be used.[10] A pregnant women with PAH should be referred to a center that is familiar with these high-risk pregnancies.[73]

Hemodynamic changes associated with anesthesia can be dangerous and, therefore, if surgery is required, patients must be referred to centers accustom to the management of PAH patients surgically.[76]

Medications with vasoreactivity given for concomitant disorders should be given with extreme caution. Vasoconstrictors, such as over-the-counter cold remedies, should be avoided. β-Blockers can have negative effects on patients with PAH because they can prevent the homeostatic changes that maintain a normal cardiac output.[10]

Medical Therapies

At present, there is no cure for PH. Prior to the development of modern pulmonary vasodilator therapies, the cornerstone of management consisted of diuretics, digoxin therapy, and warfarin therapy.[77] Current guidelines regarding when to treat state that the "consensus is to treat only when the pressure is more than 30 mm Hg measured during catheterization."[78] At this time, pulmonary vasodilator therapy and oral anticoagulation are the main tools of long-term medical therapy[79]

Medical treatment of PAH starts with diuretics and limited salt diets due to right ventricular heart failure effects, such as peripheral edema.[10]

Calcium channel blockers should be used in patients who responded to the vasodilatation challenge testing with inhaled nitrous oxide.[10] Nifedipine, 90 mg/d to 240 mg/d; up to 20 mg/d of amlodipine; or diltiazem, 360 mg/d to 900 mg/d, can be used and may improve prognosis.[80]

Prostacyclin is an arachidonic acid produced by endothelial cells that is a potent vasodilator and can inhibit platelet aggretation.[10] Epoprostenol, treprostinil, and inhaled iloprost are prostacyclin analogs used for the treatment of PAH. Epoprostenol requires an indwelling central venous catheter for continuous infusion because it has a very short half-life and carries the risk of indwelling catheters. Epoprostenol is an effective medication but is expensive and has common side effects, such as headache, flushing, jaw pain, and gastrointestinal disturbances.[81,82] Currently epoprostenol is the therapy of choice of NYHA/WHO functional class IV.[10] Treprostinil is given subcutaneously and is delivered by a pump similar to an insulin pump. Pain and inflammation at the insertion site are the most common adverse effects.[10] Iloprost can be administered by inhalation or IV routes. Each administration is approximately 30 minutes long and patients often require 6 to 9 treatments per day,[83,84] which can be time consuming for patients and caregivers. Common adverse effects are cough, flushing, jaw pain, and headache.[83]

Bosentan and ambrisentan are endothelin-1 antagonists. Endothelin-1, with its 2 isomers, endothelin A (ERTA) and endothelin B (ERTB), is a powerful vasoconstrictor and by antagonizing the receptor results in vasodilatation.[10] Bosenten is an oral agent, which acts on ERTA and ERTB and has been shown to improve patients' functional class.[85] A common adverse effect is elevated liver enzymes; therefore, monthly hepatic function testing is recommended.[10] Ambrisentan acts on the ERTA only and has shown efficacy in idiopathic PAH, CTD-associated PAH, and HIV-associated PAH.[86]

Activation of phosphodiesterase results in the metabolism of cyclic guanosine monophosphate, which signals the release of nitric oxide, a potent vasodilator. Phosphodiesterase type 5 is the most common phosphodiesterase in the pulmonary vasculature.[10] Sildenafil is an oral phosphodiesterase type 5 that is used for patients with PAH with an NYHA/WHO functional class II–IV. Common side effects are headache, flushing, and dyspepsisa.[87] Tadalafil can be used in patients who have already received bosentan.[88]

Anticoagulation

PAH is associated with increased thrombosis and disrupted coagulation and fibrinolysis, making anticoagulation an attractive and frequently used therapeutic modality.[77] Although available therapies have demonstrated efficacy at improving functionality and quality of life, PAH continues to be a progressive disease that results in eventual right ventricular failure and death.[77] Current evidence suggests that primary and/or secondary abnormalities of blood coagulation factors, antithrombotic factors, and the fibrinolytic system all contribute to a prothrombotic state.[89]

Thrombosis is a complex process characterized by interaction of endothelial cells with both soluble elements (eg, plasma coagulation proteins) and cellular elements of blood (eg, platelets).[89] In addition, patients with PAH may have venous congestion and stasis (due to the height pressure of the right atrium), and low flow of blood in the pulmonary circulation and systemic circulation (due to fall in cardiac output) subjects them to deep vein thrombosis. Pulmonary vascular bed is severely restricted in patients, and PE can be fatal due to hypoxia events.[2] Additionally, patients with PAH develop endovascular remodeling that disrupts the homeostatic interactions between platelets and the pulmonary arterial endothelium, which increases the risk for in situ thrombus formation.[90] The consideration that even a small thrombus can produce hemodynamic deterioration in a patient with a compromised pulmonary vascular bed that is unable to dilate or recruit used vasculature represents the rationale for oral anticoagulation in PAH.[91]

There are only a few studies to support anticoagulation in PAH.[10] Although the somewhat sparse evidence base is derived exclusively from idiopathic, heritable, and PAH due to anorexigens, anticoagulation has been generalized to all patient groups, given absence of contraindication.[10]

In a review article by Sauler and colleagues,[90] the investigators comment on 4 observational studies that were done to look at the correlation with idiopathic PAH and the treatment of anticoagulation. These studies evaluated the course of 120 patients with idiopathic PAH at a single center and determined that only pulmonary arterial oxygen saturation and the use of anticoagulation were prognosticators of survival. To further investigate the role of anticoagulation, 78 additional patients were treated with anticoagulation and compared with 37 patients not receiving anticoagulation. The analysis of this showed a more favorable survivorship in the warfarin-treated group. Sauler and colleagues[90] also note, however, that from a study design standpoint, the numbers were too small to reach statistical significance.

There has been one prospective observational trial of warfarin therapy in idiopathic PAH.[80] This was a single-center study that used a historical group from the National Institutes of Health Primary Pulmonary Hypertension Registry. The study evaluated 64 patients for response to high-dose calcium channel blocker administration. The decision to put patients on warfarin was based on the findings of nonuniform perfusion on a nuclear lung scan. Warfarin therapy was associated with increased survival in the group as a whole and showed a particular benefit in patients who were nonresponders to high-dose calcium channel blocker administration.[90]

Several established treatment options for PAH continue to be useful. Two retrospective analyses have reported favorable results with the oral anticoagulant warfarin.[92] Warfarin use has demonstrated a survival benefit in patients with PAH, which is why it has become standard practice to prescribe warfarin, with a goal international normalized ratio of 1.5 to 2.5 in all patients with idiopathic PAH and in patients with more advanced disease WHO functional class III–IV or those receiving therapy[93] (see **Table 3**).

Bleeding in PAH patients is important for 2 reasons: it occurs in higher rates compared with other diseases, and it may be associated with serious sequelae.[94] Anticoagulation is typically not recommended in POPH due to the risk of esophageal variceal hemorrhage. In patients with systemic sclerosis, oral anticoagulation can be difficult to manage because of their high risk of bleeding, especially from the gastrointestinal tract.[10]

The exact role of chronic thrombosis in pulmonary arteries in patients with PAH is controversial. One view suggests that thrombosis is an epiphenomenon related to stasis and endothelial dysfunction. Another view holds that chronic organized thrombotic pulmonary vascular lesions are an integral part of PVR and progression of PAH.[94] The current expert opinion is to treat patients with idiopathic PAH with warfarin anticoagulation in those without contraindications and to consider warfarin therapy in patients with acquired PAH with advanced disease, such as those receiving continuous IV therapy.[90]

REFERENCES

1. Hyduk A, Croft JB, Ayala C, et al. Pulmonary hypertension surveillance–United States, 1980-2002. MMWR Surveill Summ 2005;54(5):1–28.

2. Fallah F. Recent strategies in treatment of pulmonary arterial hypertension, a review. Glob J Health Sci 2015;7(4):307–22.

3. Fishman AP. Clinical classification of pulmonary hypertension. Clin Chest Med 2001;22(3):385–91, vii.

4. Simonneau G, Galie N, Rubin LJ, et al. Clinical classification of pulmonary hypertension. J Am Coll Cardiol 2004;43(12 Suppl S):5S–12S.

5. Olsson KM, Delcroix M, Ghofrani HA, et al. Anticoagulation and survival in pulmonary arterial hypertension: results from the comparative, prospective registry of newly initiated therapies for pulmonary hypertension (COMPERA). Circulation 2014;129(1):57–65.

6. Simonneau G, Robbins IM, Beghetti M, et al. Updated clinical classification of pulmonary hypertension. J Am Coll Cardiol 2009;54(1 Suppl):S43–54.

7. Simonneau G, Gatzoulis MA, Adatia I, et al. Updated clinical classification of pulmonary hypertension. J Am Coll Cardiol 2013;62(25 Suppl):D34–41.

8. Hatano S, Stasser T. Primary pulmonary hypertension: report on a WHO meeting, Geneva, 15–17 October 1973. Geneva (Switzerland): World Health Organization; 1975.

9. Hoeper MM, Bogaard HJ, Condliffe R, et al. Definitions and diagnosis of pulmonary hypertension. J Am Coll Cardiol 2013;62(25 Suppl):D42–50.

10. Montani D, Gunther S, Dorfmuller P, et al. Pulmonary arterial hypertension. Orphanet J Rare Dis 2013;8:97.

11. Delcroix M, Howard L. Pulmonary arterial hypertension: the burden of disease and impact on quality of life. Eur Respir Rev 2015;24(138):621–9.

12. Benza RL, Miller DP, Gomberg-Maitland M, et al. Predicting survival in pulmonary arterial hypertension: insights from the registry to evaluate early and long-term pulmonary arterial hypertension disease management (REVEAL). Circulation 2010;122(2):164–72.

13. Humbert M, Sitbon O, Chaouat A, et al. Pulmonary arterial hypertension in France: results from a national registry. Am J Respir Crit Care Med 2006; 173(9):1023–30.

14. D'Alonzo GE, Barst RJ, Ayres SM, et al. Survival in patients with primary pulmonary hypertension. Results from a national prospective registry. Ann Intern Med 1991;115(5):343–9.

15. Machado RD, Eickelberg O, Elliott CG, et al. Genetics and genomics of pulmonary arterial hypertension. J Am Coll Cardiol 2009;54(1 Suppl):S32–42.

16. Harrison RE, Flanagan JA, Sankelo M, et al. Molecular and functional analysis identifies ALK-1 as the predominant cause of pulmonary hypertension related to hereditary haemorrhagic telangiectasia. J Med Genet 2003;40(12):865–71.

17. Chaouat A, Coulet F, Favre C, et al. Endoglin germline mutation in a patient with hereditary haemorrhagic telangiectasia and dexfenfluramine associated pulmonary arterial hypertension. Thorax 2004;59(5):446–8.

18. Nasim MT, Ogo T, Ahmed M, et al. Molecular genetic characterization of SMAD signaling molecules in pulmonary arterial hypertension. Hum Mutat 2011; 32(12):1385–9.

19. Cogan JD, Pauciulo MW, Batchman AP, et al. High frequency of BMPR2 exonic deletions/duplications in familial pulmonary arterial hypertension. Am J Respir Crit Care Med 2006;174(5):590–8.

20. Aldred MA, Vijayakrishnan J, James V, et al. BMPR2 gene rearrangements account for a significant proportion of mutations in familial and idiopathic pulmonary arterial hypertension. Hum Mutat 2006;27(2):212–3.

21. Sztrymf B, Coulet F, Girerd B, et al. Clinical outcomes of pulmonary arterial hypertension in carriers of BMPR2 mutation. Am J Respir Crit Care Med 2008;177(12): 1377–83.

22. Elliott CG, Glissmeyer EW, Havlena GT, et al. Relationship of BMPR2 mutations to vasoreactivity in pulmonary arterial hypertension. Circulation 2006;113(21): 2509–15.

23. Rosenzweig EB, Morse JH, Knowles JA, et al. Clinical implications of determining BMPR2 mutation status in a large cohort of children and adults with pulmonary arterial hypertension. J Heart Lung Transplant 2008;27(6):668–74.

24. Ma L, Roman-Campos D, Austin ED, et al. A novel channelopathy in pulmonary arterial hypertension. N Engl J Med 2013;369(4):351–61.

25. Austin ED, Ma L, LeDuc C, et al. Whole exome sequencing to identify a novel gene (caveolin-1) associated with human pulmonary arterial hypertension. Circ Cardiovasc Genet 2012;5(3):336–43.

26. Boutet K, Frachon I, Jobic Y, et al. Fenfluramine-like cardiovascular side-effects of benfluorex. Eur Respir J 2009;33(3):684–8.

27. Savale L, Chaumais MC, Cottin V, et al. Pulmonary hypertension associated with benfluorex exposure. Eur Respir J 2012;40(5):1164–72.

28. Kieler H, Artama M, Engeland A, et al. Selective serotonin reuptake inhibitors during pregnancy and risk of persistent pulmonary hypertension in the newborn: population based cohort study from the five Nordic countries. BMJ 2012;344: d8012.

29. Rasheed W, Flaim B, Seymour JF. Reversible severe pulmonary hypertension secondary to dasatinib in a patient with chronic myeloid leukemia. Leuk Res 2009;33(6):861–4.

30. Caravita S, Secchi MB, Wu SC, et al. Sildenafil therapy for interferon-beta-1a-induced pulmonary arterial hypertension: a case report. Cardiology 2011; 120(4):187–9.

31. Dhillon S, Kaker A, Dosanjh A, et al. Irreversible pulmonary hypertension associated with the use of interferon alpha for chronic hepatitis C. Dig Dis Sci 2010; 55(6):1785–90.

32. Souza R, Humbert M, Sztrymf B, et al. Pulmonary arterial hypertension associated with fenfluramine exposure: report of 109 cases. Eur Respir J 2008;31(2): 343–8.

33. Walker AM, Langleben D, Korelitz JJ, et al. Temporal trends and drug exposures in pulmonary hypertension: an American experience. Am Heart J 2006;152(3): 521–6.

34. Chambers CD, Hernandez-Diaz S, Van Marter LJ, et al. Selective serotonin-reuptake inhibitors and risk of persistent pulmonary hypertension of the newborn. N Engl J Med 2006;354(6):579–87.

35. Yang X, Mardekian J, Sanders KN, et al. Prevalence of pulmonary arterial hypertension in patients with connective tissue diseases: a systematic review of the literature. Clin Rheumatol 2013;32(10):1519–31.

36. Valerio CJ, Schreiber BE, Handler CE, et al. Borderline mean pulmonary artery pressure in patients with systemic sclerosis: transpulmonary gradient predicts risk of developing pulmonary hypertension. Arthritis Rheum 2013;65(4):1074–84.

37. Asherson RA, Higenbottam TW, Dinh Xuan AT, et al. Pulmonary hypertension in a lupus clinic: experience with twenty-four patients. J Rheumatol 1990;17(10): 1292–8.

38. Burdt MA, Hoffman RW, Deutscher SL, et al. Long-term outcome in mixed connective tissue disease: longitudinal clinical and serologic findings. Arthritis Rheum 1999;42(5):899–909.

39. Jais X, Launay D, Yaici A, et al. Immunosuppressive therapy in lupus- and mixed connective tissue disease-associated pulmonary arterial hypertension: a retrospective analysis of twenty-three cases. Arthritis Rheum 2008;58(2):521–31.

40. Tanaka E, Harigai M, Tanaka M, et al. Pulmonary hypertension in systemic lupus erythematosus: evaluation of clinical characteristics and response to immuno-suppressive treatment. J Rheumatol 2002;29(2):282–7.

41. Humbert M, Sitbon O, Chaouat A, et al. Survival in patients with idiopathic, famil-ial, and anorexigen-associated pulmonary arterial hypertension in the modern management era. Circulation 2010;122(2):156–63.

42. Tyndall AJ, Bannert B, Vonk M, et al. Causes and risk factors for death in systemic sclerosis: a study from the EULAR Scleroderma Trials and Research (EUSTAR) database. Ann Rheum Dis 2010;69(10):1809–15.

43. Sitbon O, Lascoux-Combe C, Delfraissy JF, et al. Prevalence of HIV-related pul-monary arterial hypertension in the current antiretroviral therapy era. Am J Respir Crit Care Med 2008;177(1):108–13.

44. Sitbon O, Yaici A, Cottin V. The changing picture of patients with pulmonary arte-rial hypertension in France. Eur Respir J 2011;38(Suppl):675–6.

45. Krowka MJ, Miller DP, Barst RJ, et al. Portopulmonary hypertension: a report from the US-based REVEAL Registry. Chest 2012;141(4):906–15.

46. Wood P. The Eisenmenger syndrome or pulmonary hypertension with reversed central shunt. Br Med J 1958;2(5099):755–62.

47. Eisenmenger V. Die angeborene defecte der kammersheidewand das herzen. Z Klin Med 1897;132:131.

48. de Cleva R, Herman P, Pugliese V, et al. Prevalence of pulmonary hypertension in patients with hepatosplenic Mansonic schistosomiasis–prospective study. Hepa-togastroenterology 2003;50(54):2028–30.

49. Oudiz RJ. Pulmonary hypertension associated with left-sided heart disease. Clin Chest Med 2007;28(1):233–41, x.

50. Thabut G, Dauriat G, Stern JB, et al. Pulmonary hemodynamics in advanced COPD candidates for lung volume reduction surgery or lung transplantation. Chest 2005;127(5):1531–6.

51. Seeger W, Adir Y, Barbera JA, et al. Pulmonary hypertension in chronic lung dis-eases. J Am Coll Cardiol 2013;62(25 Suppl):D109–16.

52. Oswald-Mammosser M, Weitzenblum E, Quoix E, et al. Prognostic factors in COPD patients receiving long-term oxygen therapy. Importance of pulmonary ar-tery pressure. Chest 1995;107(5):1193–8.

53. Ismail K, Roberts K, Manning P, et al. OSA and pulmonary hypertension: time for a new look. Chest 2015;147(3):847–61.

54. Marrone O, Bellia V, Ferrara G, et al. Transmural pressure measurements. Impor-tance in the assessment of pulmonary hypertension in obstructive sleep apneas. Chest 1989;95(2):338–42.

55. Sajkov D, Wang T, Saunders NA, et al. Continuous positive airway pressure treat-ment improves pulmonary hemodynamics in patients with obstructive sleep ap-nea. Am J Respir Crit Care Med 2002;165(2):152–8.

56. Tapson VF, Humbert M. Incidence and prevalence of chronic thromboembolic pulmonary hypertension: from acute to chronic pulmonary embolism. Proc Am Thorac Soc 2006;3(7):564–7.

57. Pengo V, Lensing AW, Prins MH, et al. Incidence of chronic thromboembolic pul-monary hypertension after pulmonary embolism. N Engl J Med 2004;350(22):2257–64.

58. Gladwin MT, Sachdev V, Jison ML, et al. Pulmonary hypertension as a risk factor for death in patients with sickle cell disease. N Engl J Med 2004;350(9):886–95.

59. Castro O, Hoque M, Brown BD. Pulmonary hypertension in sickle cell disease: cardiac catheterization results and survival. Blood 2003;101(4):1257–61.

60. Aessopos A, Stamatelos G, Skoumas V, et al. Pulmonary hypertension and right heart failure in patients with beta-thalassemia intermedia. Chest 1995;107(1): 50–3.

61. Smedema JP, Louw VJ. Pulmonary arterial hypertension after splenectomy for hereditary spherocytosis. Cardiovasc J Afr 2007;18(2):84–9.

62. Jais X, Till SJ, Cynober T, et al. An extreme consequence of splenectomy in dehydrated hereditary stomatocytosis: gradual thrombo-embolic pulmonary hypertension and lung-heart transplantation. Hemoglobin 2003;27(3):139–47.

63. Stuard ID, Heusinkveld RS, Moss AJ. Microangiopathic hemolytic anemia and thrombocytopenia in primary pulmonary hypertension. N Engl J Med 1972; 287(17):869–70.

64. Bunn HF, Nathan DG, Dover GJ, et al. Pulmonary hypertension and nitric oxide depletion in sickle cell disease. Blood 2010;116(5):687–92.

65. Miller AC, Gladwin MT. Pulmonary complications of sickle cell disease. Am J Respir Crit Care Med 2012;185(11):1154–65.

66. Badesch DB, Raskob GE, Elliott CG, et al. Pulmonary arterial hypertension: baseline characteristics from the REVEAL Registry. Chest 2010;137(2):376–87.

67. Rich S, Dantzker DR, Ayres SM, et al. Primary pulmonary hypertension. A national prospective study. Ann Intern Med 1987;107(2):216–23.

68. Haddad RN, Mielniczuk LM. An evidence-based approach to screening and diagnosis of pulmonary hypertension. Can J Cardiol 2015;31(4):382–90.

69. Coghlan JG, Denton CP, Grunig E, et al. Evidence-based detection of pulmonary arterial hypertension in systemic sclerosis: the DETECT study. Ann Rheum Dis 2014;73(7):1340–9.

70. Tongers J, Schwerdtfeger B, Klein G, et al. Incidence and clinical relevance of supraventricular tachyarrhythmias in pulmonary hypertension. Am Heart J 2007;153(1):127–32.

71. Kovacs G, Berghold A, Scheidl S, et al. Pulmonary arterial pressure during rest and exercise in healthy subjects: a systematic review. Eur Respir J 2009;34(4): 888–94.

72. Badesch DB, Champion HC, Sanchez MA, et al. Diagnosis and assessment of pulmonary arterial hypertension. J Am Coll Cardiol 2009;54(1 Suppl):S55–66.

73. Galie N, Hoeper MM, Humbert M, et al. Guidelines for the diagnosis and treatment of pulmonary hypertension: the Task Force for the Diagnosis and Treatment of Pulmonary Hypertension of the European Society of Cardiology (ESC) and the European Respiratory Society (ERS), endorsed by the International Society of Heart and Lung Transplantation (ISHLT). Eur Heart J 2009;30(20):2493–537.

74. Sitbon O, Humbert M, Simonneau G. Primary pulmonary hypertension: current therapy. Prog Cardiovasc Dis 2002;45(2):115–28.

75. Bonnin M, Mercier FJ, Sitbon O, et al. Severe pulmonary hypertension during pregnancy: mode of delivery and anesthetic management of 15 consecutive cases. Anesthesiology 2005;102(6):1133–7 [discussion: 1135A–6A].

76. Price LC, Montani D, Jais X, et al. Noncardiothoracic nonobstetric surgery in mild-to-moderate pulmonary hypertension. Eur Respir J 2010;35(6):1294–302.

77. Robinson JC, Pugliese SC, Fox DL, et al. Anticoagulation in pulmonary arterial hypertension. Curr Hypertens Rep 2016;18(6):47.

78. Fauzi AR. Primary pulmonary hypertension. World Health Organization. Med J Malaysia 2000;55(4):529–37 [quiz: 538].

79. Kneussl MP, Lang IM, Brenot FP. Medical management of primary pulmonary hypertension. Eur Respir J 1996;9(11):2401–9.

80. Rich S, Kaufmann E, Levy PS. The effect of high doses of calcium-channel blockers on survival in primary pulmonary hypertension. N Engl J Med 1992; 327(2):76–81.

81. Sitbon O, Humbert M, Nunes H, et al. Long-term intravenous epoprostenol infusion in primary pulmonary hypertension: prognostic factors and survival. J Am Coll Cardiol 2002;40(4):780–8.

82. Robbins IM, Christman BW, Newman JH, et al. A survey of diagnostic practices and the use of epoprostenol in patients with primary pulmonary hypertension. Chest 1998;114(5):1269–75.

83. Olschewski H, Simonneau G, Galie N, et al. Inhaled iloprost for severe pulmonary hypertension. N Engl J Med 2002;347(5):322–9.

84. Hoeper MM, Schwarze M, Ehlerding S, et al. Long-term treatment of primary pulmonary hypertension with aerosolized iloprost, a prostacyclin analogue. N Engl J Med 2000;342(25):1866–70.

85. Channick RN, Simonneau G, Sitbon O, et al. Effects of the dual endothelin-receptor antagonist bosentan in patients with pulmonary hypertension: a randomised placebo-controlled study. Lancet 2001;358(9288):1119–23.

86. Galie N, Olschewski H, Oudiz RJ, et al. Ambrisentan for the treatment of pulmonary arterial hypertension: results of the ambrisentan in pulmonary arterial hypertension, randomized, double-blind, placebo-controlled, multicenter, efficacy (ARIES) study 1 and 2. Circulation 2008;117(23):3010–9.

87. Galie N, Ghofrani HA, Torbicki A, et al. Sildenafil citrate therapy for pulmonary arterial hypertension. N Engl J Med 2005;353(20):2148–57.

88. Galie N, Brundage BH, Ghofrani HA, et al. Tadalafil therapy for pulmonary arterial hypertension. Circulation 2009;119(22):2894–903.

89. Berger G, Azzam ZS, Hoffman R, et al. Coagulation and anticoagulation in pulmonary arterial hypertension. Isr Med Assoc J 2009;11(6):376–9.

90. Sauler M, Fares WH, Trow TK. Standard nonspecific therapies in the management of pulmonary arterial hypertension. Clin Chest Med 2013;34(4):799–810.

91. Fuso L, Baldi F, Di Perna A. Therapeutic strategies in pulmonary hypertension. Front Pharmacol 2011;2:21.

92. Stringham R, Shah NR. Pulmonary arterial hypertension: an update on diagnosis and treatment. Am Fam Physician 2010;82(4):370–7.

93. Bishop BM, Mauro VF, Khouri SJ. Practical considerations for the pharmacotherapy of pulmonary arterial hypertension. Pharmacotherapy 2012;32(9): 838–55.

94. Said K. Anticoagulation in pulmonary arterial hypertension: contemporary data from COMPERA registry. Glob Cardiol Sci Pract 2014;2014(2):48–52.

Preventative Cardiology

Andrew Mackie, MPAS, PA-C*, Trent Honda, PhD, MMS, PA-C

KEYWORDS

- Prevention • Cardiovascular disease • Atherosclerosis • Risk assessment

KEY POINTS

- Cardiovascular disease is the most common cause of death in the United States and around one-fourth of the American population lives with some form of the disease.
- There are a large number of modifiable factors known to affect an individual's risk of disease.
- Recent years have seen the emergence of high-quality tools to help clinicians determine patients' cardiovascular risk, as well as several evidence-based interventions that can appreciably decrease risk.

I will prevent disease whenever I can, for prevention is preferable to cure.
From the 1964 modernized version of the Hippocratic Oath.[1,2]

INTRODUCTION

In the early twentieth century, cardiovascular disease was not recognized as a common cause of death. Accordingly, the first edition of *Principles and Practice of Medicine* by Sir William Osler, written in 1895, did not even mention angina. In a subsequent edition in 1912, Sir Osler does make mention of angina but still describes it as a "rare disease in hospitals."[3] One major explanation for this omission was that cardiovascular illnesses were obscured by much more common, competing infectious diseases, such as pneumonia, tuberculosis, and diarrheal illnesses (**Fig. 1**). With advances in medicine and the advent of antibiotics in the early twentieth century, the risk of death from infectious diseases decreased dramatically in the developed world with a resulting increase in average life expectancy from around 50 years in the early twentieth century to nearly 80 years in 2010 (**Fig. 2**).

This decrease in infectious disease deaths was matched with a concomitant increase in death from cardiovascular disease. This increase began around 1920 and peaked in the late 1960s (**Fig. 3**).[4] Although the ultimate cause of this increase in cardiovascular disease is unknown, several theories have been proposed. One theory is that, with the increase in longevity, people survived long enough for cardiovascular disease to

Physician Assistant Program, Bouvé College of Health Sciences, Northeastern University, 202 Robinson Hall, 360 Huntington Avenue, Boston, MA 02115, USA
* Corresponding author.
E-mail address: a.mackie@northeastern.edu

Physician Assist Clin 2 (2017) 743–758
http://dx.doi.org/10.1016/j.cpha.2017.06.010
2405-7991/17/© 2017 Elsevier Inc. All rights reserved.

physicianassistant.theclinics.com

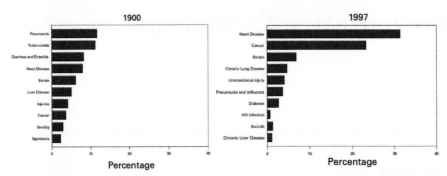

Fig. 1. United States' 10 leading causes of death as a percentage of all deaths. (*From* Centers for Disease Control and Prevention (CDC). Control of infectious diseases. MMWR Morb Mortal Wkly Rep 1999;48(29):621–9.)

become clinically evident.[5] Another potential significant factor in the increase in mortality from cardiovascular disease may be attributable to a parallel, tremendous growth in the rate of smoking. Cigarette smoking, which was uncommon before 1900, became ubiquitous in the United States in the mid-twentieth century, peaking at 42% of the population in 1965.[6] Following the 1964 Surgeon General's report on the dangers of smoking, there has been a subsequent decline in the proportion of Americans who smoke, with the most recent data demonstrating a decrease to 15.1% in 2015 (**Fig. 4**).[7]

Cardiovascular disease caused 17.5 million deaths worldwide in 2012.

Today, cardiovascular disease is by far the leading cause of mortality worldwide, directly causing more than 17.5 million deaths globally in 2012 and more than 614,000 deaths in the United States in 2014 alone.[8,9] Identifying ways to prevent

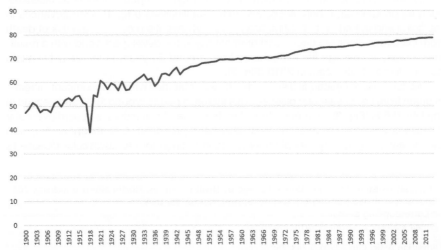

Fig. 2. Average life expectancy, 1900 to 2013. (*From* Chong Y, Tejada Vera B, et al. Deaths in the United States, 1900–2013. Hyattsville, MD: National Center for Health Statistics; 2015.)

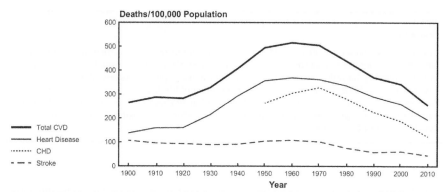

Fig. 3. Death rates (not age-adjusted) for cardiovascular diseases, United States, 1900 to 2010. CHD, coronary heart disease; CVD, cardiovascular disease; NCHS, National Center for Health Statistics. (*Courtesy of* Vital Statistics of the United States, NCHS; and *Data from* NHLBI Fact Book, Fiscal Year 2012. Available at: https://www.nhlbi.nih.gov/about/documents/factbook/2012/chapter4#4_3. Accessed July 7, 2017.)

cardiovascular morbidity and mortality is, therefore, of tremendous clinical and population health importance.

This article focuses on the prevention of atherosclerotic cardiovascular disease (ASCVD). In particular, it considers:

- Physiology and natural history of cardiovascular disease
- Identifying and quantifying cardiovascular risk
- Strategies for risk prevention.

An illustrative patient's case is considered in this article. **Box 1** outlines his initial presentation. Although this patient is healthy, his presentation provides an

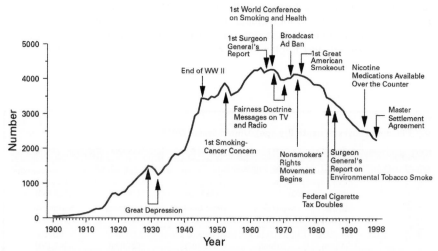

Fig. 4. Annual adult per capita cigarette consumption and major smoking and health events, United States, 1900 to 1998. (*Data from* Centers for Disease Control and Prevention (CDC).Tobacco use–United States, 1900-1999. MMWR Morb Mortal Wkly Rep 1999; 48(43);986–93.)

> **Box 1**
> **Scenario 1**
>
> The illustrative patient, a 40-year old man comes to the primary care office for the first time since his twenties. He has no complaints and is just interested in a check-up. His blood pressure is 123/72 mm Hg, his pulse rate is 80 beats per minute, his respiratory rate is 12 per minute, and his body mass index is 24 kg/m². Blood work from a recent life-insurance application indicates a hemoglobin A1C (HbA1c) of 5.4%, a total cholesterol of 143 mg/dL, and a high-density lipoprotein (HDL) of 51 mg/dL. He admits to a 5 pack-year history of smoking but states he "hasn't touched a cigarette for half a year."

opportunity to consider what can be done to ensure his continued good health in the future. Because chronic diseases, such as cardiovascular disease, have long latent periods, his health at this moment and his health trajectory must be considered. In addition, it is necessary to recognize that the nature of threats to his health will change throughout his lifetime. Once these potential threats are understood, interventions that may mitigate, or even prevent, these risks from resulting in clinical disease can be considered.

Table 1 lists the top 3 most common causes of death in the United States, stratified by age. Although cardiovascular disease is only the third leading cause of death in this patient's age group, it is instructive to note that relatively few people actually die in their early forties. The incidence rate of death between the ages of 35 and 40 years in the United States is only 147 per 100,000 but is nearly 10 times higher in those older than 65 years (1454/100,000 population).[10] Heart disease is the most common cause of death in those over age 65, which is also the group with the highest absolute risk of death. This does not, however, mean that cardiovascular disease is only a disease of patients older than 65 years. The development of atherosclerosis, the vascular lesions pathognomonic for cardiovascular disease, progresses over one's lifetime. In fact, studies in young men killed in the Korean and the Vietnam Wars found grossly visible coronary artery disease in individuals as young as 18 years old.[11,12] Therefore, because cardiovascular disease has such a long, preclinical period, prevention must be considered and implemented decades before it becomes a cause of death.

Table 1
Top 3 leading causes of death (by age), United States (2014)

Age	Rank	Young adults (age 25–44)		Middle aged adults (age 45–64)	Older adults (age ≥65)	Overall (total, all ages)
Leading cause of death (total no.)	1	Unintentional injury (33,405)		Malignancy (160,116)	Heart Disease (489,722)	Heart Disease (614,348)
	2	Suicide (6,569)	Malignancy (11,267)	Heart Disease (114,264)	Malignancy (413,885)	Malignancy (591,699)
	3	Homicide (4,159)	Heart Disease (10,368)	Unintentional injury (33,405)	COPD (124,693)	COPD (147,101)

Abbreviation: COPD, chronic obstructive pulmonary disease.
  Modified from https://www.cdc.gov/injury/images/lc-charts/leading_causes_of_death_age_group_2014_1050w760h.gif. Accessed July 7, 2017.

Coronary artery disease development begins as early as the second decade of life.

PATHOGENESIS OF ATHEROSCLEROSIS

It is informative to review the pathobiology of the underlying process of atherosclerosis. Atherosclerosis is a pathologic process in blood vessels resulting from a complex interplay between the vascular endothelium and circulating blood elements.[13] Arteries have 3 main layers: the intima, the media, and the adventitia (**Fig. 5**). The intima is the innermost layer abutting the blood column and is composed of a single sheet of endothelial cells.

A variety of irritants, including inflammatory mediators, elevated cholesterol levels, hypertension, and smoking, can lead to changes in endothelial cells which promote intimal vessel damage.[14]

Systemic inflammation is a key component of the pathophysiology of atherosclerosis.

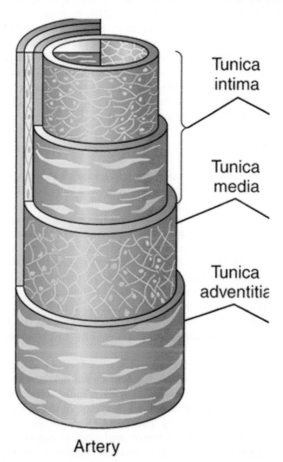

Tunica
intima

Tunica
media

Tunica
adventitia

Artery

Fig. 5. Arterial wall. (*From* McCance K, Huether S. Alterations in blood flow. In: McCance K, Huether S, editors. Pathophysiology. 6th edition. Elsevier: Philadelphia; 2010.)

Intimal injury alters vascular endothelial cell permeability, allowing enhanced uptake of low-density lipoproteins (LDLs), which then deposit in the arterial wall.[15] In addition, although endothelial cells normally resist attachment of leukocytes, inflammation resulting from this damage increases expression of endothelial adhesion molecules. This allows blood monocytes[16] to attach and then be endocytosed into the cell where they differentiate into macrophages.[13] Once macrophages have entered the intima, they engulf the LDL particles and become foam cells.[17] The foam cells subsequently die, leading to a further increase in local inflammatory mediators. This inflammation further damages the intima and leads to monocyte chemotaxis, perpetuating the cycle of vascular injury while building a fatty deposit in the wall of the vessel. In addition, calcium deposition occurs during the development of atheromas.[18]

The process of atherosclerosis continues as smooth muscle cells in the arterial media then migrate to the fatty deposit and promote synthesis of matrix molecules such as collagen.[19] This layer of collagen forms a fibrous cap over the lipid-rich core (**Fig. 6**).

If the fibrous cap is thin and ruptures or develops fissures, the thrombogenic lipid core is exposed to the blood stream, leading to platelet adhesion, activation, and aggregation. The clotting cascade is concurrently activated, leading to the formation of a thrombus in the arterial lumen. This manifests clinically as acute coronary syndromes, such as myocardial infarction or unstable angina. If the fibrous cap becomes thicker over time, despite accumulation of a substantial intraluminal lipid pools, the vessel will undergo remodeling, initially dilating to maintain the lumen diameter. Ultimately, remodeling cannot adequately compensate, and the lumen becomes narrowed, leading to a stable lesion that restricts the ability to deliver adequate blood flow to the myocardium. This manifests clinically as anginal symptoms, which often initially occur with exertion but may, over time, occur even at rest.

IDENTIFICATION OF RISK FACTORS

In 1947, in response to the emergence of cardiovascular disease as the leading cause of death nationwide, the Framingham Heart Study was initiated. This large, national, prospective cohort study was designed to investigate risk factors for cardiovascular disease. By 1957, the study had identified high blood pressure, being overweight, and hypercholesterolemia as significant risk factors for cardiovascular disease. It also identified men and older individuals as being at particularly high risk.[20] Over time, Framingham identified several both nonmodifiable and modifiable risk factors for heart disease (**Table 2**). Both of these risk factor categories inform clinical decision-making around preventative cardiology. Knowledge of nonmodifiable risk factors provides the clinician with information about baseline risk in an individual and how it changes throughout time. Knowledge of modifiable risk factors provides actionable points that can be addressed to prevent future cardiovascular morbidity and mortality.

Although the Framingham cohort consisted mostly of white and middle-income participants, other important studies have identified similar risk factors in other populations. Two examples, which aimed for a more diverse ethnic representation in patient populations, include the Multiethnic Study of Atherosclerosis (MESA) and The Hispanic Community Health study. The MESA study began in 2000 with recruitment of African American, Chinese, Hispanic, and white populations.[26] The Hispanic Community Health Study started in 2006 and has enrolled more than 15,000 subjects.[27] Both of these cohorts will contribute to a better understanding of differences in risk among diverse populations.

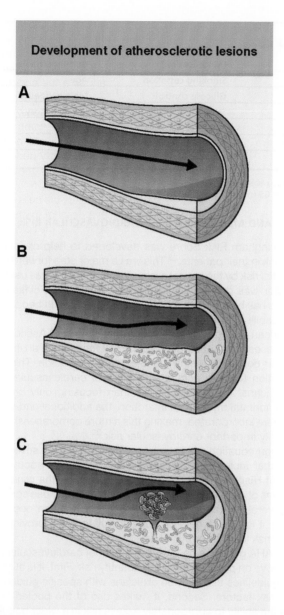

Fig. 6. Cross-section of the stages of atherosclerotic plaque formation. (*A*) Endothelial dysfunction preceding the formation of atherosclerotic lesions, characterized by increased endothelial permeability, expression of vascular adhesion molecules, and migration of leukocytes into the arterial wall. (*B*) Early atherosclerotic lesion with lipid-rich core, debris, leukocytes, and a fibrous cap. (*C*) Ruptured fibrous cap leading to superficial thrombosis with or without distal embolization. (*From* Windecker S. Acute coronary syndromes. In Albert RK, Slutsky AS, Ranieri VM, et al, editors. A clinical critical care medicine. Elsevier: Philadelphia; 2006.)

Table 2
Conventional risk factors

Modifiable[a]	(Modification)	Non-modifiable
Smoking[21]	Smoking cessation	Age
Diabetes	Glucose control	Male gender
Dyslipidemia[22]	Statins	Family history of premature CHD[b]
Hypertension[23]	Antihypertensives	
Central obesity[24]	Diet, exercise	
Inactivity[25]	Exercise	

[a] Relevant guideline referenced.
[b] Men 55 or women 65 in 1st degree relative.

QUANTIFICATION AND MEASUREMENT OF CARDIOVASCULAR RISK

In 1998, the Framingham Risk Score was developed to help clinicians quantify the 10-year cardiac risk in their patients.[28] This was a major step forward in terms of identification of potential risk by the typical clinician. Although this was useful, the Framingham risk calculator was derived from a mainly white middle-class population from New England. This has been identified as a major shortcoming because it significantly limits its generalizability to the larger population.

The 2013 American College of Cardiology/American Heart Association (ACC/AHA) guideline on the assessment of cardiovascular risk focused on an improving risk prediction in the wider population using a pooled cohort equation. This incorporates an expanded population to more accurately represent cardiovascular risks in women and African Americans. In addition, rather than focusing only on cardiac events, such as fatal and nonfatal myocardial infarction, the additional end-points of nonfatal and fatal stroke were incorporated, making this a more comprehensive tool in terms of quantifying clinically important cardiovascular risk.[29]

The pooled cohort equation risk calculator was derived from several different study populations[30–34] that included white and African American populations. It did not include patients of Hispanic or Asian ethnicity. Therefore, the clinician must understand the limitations of applying it to populations other than those specifically included because either overestimation or underestimation of risk can occur. Recent[35] and future studies will, it is hoped, help produce calculators that provide valid estimates of cardiovascular risk in other populations.

The 2013 ACC/AHA guideline on the assessment of cardiovascular risk has several features that improve on previous efforts to quantify risk. First, it is aligned with several relevant clinical guidelines that provide clinicians with specific guidance for management of various risk factors. Second, it makes use of the pooled cohort equation, which increases the ability to appropriately assess risk in a wider population than previously available. Third, it is based on clinically meaningful hard endpoints that consist not only of coronary heart disease but also cerebral vascular disease. These end points include both nonfatal myocardial infarction or coronary heart disease death and fatal or nonfatal stroke. Finally, these guidelines are evidence-based and provide specifics regarding both the strength of the recommendations and the level of evidence that supports them.

This guideline recommends first calculating risk from a patient between the ages of 20 and 40 years, with lifestyle guidance if the patient is found to be low risk.[29] After the age of 40 years, risk calculation is recommended every 4 to 6 years, with application of the relevant guidelines if intermediate or high risk is found. In addition, patients who belong in a borderline risk range (5%–7.5% 10-year risk) may be considered for further evaluation to determine if their risk warrants upward revision. Novel risk factors that were determined to have adequate evidence for this group included high-sensitivity C-reactive protein, coronary artery calcium score, and ankle brachial index. The presence of any of these may influence initiation of primary prevention in a patient after a shared decision-making discussion. **Fig. 7** provides an approach for using this risk calculator.

STRATEGIES FOR RISK PREVENTION

Atherosclerosis has several characteristics that make it very well suited to preventative efforts. First, it is a common disease. This is important because prevention efforts are only cost-effective if they are oriented at a high-risk population. For example, if the prevalence of a hypothetical disease was 0.01% in a population of 100,000 and a preventative medicine program achieved a 50% reduction in prevalence over a 10-year period, this would only meaningfully affect 5 people. However, with a disease as prevalent as cardiovascular disease, with approximately 26% of Americans in 2016 living with some form of the disease, the number of people in the same population of 100,000 who would be meaningfully affected by the exact same preventative measures would be 13,000.[36]

Second, cardiovascular disease has a long latency period. This, in the context of established, modifiable risk factors, allows for targeting of interventions to those at greatest risk well before cardiovascular events occur. As the risk factors associated with ASCVD were identified, efforts to mitigate these factors became possible. For example, bile-acid sequestrants were introduced in the 1960s. Initial efforts to lower cholesterol with bile-acid sequestrants and other agents failed to demonstrate clinical benefit.[37] However, in 1994, the Scandinavian Simvastatin Survival Study (4S) was published and established improved survival using a statin.[38] Since the 4S was

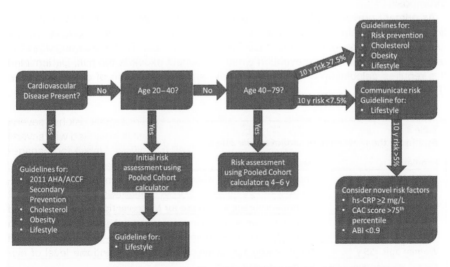

Fig. 7. Risk assessment and intervention flow chart. ABI, ankle brachial index; CAC, coronary artery calcium; hs-CRP, high-sensitivity C-reactive protein. (*From* Goff Jr DC, Lloyd-Jones DM, Bennett G, et al. 2013 ACC/AHA Guideline on the Assessment of Cardiovascular Risk. A Report of the American College of Cardiology/American Heart Association Task Force on Practice Guidelines. Circulation 2014;129(25 Suppl 2):S49–73.)

published, there have been meta-analyses of differing intensity of statin therapy[39] and even low-risk[40] populations demonstrated the benefit of statins in reducing cardiovascular risk. Statins provide an excellent example of the impact made by both primary and secondary intervention when specific risk factors can be targeted.[41]

Additional studies have demonstrated the benefit of treating hypertension. It is estimated that in excess of 40.6% (95% CI 24.5%–54.6%) of cardiovascular disease in the population is attributable to hypertension, and several studies have demonstrated that the cardiovascular risk conferred by hypertension decreases with successful treatment. For instance, a landmark study published in *The Lancet* showed hypertension treatment decreases the risk of stroke in patients older than 60 years by 42% and decreases the occurrence of adverse cardiac events by 26%.[42–44]

Although the benefits of glucose control in diabetic patients have long been shown to decrease the risk of microvascular complications, until recently, supportive evidence for reduction in macrovascular complications has been elusive.[45] Several newer studies have shown benefits for some pharmacologic interventions for macrovascular outcomes. These include the glucagon-like peptide (GLP)-1 analog liraglutide[46] and sodium-glucose cotransporter (SGLT)-2 inhibitors.[47] Additional studies of these agents are needed to completely elucidate the long-term efficacy for cardiovascular prevention.

As previously noted, platelets play a key role in acute coronary syndromes; therefore, antiplatelet agents play a central role in both primary and secondary prevention of these episodes. Several therapeutic options are now available but aspirin has been studied most extensively.[48]

Aspirin for secondary prevention was first found to confer a mortality benefit in the International Study of Infarct Survival (ISIS) 2 trial in 1988, which studied more than 17,000 subjects who had suffered a myocardial infarction.[49] This has subsequently been confirmed in several trials and meta-analyses.[48] It has also been used in combination with other antiplatelet agents after coronary angioplasty to prevent in-stent thrombosis.[50]

As primary prevention, low-dose aspirin (eg, 81 mg) daily can reduce the risk of a first myocardial infarction or stroke but demonstration of a clear mortality benefit has not been consistent.[48] Current US Preventive Services Task Force endorses the use of aspirin for primary prevention when the benefit exceeds the risk. Determining this requires calculation of the patient's risk, and consideration of age and gender (**Table 3**).[51]

Table 3
Aspirin for the prevention of cardiovascular disease

Population	Recommendation
Men age 45–79	Encourage aspirin use when potential CVD benefit (MIs prevented) outweighs potential harm of GI hemorrhage.
Men age <45	Do not encourage aspirin use for MI prevention.
Women age 55–79 y	Encourage aspirin use when potential CVD benefit (strokes prevented) outweighs potential harm of GI hemorrhage.
Women age <55 y	Do not encourage aspirin use for stroke prevention.
Men & Women age ≥80 y	No Recommendation

Abbreviations: GI, gastrointestinal; MI, myocardial infarction.
Adapted from Agency for Healthcare Research and Quality, guide to clinical preventative services, recommendation for adults. Available at: https://www.ahrq.gov/professionals/clinicians-providers/guidelines-recommendations/guide/section2.html#aspirin. Accessed July 7, 2017.

In addition to the aforementioned pharmacologic interventions, lifestyle modifications (**Table 4**), such as increasing physical activity, improving diet, and smoking cessation, have also been found to be effective.[52–54] A healthy diet is described by the Guideline on Lifestyle as comprising "vegetables, fruits, whole grains, low-fat dairy products, poultry, fish, legumes, nontropical vegetable oils, and nuts; and limited intake of sweets, sugar-sweetened beverages, and red meats."[55] For exercise, a total of 150 minutes per week of moderate intensity active is recommended. Interventions to facilitate smoking cessation are described elsewhere.[21–25]

CONNECTING RISK ASSESSMENT AND PREVENTION STRATEGIES TO INTERVENTIONS

When approaching efforts to prevent ASCVD, it is useful to consider different levels of prevention, depending on what time in the natural history of the disease intervention is made. These are referred to as primordial, primary, and secondary prevention.

Primordial intervention refers to efforts to prevent development of cardiovascular risk factors in a population.[56] An example is public health efforts to curb smoking via educational efforts, taxes to discourage tobacco use, and banning advertisements that encourage young people to smoke. An advantage of the approach is early intervention, either by preventing or by substantially modifying development of the disease in a large segment of the population. Disadvantages include the need to target the entire population, with the attendant cost being higher than with a more targeted approach. In addition, the usual vehicle for these efforts is a change in public policy, which is generally a difficult proposition and is often outside of the immediate control of the clinician. For the primary care provider, however, primordial intervention can be easily incorporated in office visits via anticipatory guidance and patient education on modifiable risk factors, even in the pediatric population[57,58] (**Box 2**).

If the illustrative patient's risk factors did not change in 10 years, his 10-year risk would increase by a factor of 4% to 2%. This increase represents the nonmodifiable effect of age.

Primary prevention refers to interventions aimed at reducing the possibility of developing an event in someone who already has risk factors. An advantage of primary prevention is that it allows clinicians to target interventions to high-risk patients. Because only a few individuals in a population are treated, this helps ensure that interventions

---

Table 4
Interventions shown to decrease cardiovascular risk

Lifestyle	Pharmacologic[a]
>150 min of physical activity per week	Statin therapy
Mediterranean type diet[b]	Hypertension management
Smoking cessation	Diabetes management[c]
Decreasing alcohol consumption	Aspirin therapy
Weight management	

[a] Benefits are established in some, but not all, patient populations.
[b] Moderate in total fat (32% to 35% of total calories), relatively low in saturated fat (9% to 10% of total calories), high in fiber (27 to 37 g/d), and high in polyunsaturated fatty acids (particularly omega-3s).
[c] Suggested by recent studies.

Box 2:
Primordial prevention

The illustrative patient is 40 years old and relatively healthy, but had previously been a smoker. His brother, who is 10 years younger, has never smoked for a variety of reasons. His brother was born in 1987 and when he was 11 years old in 1999 the Master Settlement Agreement between tobacco companies and 46 state attorneys general was litigated.[59] In part, this provided money for antismoking educational efforts, which countered forces that only a few years earlier contributed to his older brother starting to smoke. When he was 17 years old, smoking was banned in restaurants in his state and by that time there were also large increases in the tobacco excise tax in his state that presented a substantial economic barrier to developing nicotine addiction.

---

are cost-effective. It also results in a greater per-person risk reduction than primordial prevention. Disadvantages include the need to screen a relatively large number of patients to see if they are candidates for primary prevention, the cost of ancillary testing for cholesterol and other blood tests, and that the intervention may simply delay rather than prevent the event. For the primary care provider, this includes identifying those with risk factors (eg, poor diet, inactivity, smoking, high alcohol intake) and providing education, interventions (often pharmacologic), and strategies to reduce risk factor exposure[60] (**Box 3** and **4**).

Secondary prevention is used in patients who have already suffered an event in an effort to reduce the risk of recurrence. Targeting patients who have already suffered an event reduces the total number of patients requiring treatment, resulting in a more focused intervention. Disadvantages are that postevent therapies are less effective when applied so far along in the disease process, it benefits a relatively small number of patients, and it occurs after sustaining morbidity from the initial event. An example of this for the primary care provider would be optimizing beta blockade after a myocardial infarction.[61]

Box 3
Primary prevention

The illustrative patient again in 10 years, at age 50 years. His blood pressure has increased to 144/88 mm Hg. Blood work now demonstrates an HbA1c of 6.6%, total cholesterol 210 mg/dL, and HDL 38 mg/dL.

   The patient now has a 10-year cardiovascular risk of 11%. If his risk factors were optimized, however, his risk would be 2%.

   • He is currently diabetic, and has hypertension and suboptimal serum lipids. In addition to the lifestyle interventions outlined in **Box 1**, this patient would benefit from diabetes and hypertension management, as well as statin therapy. The ACC/AHA 2016 cholesterol guidelines recommend high-intensity statin therapy for all patients with a 10-year cardiovascular risk greater than 7.5%. Additionally, patients with 10-year risks greater than 10% would likely benefit from daily aspirin therapy.
   • If this patient were African American, his 10-year cardiovascular risk would be 13% and would decrease to less than 4% with risk factor optimization.
   • If this patient were female, her 10-year cardiovascular risk would be only 5%, with the risk falling to less than 1% with risk factor optimization.

Nonmodifiable risk factors have a significant effect on the 10-year cardiovascular risk. What is significant for all of these scenarios, however, is that optimizing modifiable risk factors leads to significantly decreased risk in all demographics.

Box 4
Secondary prevention

Eight years later, the illustrative patient is now a 58-year-old white man with diabetes, dyslipidemia, and hypertension on treatment. His last HbA1c was 8.9%, blood pressure was adequately controlled at 128/78, and his total cholesterol was 180 mg/dL with an HDL of 35 mg/dL. The provider gives positive feedback to this patient for adherence to his antihypertensive and cholesterol medication but also notes that his diabetes is suboptimally controlled. In addition, the patient admits he has started smoking "a few cigarettes here and there," and his weight has increased 15 pounds since his last visit 1 year ago. The provider counsels him on smoking, recommends a nicotine patch, and adds a second oral agent to his diabetes regimen.

Three months later he develops crushing substernal chest pain and presents to the emergency department where he is diagnosed with an ST segment elevation inferior wall myocardial infarction. He undergoes primary angioplasty and stent placement to his right coronary artery and is noted to have 30% stenoses in his other 2 coronaries.

Two weeks after discharge he presents to the provider on dual antiplatelet therapy, a high-dose statin, an angiotensin receptor blocker, and a beta blocker. The provider notes that the patient was discharged on insulin and has an appointment to see an endocrinologist in the near future.

The focus must now shift toward secondary prevention to avoid an additional cardiac event. The patient is also at risk for peripheral vascular disease and cerebral vascular disease, and will need primary prevention for these. Fortunately these efforts overlap.

SUMMARY

Cardiovascular disease is the most common cause of death in the United States and around one-fourth of the American population live with some form of the disease. Fortunately, there are a large number of modifiable factors known to affect an individual's risk of disease. This, coupled with its high prevalence and long latency period make cardiovascular disease prevention a cornerstone of public health and clinical practice. Recent years have seen the emergence of high-quality tools to help clinicians determine patients' cardiovascular risk, as well as several evidence-based interventions that can appreciably decrease risk. Incorporating these tools into the evaluation and management of patients throughout their lifetime can help to mitigate the clinical and public health burden of cardiovascular disease in the United States.

REFERENCES

1. Lasagna L. Would Hippocrates rewrite his oath? New York Times (1923-Current file) 1964. SM11.
2. Eva KW. Trending in 2014: Hippocrates. Med Educ 2014;48(1):1–3.
3. Grimes DS. An epidemic of coronary heart disease. QJM 2012;105(6):509–18.
4. National Heart L, and Blood Institute, NIH. NHLBI Fact Book, Fiscal Year 2012. 2012. Available at: https://www.nhlbi.nih.gov/files/docs/factbook/FactBook2012.pdf. Accessed January 2, 2017.
5. Dalen JE, Alpert JS, Goldberg RJ, et al. The epidemic of the 20(th) century: coronary heart disease. Am J Med 2014;127(9):807–12.
6. Alberg AJ, Shopland DR, Cummings KM. The 2014 Surgeon General's report: commemorating the 50th Anniversary of the 1964 Report of the Advisory

Committee to the US Surgeon General and updating the evidence on the health consequences of cigarette smoking. Am J Epidemiol 2014;179(4):403–12.

7. Clarke TC, Ward BW, Freeman G, et al. Early release of selected estimates based on data from the January– March 2015 National Health Interview Survey. National Center for Health Statistics; 2015.

8. Organization WH. Cardiovascular diseases. Fact sheet 2016. Available at: http://www.who.int/mediacentre/factsheets/fs317/en/. Accessed January 2, 2017.

9. Centers for Disease Control and Prevention NCfIPaC. Leading causes of death by age group 2014. 2005. Available at: https://www.cdc.gov/injury/wisqars/pdf/leading_causes_of_death_by_age_group_2014-a.pdf. Accessed January 2, 2017.

10. Kenneth D, Kochanek MA, Sherry L, et al. Deaths: Final Data for 2014. Natl Vital Stat Rep 2016;65(4).

11. McNamara JJ, Molot MA, Stremple JF, et al. Coronary artery disease in combat casualties in Vietnam. JAMA 1971;216(7):1185–7.

12. Enos WF, Holmes RH, Beyer J. Coronary disease among United States soldiers killed in action in Korea; preliminary report. J Am Med Assoc 1953;152(12):1090–3.

13. Libby P, Theroux P. Pathophysiology of coronary artery disease. Circulation 2005; 111(25):3481–8.

14. Klabunde R. Cardiovascular physiology concepts. Philadelphia: Lippincott Williams & Wilkins; 2011.

15. Ross R. Cell biology of atherosclerosis. Annu Rev Physiol 1995;57:791–804.

16. Ghattas A, Griffiths HR, Devitt A, et al. Monocytes in coronary artery disease and atherosclerosis. Where Are We Now? J Am Coll Cardiol 2013;62(17):1541–51.

17. Xu S, Bendeck M, Gotlieb AI. Vascular pathobiology. In: Buja LM, Butany J, editors. Cardiovascular pathology. 4th edition. St Louis (MO): Elsevier Science; 2015. p. 85–124.

18. Libby P. Changing concepts of atherogenesis. J Intern Med 2000;247(3):349–58.

19. Faxon DP, Fuster V, Libby P, et al. Atherosclerotic Vascular Disease Conference: Writing Group III: pathophysiology. Circulation 2004;109(21):2617–25.

20. Dawber TR, Moore FE, Mann GV. Coronary heart disease in the Framingham study. Am J Public Health Nations Health 1957;47(4 Pt 2):4–24.

21. Siu AL. Behavioral and pharmacotherapy interventions for tobacco smoking cessation in adults, including pregnant women: U.S. Preventive Services Task Force Recommendation Statement. Ann Intern Med 2015;163(8):622–34.

22. Stone NJ, Robinson JG, Lichtenstein AH, et al. 2013 ACC/AHA guideline on the treatment of blood cholesterol to reduce atherosclerotic cardiovascular risk in adults: a report of the American College of Cardiology/American Heart Association Task Force on Practice Guidelines. Circulation 2014;129(25 Suppl 2):S1–45.

23. James PA, Oparil S, Carter BL, et al. 2014 evidence-based guideline for the management of high blood pressure in adults: report from the panel members appointed to the Eighth Joint National Committee (JNC 8). JAMA 2014;311(5): 507–20.

24. Jensen MD, Ryan DH, Apovian CM, et al. 2013 AHA/ACC/TOS Guideline for the Management of Overweight and Obesity in Adults. A Report of the American College of Cardiology/American Heart Association Task Force on Practice Guidelines and The Obesity Society. J Am Coll Cardiol 2014;129(25 suppl 2):S102–38.

25. Eckel RH, Jakicic JM, Ard JD, et al. 2013 AHA/ACC guideline on lifestyle management to reduce cardiovascular risk: a report of the American College of Cardiology/American Heart Association Task Force on Practice Guidelines. Circulation 2014;129(25 Suppl 2):S76–99.

26. Bild DE, Bluemke DA, Burke GL, et al. Multi-Ethnic Study of Atherosclerosis: objectives and design. Am J Epidemiol 2002;156(9):871–81.

27. Sorlie PD, Aviles-Santa LM, Wassertheil-Smoller S, et al. Design and implementation of the Hispanic Community Health Study/Study of Latinos. Ann Epidemiol 2010;20(8):629–41.

28. Wilson PWF, D'Agostino RB, Levy D, et al. Prediction of coronary heart disease using risk factor categories. Circulation 1998;97(18):1837–47.

29. Goff DC Jr, Lloyd-Jones DM, Bennett G, et al. 2013 ACC/AHA guideline on the assessment of cardiovascular risk: a report of the American College of Cardiology/American Heart Association Task Force on Practice Guidelines. J Am Coll Cardiol 2014;63(25 Pt B):2935–59.

30. The Atherosclerosis Risk in Communities (ARIC) Study: design and objectives. The ARIC investigators. Am J Epidemiol 1989;129(4):687–702.

31. Fried LP, Borhani NO, Enright P, et al. The cardiovascular health study: design and rationale. Ann Epidemiol 1991;1(3):263–76.

32. Friedman GD, Cutter GR, Donahue RP, et al. Cardia: study design, recruitment, and some characteristics of the examined subjects. J Clin Epidemiol 1988; 41(11):1105–16.

33. Dawber TR, Kannel WB, Lyell LP. An approach to longitudinal studies in a community: the Framingham Study. Ann N Y Acad Sci 1963;107:539–56.

34. Kannel WB, Feinleib M, McNamara PM, et al. An investigation of coronary heart disease in families. The Framingham offspring study. Am J Epidemiol 1979; 110(3):281–90.

35. Yang X, Li J, Hu D, et al. Predicting the 10-Year Risks of Atherosclerotic Cardiovascular Disease in Chinese Population: The China-PAR Project (Prediction for ASCVD Risk in China). Circulation 2016;134(19):1430–40.

36. Writing Group M, Mozaffarian D, Benjamin EJ, et al. Heart disease and stroke statistics-2016 update: a report from the American Heart Association. Circulation 2016;133(4):e38–360.

37. LaRosa JC. Unresolved issues in early trials of cholesterol lowering. Am J Cardiol 1995;76(9):5C–9C.

38. Scandinavian Simvastatin Survival Study Group. Randomised trial of cholesterol lowering in 4444 patients with coronary heart disease: the Scandinavian Simvastatin Survival Study (4S). Lancet 1994;344(8934):1383–9.

39. Baigent C, Blackwell L, Emberson J, et al. Efficacy and safety of more intensive lowering of LDL cholesterol: a meta-analysis of data from 170,000 participants in 26 randomised trials. Lancet 2010;376(9753):1670–81.

40. Mihaylova B, Emberson J, Blackwell L, et al. The effects of lowering LDL cholesterol with statin therapy in people at low risk of vascular disease: meta-analysis of individual data from 27 randomised trials. Lancet 2012;380(9841):581–90.

41. Alcocer L. Statins for everybody? New evidence on the efficacy and safety of the inhibitors of HMG Co-A reductase. Am J Ther 2003;10(6):423–8.

42. Go AS, Mozaffarian D, Roger VL, et al. Heart Disease and Stroke Statistics—2014 Update. Circulation 2014;129(3):e28.

43. Wright JT Jr, Williamson JD, Whelton PK, et al. A randomized trial of intensive versus standard blood-pressure control. N Engl J Med 2015;373(22):2103–16.

44. Staessen JA, Fagard R, Thijs L, et al. Randomised double-blind comparison of placebo and active treatment for older patients with isolated systolic hypertension. The Systolic Hypertension in Europe (Syst-Eur) Trial Investigators. Lancet 1997;350(9080):757–64.

45. Action to Control Cardiovascular Risk in Diabetes Study Group. Effects of Intensive Glucose Lowering in Type 2 Diabetes. N Engl J Med 2008;358(24):2545–59.

46. Marso SP, Daniels GH, Brown-Frandsen K, et al. Liraglutide and cardiovascular outcomes in type 2 diabetes. N Engl J Med 2016;375(4):311–22.

47. Wu JH, Foote C, Blomster J, et al. Effects of sodium-glucose cotransporter-2 inhibitors on cardiovascular events, death, and major safety outcomes in adults with type 2 diabetes: a systematic review and meta-analysis. Lancet Diabetes Endocrinol 2016;4(5):411–9.

48. Ittaman SV, VanWormer JJ, Rezkalla SH. The role of aspirin in the prevention of cardiovascular disease. Clin Med Res 2014;12(3–4):147–54.

49. Baigent C, Collins R, Appleby P, et al. ISIS-2: 10 year survival among patients with suspected acute myocardial infarction in randomised comparison of intravenous streptokinase, oral aspirin, both, or neither. The ISIS-2 (Second International Study of Infarct Survival) Collaborative Group. BMJ 1998;316(7141):1337–43.

50. Sharma A, Lavie CJ, Sharma SK, et al. Duration of dual antiplatelet therapy after drug-eluting stent implantation in patients with and without acute coronary syndrome: a systematic review of randomized controlled trials. Mayo Clin Proc 2016;91(8):1084–93.

51. US Preventive Services Task Force Guides to Clinical Preventive Services. The guide to clinical preventive Services 2014: recommendations of the U.S. Preventive Services Task force. Rockville (MD): Agency for Healthcare Research and Quality (US); 2014.

52. Li J, Siegrist J. Physical activity and risk of cardiovascular disease–a meta-analysis of prospective cohort studies. Int J Environ Res Public Health 2012; 9(2):391–407.

53. Hartley L, Igbinedion E, Holmes J, et al. Increased consumption of fruit and vegetables for the primary prevention of cardiovascular diseases. Cochrane Database Syst Rev 2013;(6):CD009874.

54. Rees K, Hartley L, Flowers N, et al. 'Mediterranean' dietary pattern for the primary prevention of cardiovascular disease. Cochrane Database Syst Rev 2013;(8):CD009825.

55. Eckel RH, Jakicic JM, Ard JD, et al. 2013 AHA/ACC Guideline on Lifestyle Management to Reduce Cardiovascular Risk. A Report of the American College of Cardiology/American Heart Association Task Force on Practice Guidelines. Circulation 2014;129(25 suppl 2):S76–99.

56. Claas SA, Arnett DK. The role of healthy lifestyle in the primordial prevention of cardiovascular disease. Curr Cardiol Rep 2016;18(6):56.

57. Sussman S. A lifespan developmental-stage approach to tobacco and other drug abuse prevention. ISRN Addiction 2013;2013:745783.

58. Tian J, An X, Fu M. Pediatric cardiovascular risk factors: a review. Minerva Pediatr 2016;69(3):225–9.

59. Jones WJ, Silvestri GA. The master settlement agreement and its impact on tobacco use 10 years later: lessons for physicians about health policy making. Chest 2010;137(3):692–700.

60. Estruch R, Ros E, Salas-Salvadó J, et al. Primary prevention of cardiovascular disease with a Mediterranean diet. N Engl J Med 2013;368(14):1279–90.

61. Howard PA, Ellerbeck EF. Optimizing beta-blocker use after myocardial infarction. Am Fam Physician 2000;62(8):1853–60, 1865–6.

Moving?

Make sure your subscription moves with you!

To notify us of your new address, find your **Clinics Account Number** (located on your mailing label above your name), and contact customer service at:

Email: journalscustomerservice-usa@elsevier.com

800-654-2452 (subscribers in the U.S. & Canada)
314-447-8871 (subscribers outside of the U.S. & Canada)

Fax number: 314-447-8029

Elsevier Health Sciences Division
Subscription Customer Service
3251 Riverport Lane
Maryland Heights, MO 63043

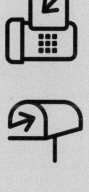

*To ensure uninterrupted delivery of your subscription, please notify us at least 4 weeks in advance of move.

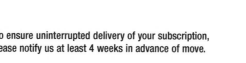

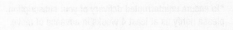

Printed and bound by CPI Group (UK) Ltd, Croydon, CR0 4YY

03/10/2024

01040398-0003